ADVANCE PRAISE FOR NOVEMBER P[...] AND *NOVEMBER PROJECT: THE B[...]*

D0691240

"Ask a crossfitter about their workout and they'll tell you about the WOD. Ask a[...] they'll tell you about the cool person they just met."

—Chris "Rhymes with Chrysler" Hueisler, 36, national RunWestin concierge, Belmont, Mass., Boston tribe

"A class at the gym is to November Project what riding in the back of a taxi is to space travel. There is nothing in the world of fitness, motivation, and sheer energy that compares to showing up at 6:27 a.m. with hundreds of screaming people ready to train in the cold, rain, snow, ice, sun, heat, and beauty of a city that is still asleep."

—Casey Neistat, 34, filmmaker and entrepreneur, 3:02 marathoner, New York City, Boston tribe

"OK, so they don't want to be called a 'running group.' Fine. But through running, November Project is changing the world, one tribe at a time. Their method is both radical and simple, equally profane and profound: Show up, work harder than you ever would alone, and have more fun than you thought was legal in public places. If you haven't shown up, you absolutely should. Until then, this utterly original book is the next best thing."

—David Willey, 48, editor-in-chief, *Runner's World* magazine, Emmaus, Penn., Boston and New York tribes

"I want to hug EVERYONE now. I was on a job interview last week, and when it was over, I had to remind myself I shouldn't hug my interviewer. It's instinct now to high five every runner I see. It's like I shit rainbows. This is what NP has done to me."

—Emilie Mandaric, 30, speech therapist, Allston, Mass., Boston tribe

"I brought my dad to a workout and hugged him for the first time in 15 years. Thank you, November Project."

—Anonymous

"Thanks to NP, I went from a 10ker to a marathoner. But that's not just because my fitness levels increased, it's because my fitness self-esteem increased. I never would have thought that running a marathon was possible, but now I think that any athletic endeavor I train for and am supported through is completely within my reach."

—Molly Ryan, 27, public health professional, Medford, Mass., Boston tribe

"I wish that you guys would leave me the fuck alone. I don't want to give you a quote for your cult fitness book!"

—Karate Kid, 47, Reseda, Calif., adult karate enthusiast

"I was once an elite athlete who pushed his limits for 3 or 4 workouts every day and set his sights on epic adventures. Now, I have a business, a wife, and two young kids. I'm lucky to train twice a week. Although I no longer aim for the biggest waves, longest routes, or the deepest burn, I still want to be fit enough to get out there. November Project is the perfect remedy. It's flexible, inclusive, and fun. It gives me the athletic base to bag peaks, taste trail, and ride currents on the weekends with my young family."

—Adam Kreek, 35, 2008 Olympic gold medalist (rowing), motivational speaker, Victoria, B.C., Victoria tribe

"The level of commitment November Project requires, the lack of excuses and bullshit, and the waking up at 5:30 a.m. weeds out all the crappy people, and you are left with some of the best, kindest, most vibrant souls you will ever meet in this life."

—Rebecca Daniels, 33, photographer, San Francisco, San Francisco tribe

"Since I started NP, I have PRed every single distance that I've raced. The PRs have been significant, too. I've also seen my strength increase and have actual muscles in my arms!"

—Pete Navatto, 41, New York State senior court officer, Oceanside, N.Y., New York City tribe

"The best rowing moments are when everyone in the boat is working their ass off to make their teammates go fast, when my 100 percent effort and yours become ours. There's more speed in digging deep together, and there's also this incredible joy. Or in November Project speak, Fuck Yeah! So Just Show Up (Olympic rowing experience not required)."

—Esther Lofgren, 31, 2012 Olympic gold medalist (rowing) and world record holder, Alexandria, Va., Boston tribe

"I'm getting back to times I ran as a kid, which I thought were long out of reach. There was a time growing up when you tried so hard to figure out who you were. Then you enter the working world and a sense of settling down and conformity and routine can set in. NP has helped shine a light on that sense of self-discovery again."

—Michael Kearns, 39, construction management, Sturbridge, Mass., Boston tribe

"I was promised FREE fitness. So I showed up. Then I started having to do more laundry to have clean gear. Then I needed warm-weather gear. Then I needed new shoes that could handle distances. Then I needed new sizes since I was actually in shape. Now I'm out there buying shelving to hold it all. Brogan Graham, I'm sending you receipts to expense all this. #worthit"

—Patrick Burke, 32, NHL player safety director and cofounder of You Can Play, New York City, Boston and New York City tribes

"I can't fucking stop these people. I'm at every single workout and yet nobody seems to care that I'm even around."

—Gravity

"New requirements for any place I live in the future: There must be a tribe. What a bunch of brilliant, beautiful weirdos. I've finally found my people."

—Chris Mosier, 35, LGBT advocate, first transgender athlete on Team USA (duathalon), New York City, New York City tribe

"The whole thing's fuckin' weird."

—Dean Karnazes, 53, renowned ultra runner and *New York Times* bestselling author, Milwaukee, Madison, San Francisco, and Boston tribes

"The reason I joined the Tribe was the unique combination of fitness, community, respect, love, and most importantly inclusion. I love getting hugged by total strangers at 6:25 am. My fav hashtag: #JustShowUp."

—Bart Yasso, 60, chief running officer, *Runner's World* magazine, Emmaus, Penn., Philadelphia tribe

"November Project is good! Good! Good! Good!"

—Micah L'Esperance-Chouillard, 3, Brookline, Mass., Boston tribe

"I felt welcomed, I felt at home, I felt part of something, I felt happy, I felt like I had just taken a slug of Zoloft."

—Molly Rossignol, 46, family doctor, Madison, Wisc., Madison tribe

NOVEMBER PROJECT

PROJECT

THE BOOK

FREE lifetime membership to

NOVEMBER PROJECT

workouts with the purchase of this book

NOVEMBER PROJECT

PROJECT

THE BOOK

INSIDE THE FREE, GRASSROOTS FITNESS MOVEMENT THAT'S TAKING OVER THE WORLD

BROGAN GRAHAM & BOJAN MANDARIC WITH CALEB DANILOFF

RODALE.

RODALE *wellness*

Live happy. Be healthy. Get inspired.

Sign up today to get exclusive access to our authors, exclusive bonuses, and the most authoritative, useful, and cutting-edge information on health, wellness, fitness, and living your life to the fullest.

Visit us online at RodaleWellness.com
Join us at RodaleWellness.com

Mention of specific companies, organizations, or authorities in this book does not imply endorsement by the author or publisher, nor does mention of specific companies, organizations, or authorities imply that they endorse this book, its author, or the publisher.

Copyright © 2016 by Brogan Graham, Bojan Mandaric, and Caleb Daniloff

All rights reserved. No part of this publication may be reproduced or transmitted in any form or by any means, electronic or mechanical, including photocopying, recording, or any other information storage and retrieval system, without the written permission of the publisher.

Rodale books may be purchased for business or promotional use or for special sales. For information, please write to: Special Markets Department, Rodale Inc., 733 Third Avenue, New York, NY 10017.

Printed in the United States of America

Rodale Inc. makes every effort to use acid-free ∞, recycled paper ♺.

Book design by Phil Yarnall / SMAY Design

The Harvard Stadium plan shown on pages 3–4 and 12 was provided courtesy of the Newton Free Library Digital Collection, from the book Blue Book of Newton, Boston, (Mass.): Edward A. Jones, 1891-, 1917 Harvard Stadium Map.

Library of Congress Cataloging-in-Publication Data is on file with the publisher.

ISBN-13: 978-1-62336-629-2   paperback

Distributed to the trade by Macmillan

2 4 6 8 10 9 7 5 3 1   paperback

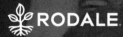

Follow us @RodaleBooks on 🐦 f 📌 📷

We enable and inspire people to improve their lives and the world around them.
rodalebooks.com

PHOTO CREDITS

All photos by Bojan Mandaric, except for the following:

Matt Anzur, 132, 197 (4th row)
Chris Arroyo, 215
Brian Babineau/Getty Images, 30
Sara Beaney, 38, 104 (top right)
Jesse Burke, front cover, xiv (all), 106, 110, 115 (top right, bottom left and right), 116 (top left and right), 118, 119 (top, bottom left and middle), 120, 121 (top, bottom right, and both bottom left), 122 (bottom), 123 (all)
Chris Capozzi, 141 (lower right)
Courtesy of Maria Cesca, 11 (right)
Evan Dana, 73, 74 (bottom left), 76
Rebecca Daniels, 153
Caleb Daniloff, 60 (both), 150, 160, 177, 204 (top), 208
JoEllen Depakakibo, 168
Courtesy of Ann Doody, all family shots in Brogan chapter
Rick Duha and Thomas Hall, 172
Endurance Challenge Event Photography, 213
Rosa Evora, 27 (bottom right), 104 (bottom right)
Stephen Felter, 49
Janel Kozlowski Fink, 191, 194 (bottom), 200
Courtesy of Nicolas Flattes, 11 (left), 214 (both by Ultrarace Photos)
Cody and Natalie Gantz, 152, 155, 162, 164, 169 (bottom)
Kate Gilly, 171 (top)
Scott Goldstein, 45 (bottom right), 186, 225
Sam Goresh, 104 (top left), 108
Brogan Graham, 4, 21, 117, 197 (2nd row)
Katie Hughes, 188, 195 (top, center, bottom left), 196 (top, bottom center, and right), 199, 202, 205, 207, 209, 211, 212
Diana Hunt, xxiii, xv
Andrea Issotti/Shutterstock, 81 (bear)
Dylan Ladds, Dooster, 6, 8, 12–13, 138 (top left)
Dylan Ladds & Ryan Scura, Dooster, 140 (top right), 192–193, 194 (top), 197 (top), 224
Dan Layo, 171 (bottom), 198
Kelvin Ma, x, 34, 78, 119 (right)
Laura McCloskey, 156, 158, 165, 166–167, 169 (top), 170
Amanda Allen Nurse, 67
Rusian Olinchuck/Getty Images, 35, 40 (map)
Emily Saul, 72
Derrick Shallcross, 228
TedX Beacon Street, 185
Sasha Teninty, 161
Zack Williamson, 98

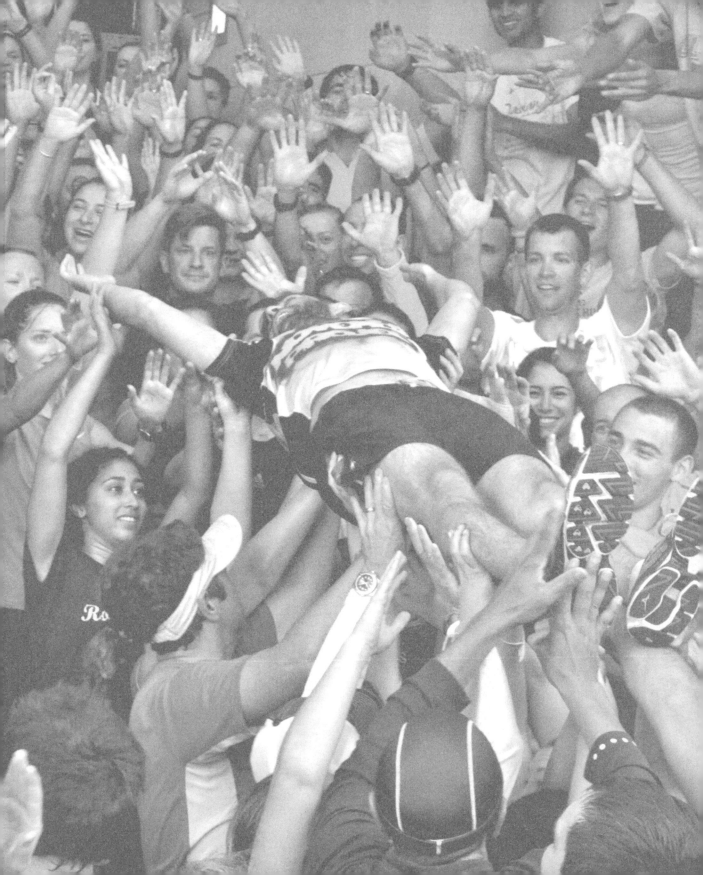

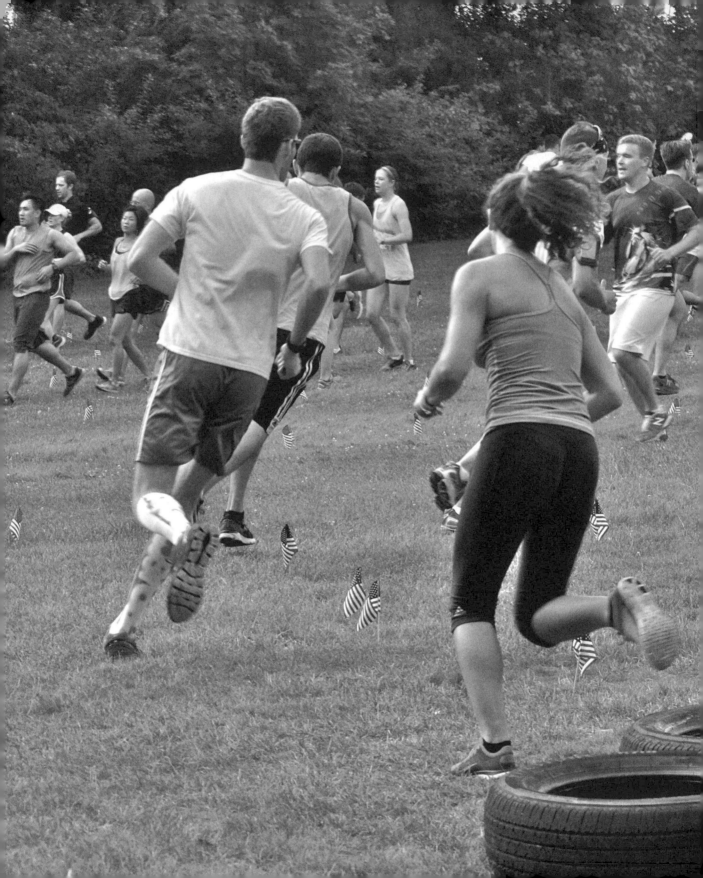

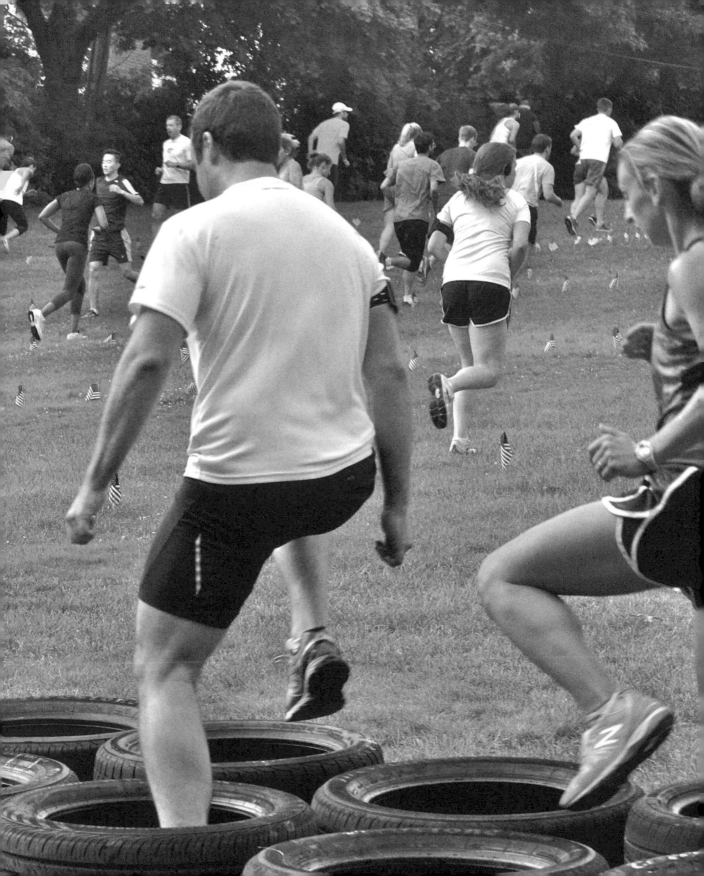

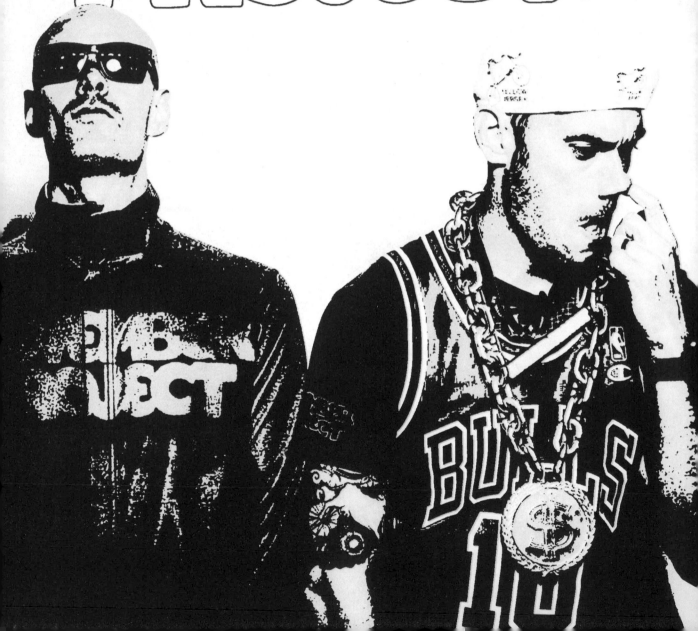

DEDICATION

To our effortlessly cool, fearless adventurer Samantha Dweck
forever, forever, forever

CONTENTS

NOVEMBER PROJECT

PART II. #WORLDTAKEOVER

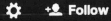

November Project
@Nov_Project

⚙ +👤 Follow

Come one, come all #novemberproject is in full swing.
Next meeting @ Harvard Stadium 05/09 @6:30am

7:05 PM - 2 May 2012

↩ 🔁 ♥ •••

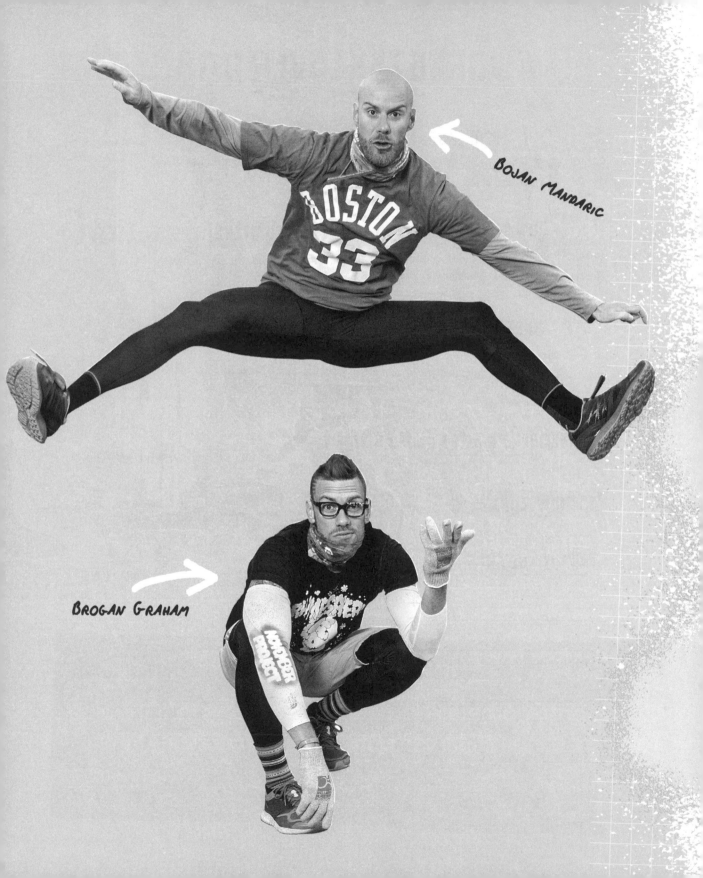

BOJAN MANDARIC

BROGAN GRAHAM

"Put Us on the Fuckin' Cover!"

BY CALEB DANILOFF

Wisconsin Notes*

- The Pour House is more or less a dive bar in downtown Boston

- BG likes assholes more than Bojan does

- A Serbian shoulder tells a life story

- Origin myths can form while you're sipping beverages

- November Project is a training ground and a lifestyle

- Hugging "makes you chill the fuck out"

- A bold suggestion is made

- A writer smiles awkwardly

* When the Madison, Wisconsin, tribe came on board, they complained about having to wade through the Boston blog posts. These just-the-facts, straight-shooters wanted the straight dope. So Wisconsin Notes was born, a CliffsNotes of sorts written for the Madison tribe.

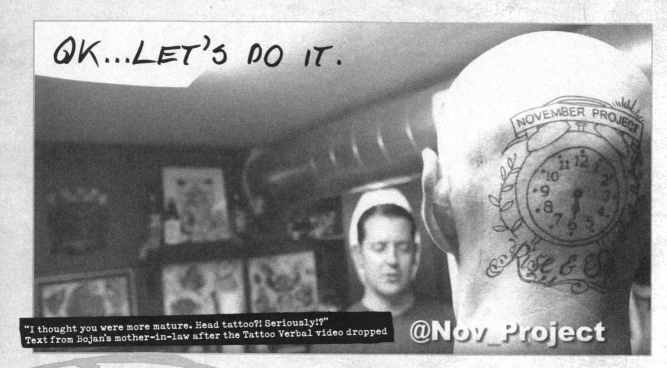

OK...LET'S DO IT.

"I thought you were more mature. Head tattoo?! Seriously!?"
Text from Bojan's mother-in-law after the Tattoo Verbal video dropped

@Nov_Project

BOSTON, MASSACHUSETTS
MAY 30, 2013

The Pour House sits at the top of Boylston Street, one of Boston's most prominent downtown thoroughfares—home to high fashion, high-tech gadgets, and high-priced steak. The 35-year-old pub is a quick grub stop during the day and a college dive bar at night, known for its wet fries, cheap brunches, and $5 Bloody Marys. With no cover and perky bartenders on two levels, Northeastern University and Berklee College of Music students, with the occasional sprinkle of tight V-necks and skirts from Boston University, pack the late-night line to get in.

It was a Thursday evening in late May when I pulled open the heavy wooden door, the warm street air rushing past me. At the bar, a couple of locals were hunched over drinks, as still as gargoyles. The booths were packed, though; the tables were crowded with sauce-splattered plates piled high with wing bones and hollowed-out hills of nachos, balled-up napkins, and greasy beer steins. A tall, bald-headed dude, about 6 feet 4, stood toward the middle of the bar in jeans and a gray T-shirt. That was my man: Bojan Mandaric. I still wasn't sure how to pronounce his name.

He was Serbian and one of the cofounders of a curious fitness outfit in Boston I'd been asked to write about for *Runner's World* magazine. Even after scrolling through their blog and some local press, I wasn't quite seeing the running story. I needed some extra color, and so I suggested we meet at the bar where the idea for the group was apparently hatched.

I'd heard of November Project a while back, but it hadn't found purchase. A local news show had aired a segment on what looked like a bunch of twenty- and thirtysomethings running a hill in Brookline, a well-to-do community just outside of Boston. Up and down, back and forth, no destination. Two former Northeastern University rowers grinned and talked knowingly, explaining that their workouts took place three mornings a week, always free. And while, technically, the group—or the tribe, as they called themselves—was "running," it didn't seem like capital-R running to me. As a former drunk who found salvation in a pair of New Balances, for me, running was all about getting from one place to another, not just geographically, but psychologically, emotionally, spiritually. The road was my bible and I worshipped every chance I got. Alone. In black (navy blue if I was feeling sassy). Not the look-at-me neon that seemed popular among these

November Project people. The only thing that resonated was the predawn routine. Sweating as the sun comes up has always sent a hot shot of glory coursing through my body and juiced the rest of my day. But their workouts ended with positivity awards and hugs. Oy vey. Millennials. Next!

I recognized the 31-year-old Mandaric from a short video entitled "The Tattoo Verbal" that he and cofounder Brogan Graham had made about getting November Project ink. It all had to do with some promise they made when they hit 300 people at a single workout. The clip showed Graham getting a huge old-school alarm clock needled onto his triceps, set to 6:30 a.m., ribboned with the words "Rise and Shine." When it was Mandaric's turn, the camera cut to the artist stenciling the same design to the back of the Serbian's bald head and ended with Mandaric calmly stating, "Okay, let's do it." I was anxious to see if he'd gone through with it.

"Bojan?"

"Yes. Caleb?"

We shook hands, and he clapped me on the back. "Good to meet you, man."

I recognized his eyes, or the look in them, rather. I'd lived in Soviet Moscow for almost 6 years in the 1980s, the son of an American journalist, and came from Russian stock. Mandaric's brown peepers had that Slavic cast: slightly brooding but curious, smile-worn but guarded. I didn't see any room for fools. The Serbs and Russians were like childhood cousins who'd spent their summers together in the country climbing trees, raiding vegetable gardens, and tying cans to the tails of cats. I was always glad for some connection to shrink the space between me and my subject, in this case about 6 vertical inches and 4 across the chest.

"I'm looking for the skull tat," I said, craning my neck to peer up behind his ear.

"Oh, ha, that part was a joke. You kidding? I'm not getting my fuckin' dome inked. Come on, let's bounce downstairs, see if BG's there."

I didn't have time to decide whether I felt disappointed or dumb for not getting the joke because Mandaric's English had knocked me back. It was impeccable, loose, fluid. I expected a blockish, yawning Slavic-style accent, with an occasional grasping for the right word. Not full-on American dudeness.

I followed Mandaric down the stairs to the basement bar, watching him dip his very blank pate to the left to avoid the overhang. No sign of Graham. We took a spot at the bar. From the tattoo video, I knew Graham was wicked tall, too. Square jaw, fit as fuck, veiny biceps, wrap-around sunglasses. Definitely what I'd call a Master of the Universe. Given the rowing thing and a name like Brogan, I pictured privilege and the easy swagger that comes with towering height and a back like a picnic bench. I was fully primed to dislike him. When we spoke on the phone to set up the interview and I mentioned that I'd started running Harvard Stadium a few weeks earlier, he blurted, "What's your full-tour** PR?" I had no clue what he was talking about. *What's a tour? Let alone a full one?* I was caught off guard and didn't want to seem lame. "Um, twenty sections," I'd said, rounding up and seeing no need to mention it was the little steps.

"Here he comes," Mandaric said, looking toward the stairwell.

Graham's legs came into view first. Long, bulbous shins screwed into giant clip-in bicycle shoes, like buffalo hooves. The rest of him just kept coming. I swear it took a full 30 seconds for a pair of shoulders and a helmeted head to emerge from beneath the ceiling overhang. But before I could study his face, his long arms were stretched out like condor wings and the light vanished. It wasn't just a press-and-get-out-before-it-seems-like-a-gay-thing man-hug. It lasted. I could feel his abs through my jacket like he was smuggling kindling. When he finally let go, he looked me in the eyes and said,

"BOSTON IS KNOWN FOR A LOT OF THINGS: AMERICAN HISTORY, ACADEMICS, HIGH-TECH AND SCIENCE. AND NOW IT'S GETTING KNOWN FOR FITNESS, AND ISN'T THAT PRETTY COOL."
—LARRY ANDERSON, HEAD COACH OF MIT's MEN'S BASKETBALL TEAM

** A FULL TOUR IS RUNNING UP AND DOWN ALL 37 SECTIONS OF HARVARD STADIUM, FOR A TOTAL OF 1,131 STEPS.

DOUBLE BURGER? POSSIBLE HED: MOVEABLE FEAST.
GET NAMES OF NEW RUNNERS.
ANTI LAST-KID-PICKED. GRAHAM IS ENORMOUS.

"Fuck yeah, dude. Great to meet you. This is awesome."

I smiled. "Um, yeah, you, too."

I had to step back to take him all in. According to the articles I'd read, the Wisconsin-born Graham stood either 6 feet 6 or 6 feet 7, but with his gray kettle helmet, he looked closer to 6 feet 9. Amplifying his presence was some of the straightest posture I'd ever seen, like he'd been built with cranes and welding torches. He and Mandaric fist-bumped.

"Let's grab a booth," Graham said, his voice deep and raspy. "Fuckin' starving."

Walking between the two of them, I felt like Justin Bieber with his security detail. A couple dudes playing darts near the bathrooms turned to look. We slid in, passed each other menus, and Mandaric and Graham made small talk about an old spray-paint stencil Graham found in his apartment. "Remember—it was just you and me, we were still using a *zero* for the *o*." While swiping through some of their social media posts, I had seen plenty of pics of shirts, jackets, hats, bags, even pillowcases, tagged with the words *November Project.* In one pic, a dreadlocked dude had the logo blasted across his bare chest with the hashtag #itsnotacult. A waitress appeared and they both ordered Harpoon IPAs. I asked for a water and dug out my recorder.

"So how would you explain November Project?" I asked hopefully. "Is it like a running club?"

"Nah, it's not a run club or a boot camp, but the people who train with us accidentally become runners," Graham said, flipping his phone over and placing it screen-down. "We're our own thing."

Mandaric took the baton.

"We don't like to put ourselves into a bucket," he said. "Because of the variety of athletic levels and backgrounds and the intensity and consistency of our workouts, most of our members, whether they realize it or not, are in a constant state of improvement. Some were sofa spuds just 6 months ago. Road races are the easi-est ways to measure improvement, so we do have a lot of people running. Would they call themselves runners? Sure. There are a couple run groups that have spun off from the tribe. But we're more like the urban athlete. Our members are also cyclists, cross-country skiers, rowers, yogis, crossfitters, hockey players. We're across the board."

"Urban athlete, yeah, I like that," Graham said. "People never understand November Project at first. That's always been our problem. Because there's nothing to compare it to. We call it a 'free, grassroots fitness movement,' but you really have to just show the fuck up. That's the only way you'll get it."

The waitress returned with our drinks.

"Sheila took care of you upstairs," she smiled, placing chilled pint glasses in front of Graham and Mandaric.

"Aw, look at that," Graham said. "That makes me feel like a famous person. Cheers."

According to the Google search I had done, November Project workouts had been earning a degree of fame lately, at least locally. "Flash-mob fitness!" "The fight club of running clubs!" "Hugs and fitness!" In recent months, it had added two more chapters: one in Madison, Wisconsin, run by Graham's older brother, and a second headed up by a college friend in San Francisco. I wasn't sure that counted as a movement. I told them I'd seen the *Boston Globe* newspaper story that featured pictures of Graham clad in striped pirate pants, doo-rag, and eye patch cheering on other colorfully dressed sweat hogs as they ran up the concrete steps of Harvard Stadium. (Oh yeah, I forgot to mention the costumes. I definitely didn't do costumes.)

"There are a lot of run clubs in this town, but we are definitely having the most fun," Graham said, wiping the suds off his lips with his long fingers. "We keep it weird, keep it competitive, keep it welcoming. And my Serbian friend here and I will always be there to greet you. That's our sauce."

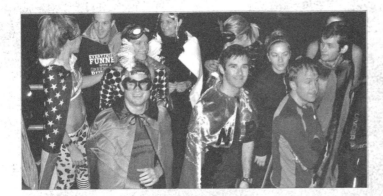

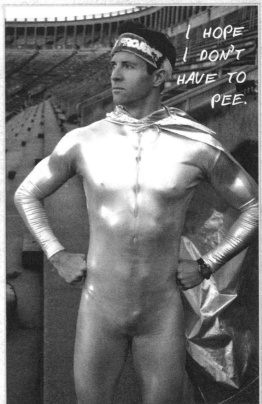

I HOPE I DON'T HAVE TO PEE.

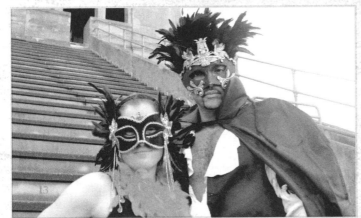

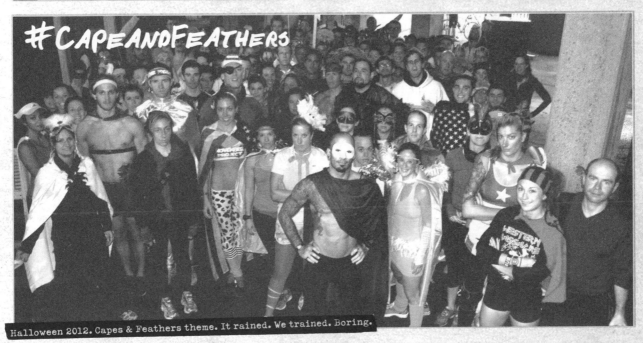

#CapeandFeathers

Halloween 2012. Capes & Feathers theme. It rained. We trained. Boring.

"So how fit do you have to be to join?" I asked, flipping a notebook page. "Could my 78-year-old mom with an artificial hip get something out of it?"

"Can she move? Shit, bring your grandmother," Graham said. "The workouts are scalable. The bad-ass racers show up to the stadium and try and knock off a 'double burger'*** in an hour. And the folks just off the couch walking 10 sections, they're going to be sucking wind just as hard. Everyone's on the same battleground. There's no front of the line or back of the line. That's where we're not at all like a run club, where the fastest and slowest never really interact. And when you have an Ironman finisher or a professional hockey player cheering you on in your first pair of running shoes, that can't help but step up your game. Plus, you get the chance to know somebody you might never have come across."

"And this is where it all began, eh," I said.

"Right at the end of that bar," Graham said, twisting his napkin into a point. "Yeah, it was, 'What are we going to do this winter?'"

Mandaric said he'd just rowed in the 2011 Head of the Charles Regatta for the Northeastern University Rowing Alumni team ("one of his 5 or 500 fuckin' gold medals," Graham piped in). But that had been several weeks earlier, and that boat wasn't moving anymore. Nor was Mandaric.

"I have a tendency, if the weather's shitty, days are shorter, I come home and I'm just not motivated," Mandaric said. "I sit on the couch and eat a delicious dinner my wife cooks and not do shit. I'd gain 20 pounds over the winter. Springtime rolls around and I kick my ass back into gear, fire on all cylinders. But this guy, he could eat half this bar and still look the way he does. He's like a fuckin' shark, like, if he stops moving, he's gonna die."

I looked at Graham, dipping a cluster of fries in

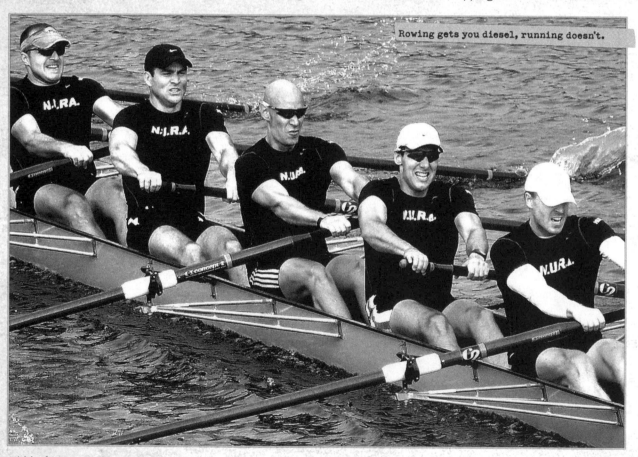

Rowing gets you diesel, running doesn't.

*** A DOUBLE BURGER IS TWO FULL TOURS, OR 74 SECTIONS.

ketchup. He gave a head nod and a smile to someone behind me. There did seem to be a palpable vibration about him, like he was always in a state of liftoff. Mandaric, a year ahead of Graham at Northeastern, had been a hot Serbian rowing recruit with supercharged technical skills who jetted straight to the varsity boat. Graham, meanwhile, a self-described "donkey," a power guy, said he was still learning the ropes on the JV squad. Hoops had been his sport in high school.

As fellow oarsmen, the men had grown tight, bonded by the sport's extreme, almost maniacal pushing of physical boundaries. Eight bodies working as one, no star players, no egos. Just a communal red-line exertion during races that often lasted less than 10 minutes, but that left rowers keeled over, wrung out like dish towels, shoes spattered with last night's dinner.

After graduation, they went their separate ways—Graham traveling, Mandaric to grad school to pursue a degree in new media. Both coached collegiate rowing for a while. When they drifted back to Boston, they'd get together occasionally over beers, trying to carve out meaningful conversation beneath loud bar music. Sunday, October 30, 2011, was one of those occasions.

"I was very specific," Mandaric said. "I don't want to pay to go to a fuckin' gym. I don't want to pay to be fit."

With a hard clink of their mugs, they pledged to show up every morning during the month of November before work to run the river, hills, or the steps of Harvard Stadium—some of their old rowing workouts. This wasn't just two beer buds getting bromantic over suds; this was accountability, a core ethic. A crew boat requires that all eight seats have asses in them. One rower calls in sick, keeps hitting the snooze bar, or can't get over last night's breakup equals a soul-crushing on-land workout for the rest of the team, each guy hating on the slacker and plotting revenge. Mandaric looked at me with his no-nonsense eyes: "I just said to him, 'You better fuckin' be there.'"

A few days later, while the sun was still hitting the snooze button, Graham was shifting from foot to foot outside his apartment in Cambridge's Central Square with his hand on a telephone pole. It was 27°F, wet snow spitting in his face. He was waiting for Mandaric, who had set off running from his place in Brighton 3 miles away. Because Mandaric had to get to work earlier than Graham, they staggered the workout. When Mandaric arrived, the pair ran back to Brighton, where Graham then turned around and dialed up his 5-K pace for a solo dash back to Central. They christened this workout the "Door to Door" and created a Google Doc where they could post their times and track improvements. They named it November Project.

"During those first months, we really got to know each other and became better friends," Mandaric said, leaning back in the booth, smoothing out his shirt. "That was a time when we were talking about life, relationships, the shit that's bothering us."

"It became very addictive," Graham recalled. "You're sitting at your desk at work afterward, proud of yourself even though you're all tucked in, kinda boring, kinda adult, using your indoor voice. But you've already had a dose of something that's pretty raw and pretty real. And when we started getting texts from our friends, asking, 'When are you gonna run next?', the wheels started to turn."

After 6 months of logging miles along the Charles, eating stadium stairs, and tackling road races in shirts stenciled with November Project (with zeros for o's), they began hyping their workouts as a joke on social media.

"I don't even remember how it went from 5 people to 50 people," Mandaric said. "The initial idea was not to grow the numbers, it's something that just happened. So we started a blog, tracked people's times, started giving away frozen pizzas for PRs. When we had enough people on Wednesdays at the stadium, we created Fridays—repeats on this monster hill in Brookline—and when we had enough people there, we created Mondays."

November Project. ☆ 📁

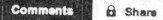

🖨 ↶ ↷ 🗐 ▾ 🖌 | $ % 123 ▾ | 10pt ▾ | B Abc A ▾ A ▾ ⊞ ▾ ≡ ▾ ⊣⊢ ▾ ⤵

fx |

	A	B	C	D	E
1	**Date**	**Day**	**Start**	**Location**	**Work**
2	11/1/2011	Tuesday	6:30:00	Harvard Stadium	37 sections
3	11/2/2011	Wednesday	6:45:00	Brighton - Central	7.61 miles
4	11/3/2011	Thursday	7:00:00	Charles River Stations	Pushups, Box Jumps, SitUps, Pullups, Supermen, wheels?
5	11/4/2011	Friday	7:00:00	South Boston Yoga	Kitty's class - YOGA
6	11/5/2011	Saturday			
7	11/6/2011	Sunday	13:30:00	Brighton - Dover	42 mile bike ride
8	11/7/2011	Monday	6:45:00	Brighton - Central	7.61 miles
9	11/8/2011	Tuesday	6:45:00	Charles River Stations	Pushups, Box Jumps, Situps, Pullups, Supermen
10	11/9/2011	Wednesday	6:30:00	Harvard Stadium	37 sections
11	11/10/2011	Thursday	7:00:00	Living Room	deck O cards
12	11/11/2011	Firday	7:00:00	Living Room Yoga?	P90X yoga
13	11/12/2011	Saturday			
14	11/13/2011	Sunday			"Chilly 1/2 Marathon."
15	11/14/2011	Monday	19:00:00	Brighton	run 20 minute out and back
16	11/15/2011	Tuesday	7:00:00	Charles River Stations	Pushups, Box Jumps, Situps, Pullups, Supermen
17	11/16/2011	Wednesday	6:15:00	Harvard	37 Sections
18	11/17/2011	Thursday		Home	deck
19	11/18/2011	Friday	6:15/6:45	Brighton - Central	7.66
20	11/19/2011	Saturday			
21	11/20/2011	Sunday	12:15:00	Brighton - Dover	bike ride 32.7 miles
22	11/21/2011	Monday	6:15/6:45	Brighton - Central	7.66
23	11/22/2011	Tuesday		Charles River Stations	
24	11/23/2011	Wednesday		Brighton	deck
25	11/24/2011	Thursday		Harvard	37 sections
	11/25/2011	Friday			

Not many of the pieces I'd read had talked about the Monday workout except to note that it was always at a different location around the city announced via social media a day or two beforehand. From maligned neighborhoods to municipal plazas to hidden parks, a surprise fitness circuit awaited members, who were expected to run there.

"I was just on Google Maps looking for green space. Bojan and I really hadn't been to a lot of these places and we'd lived here for 10 years. In our lives, where we just see our driveway and where we work and the one bar we go to—to visit a new neighborhood is fun. I'm really proud of Mondays. It's the silliest day, the exploration piece. It's really cool."

Mandaric summed it up this way: "It lets you re-fall in love with the city you live in every week."

"Tell me about the hugging. I wonder if a lot of people can't get past that."

"It's a Midwest thing," Graham said. "We say, shakers don't risk anything in life. In Boston, there's a vibe that's pretty cool, but you give someone a big bear hug and every bit of coolness drops to the floor. You forget about not feeling good enough or fast enough. And if you show up as a hardcore athlete about to throw down, it makes you chill the fuck out. Everyone finds comfort in it. People might think it's weird, that's fine. We're going to keep doing it. It's a huge dose of community. There are many things that set us apart from other run groups. We tell people if you're not into hugging, you better fuckin' fake it or you're not going to like it here." The waitress arrived to clear plates. "That burger was killer, thank you," Graham said. "I'm going to pretend you made it."

She smiled, smitten. Graham turned back to me as he handed off the plate.

I'd never thought about it that way. He almost made it seem cool, necessary even. It takes courage to embrace a stranger, and with a little bit of risk who knows what can open up? *Okay, point to you, Mr. Graham.* But still, as a Gen-Xer raised on alienation and shaped by drunken assholery, I was pretty sure I'd be fuckin' faking it.

"You got any tats?" Graham asked.

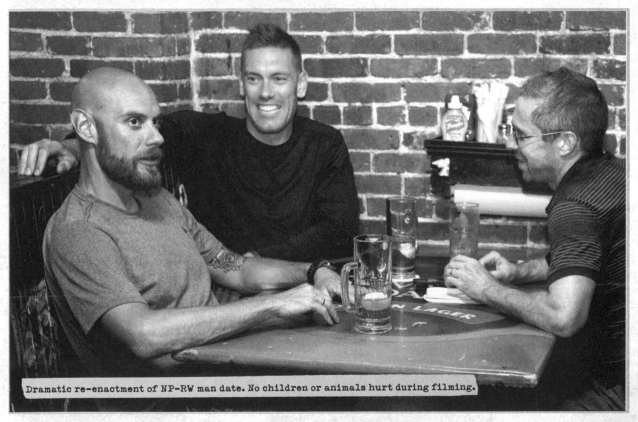

Dramatic re-enactment of NP-RW man date. No children or animals hurt during filming.

"I do, yeah," I said.

"Nice, whatd'ya got?"

I pulled up my left shirtsleeve.

"I got this one when I was 19," I said. "It's almost 25 years old."

"Here we go, here we go," Graham exclaimed. "I'm taking a picture of that one. Pull it up."

"It's a duck-billed platypus wearing a suit and smoking a cigar, carrying a briefcase with the word MOCKBA written on it. It's faded now, but that's Moscow in Russian."

"Yeah, yeah, dude, I gotta get that one," Mandaric joined in. "Where'd ya get that?"

"Ohio, during a cross-country trip."

"What city?" Graham asked.

"Don't remember. There were a lot of substances involved."

"What else you got?" he said.

I pinched down my shirt collar.

"Here we go," Graham said, leaning forward. "Here. We. Go!"

"That's a Bukowski poem," I explained.

"That's fuckin' awesome," Graham said, turning to Mandaric. "Yeahhhh, dude! You show him yours?"

Mandaric rolled up his sleeve, revealing a shoulder coated in ink.

"So that's for November Project," he started explaining, pointing to a rocket ship stamped Nov. Project. "And obviously I'm born and raised in Serbia, so the alien with the sunglasses stands for resident alien. And this is me, my wife, and my sister. The clock tower is my hometown clock tower. And my mom passed away when I was 16 so that's her initials in Cyrillic. Then when we have kids, I'm gonna fill it in with more little aliens or flying sorcerers."

"Tattoos are awesome," Graham said, "I love tattoos."

Okay, so maybe this Brogan Graham was a different breed of cat.

"I keep saying this, but ideally, I'd like to have NP in every city in the U.S. and the world," Mandaric said, picking up an earlier thread. "I don't think it's that far-fetched. After *Outside* ran their story, people reached out asking, 'How do we start one in my city?' They're realizing the potential and want to replicate it. There's no secret. Everyone can do it."

"Yeah, this is a dream community for me," Graham said. "It's active people who are always down. I could send out a tweet right now, 'Who wants to do a 5-miler starting at Pour House?' and we'd get 20 people here in 15 minutes. It's cool."

"So what makes it work?"

"When you don't pay dues, your only admission price is showing up," Graham said. "People believe in what we're doing because they feel like they own it. They're shareholders 'cause their ass is standing there."

"My philosophy is you attract people who represent your personality," Mandaric added. "If you're a good person, you're gonna surround yourself with good people. If you're an asshole, I might hang out with you once or twice, but third time I'm like, that dude's a fuckin' asshole; I don't want anything to do with him. So the people who we—"

"Hold on," Graham interrupted. "I'll hang out with assholes—like, six times. Up to ten times. Ten to fifteen times. I'll hang out with an asshole fifteen times. Because they're fun. Anyway."

I didn't hear any more. I stared at Graham, his close-cropped head, his sharp cheekbones, his ready-for-anything eyes. In college, I'd earned the nickname "Asshole" and proudly answered to it. Might we have hung out? Nah, probably not. I disdained athletic endeavors (up to and including walking to class) and reveled in the irony of wearing a high school varsity jacket that reeked of cigarette smoke and burnt breakfast meats. But suddenly, the space between us narrowed. I realized I'd stopped taking notes for the past 20 minutes. *Shit*. I checked the recorder.

#RunDeckRun.
UNDER 6 MILES AWAY, YOU GOTTA RUN.
DISCOVER CITY'S NOOKS + CRANNIES. DECK=DECK
OF CARDS

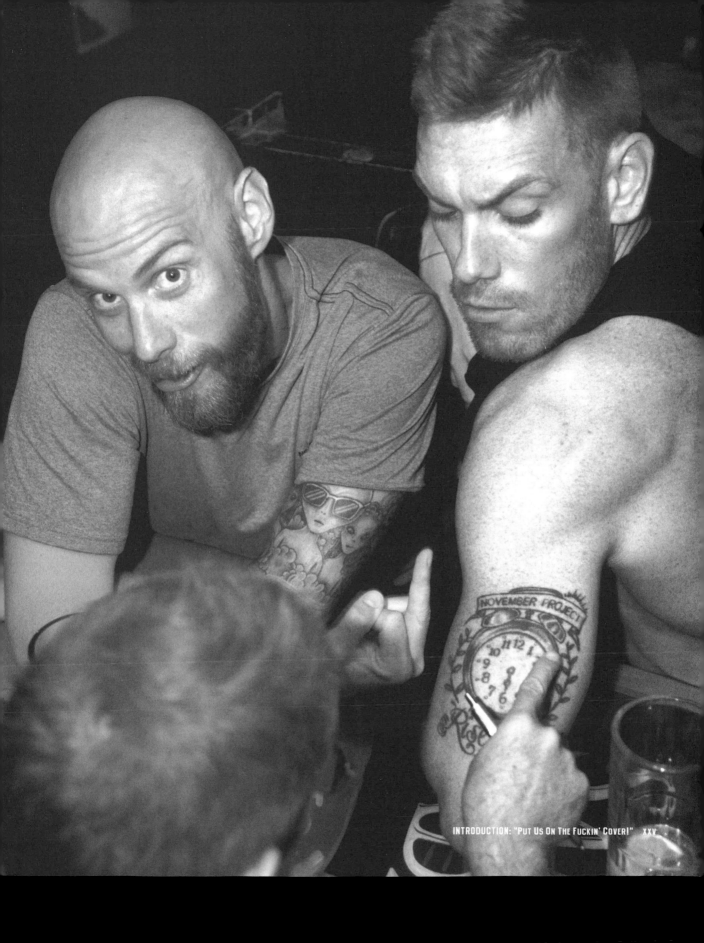

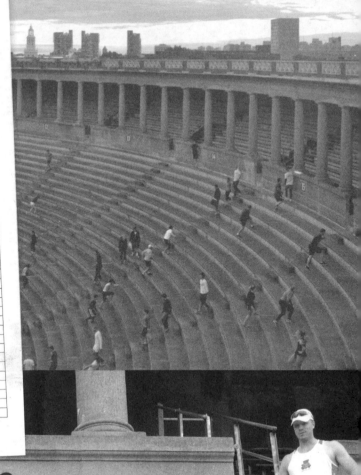
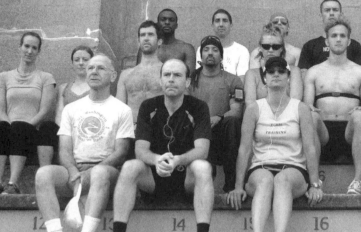
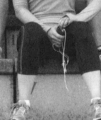
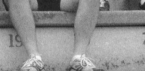

GRASSROOTS GEAR?
TALK TO GRAHAM'S GIRL.

"What surprises me, in the right way, is how proud people are of this thing," Graham continued. "It's more than being proud about being tagged in a Facebook photo which says, 'Look at me, I'm working out way before you got out of bed; I'm the shit.' A little self-pride, that's one level.

"But my girl did the Run to Remember half-marathon on Sunday, and I was standing on the corner to take her jacket as she ran by. Suddenly, I hear, 'November Project!' and a few moments later, 'Fuck yeah, NP!' It got to the point where I heard it a half dozen times in the first couple of minutes. This wasn't about Facebook or trying to recruit spectators or because I was standing there, but because they were proud. All of them were wearing grassroots gear. Of all the shit you could put on the front of your chest to race in, that's really fuckin' cool. Race day is an important thing. You set out your shirt the night before, get out your bib, your goo packets, or whatever. That's a goosebumps story for me."

Mandaric leaned back in the booth and took me in for a moment.

"So this story, it is gonna be a page, or a little box, or a full-on article?" Mandaric asked.

"They're looking for a thousand words, maybe fifteen hundred, depending."

I glanced at Graham, who seemed to be staring just beyond me or was lost in thought. I reached for the check.

"So put us on the fuckin' cover," he blurted.

Uh, what? Blank look. Watery smile.

"Why not?" he continued, wide-eyed. "Put our goofy asses on the cover. Can you imagine? People will pick it up and say, this is running; I don't have to be that skinny hot blond chick. I'm not gonna be Dean Karnazes. It'll be like those two awkward guys with tattoos. Put your fuckin' slow guys on the cover."

I didn't know what to say. The cover? The freakin' cover? I didn't know the route that led to this sacred real estate, the gatekeepers with their secret codes and formulas. I hadn't even been to a November Project workout yet, had only spoken to these guys for 90 minutes. They were either delusional, hopelessly naïve, or had balls the size of Gibraltar.

"I'm just a contributing writer and don't have much influence on what goes on the cover," I said.

Graham looked at me a moment and I thought I registered a flash of disappointment in his eyes, not in the fact that I couldn't promise them the cover, but that he was looking at someone who saw limits, who doubted his own influence, and that made him a little sad. I told myself it was just the angle of the light and looked away.

When I returned his gaze, all I could do was force a smile and say I'd see them in a few weeks, not sure when exactly. I had other pieces on my plate. I made sure to get their race PRs and was relieved to learn Graham was a Boston Qualifier. My plan now was to parachute in for the three sessions and gather enough content to notch another *Runner's World* byline in my belt. It was all about the next story, the bigger one, the one that I could really sink my teeth into. The one I was always hoping would change my life.

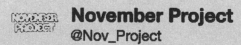 **November Project**
@Nov_Project

⚙   +⚊ Follow

"No, MOM! I can't MAIL u a shirt! U have to join the tribe to get a one! And it's not GrassrootsSHIRT! It's #GrassrootsGEAR!" @nov_projectprob

2 Apr 2013

World Takeover Leaps to the Cover of @RunnersWorld Magazine

🕐 6th November 2013   👤 brogan   🗂 Blog   💬 0 Comments

BOOOOOOOOOOOOM! The cover story for the December issue of *Runner's World* is nearly 100 percent November Project and 400 percent real! It's been spotted now in the hands of November Project members in all seven locations and, as of yesterday, at least one airport bookstore near you. As much as this *RW* tale highlights the Boston experience, it's important to know that we, as a seven-city mob, are growing fast in all the right ways. Getting this type of recap of who we are and what we stand for is huge . . . giant . . . no, it's . . . it's . . . it's unlike anything we've seen in our 2-year lifespan. Today's post captures all seven tribes enjoying the love from *Runner's World* and their inside scoop. Open wide and make room for this power-hype burrito of WEDNESDAY love-sauce coming your way! **The tribe is seemingly taking over.**

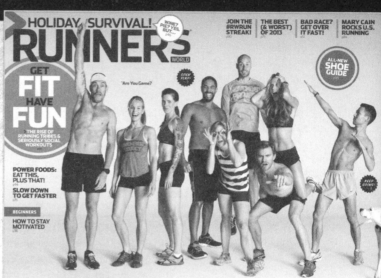

Though many folks from the "normal media" have come and gone, staying just long enough to drop the right lingo and understand our workouts, this is not the case with *Runner's World*. Caleb Daniloff, the writer for the December issue cover story, will not be put in this classification. He's officially hooked and rarely misses a workout throughout the week.

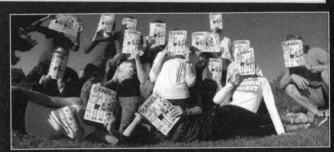

Another special thanks to David Willey (*RW* editor and NP member) for believing in the good of our community and pushing our story in a year of dramatic ups and downs. The article has been spotted on the shelves! Let's see just how far this November Project love-beast can reach. Onward.

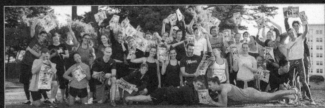

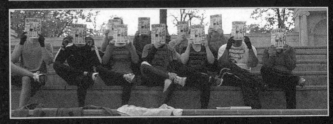

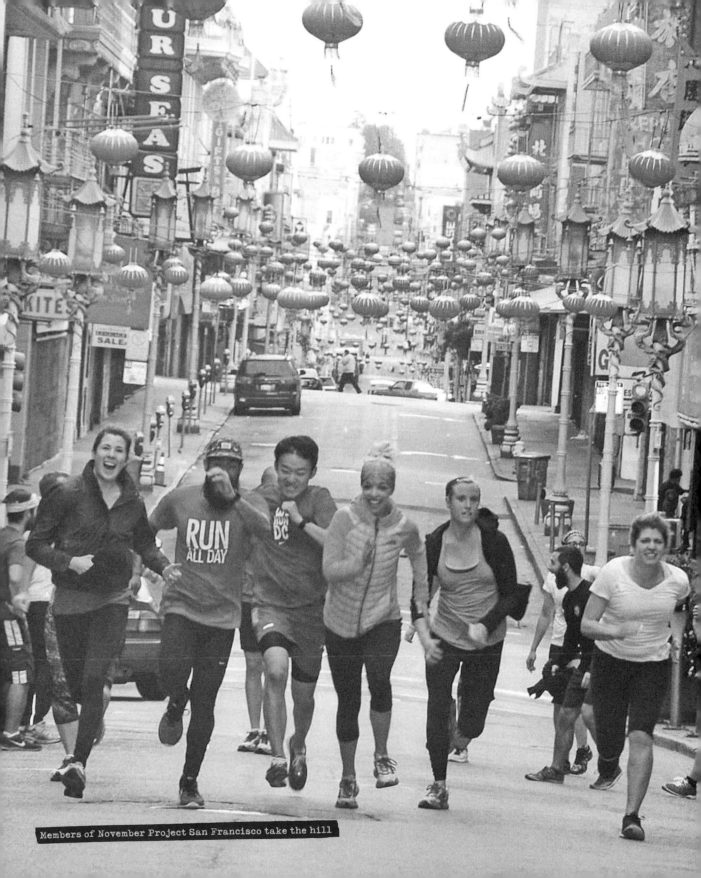

Members of November Project San Francisco take the hill

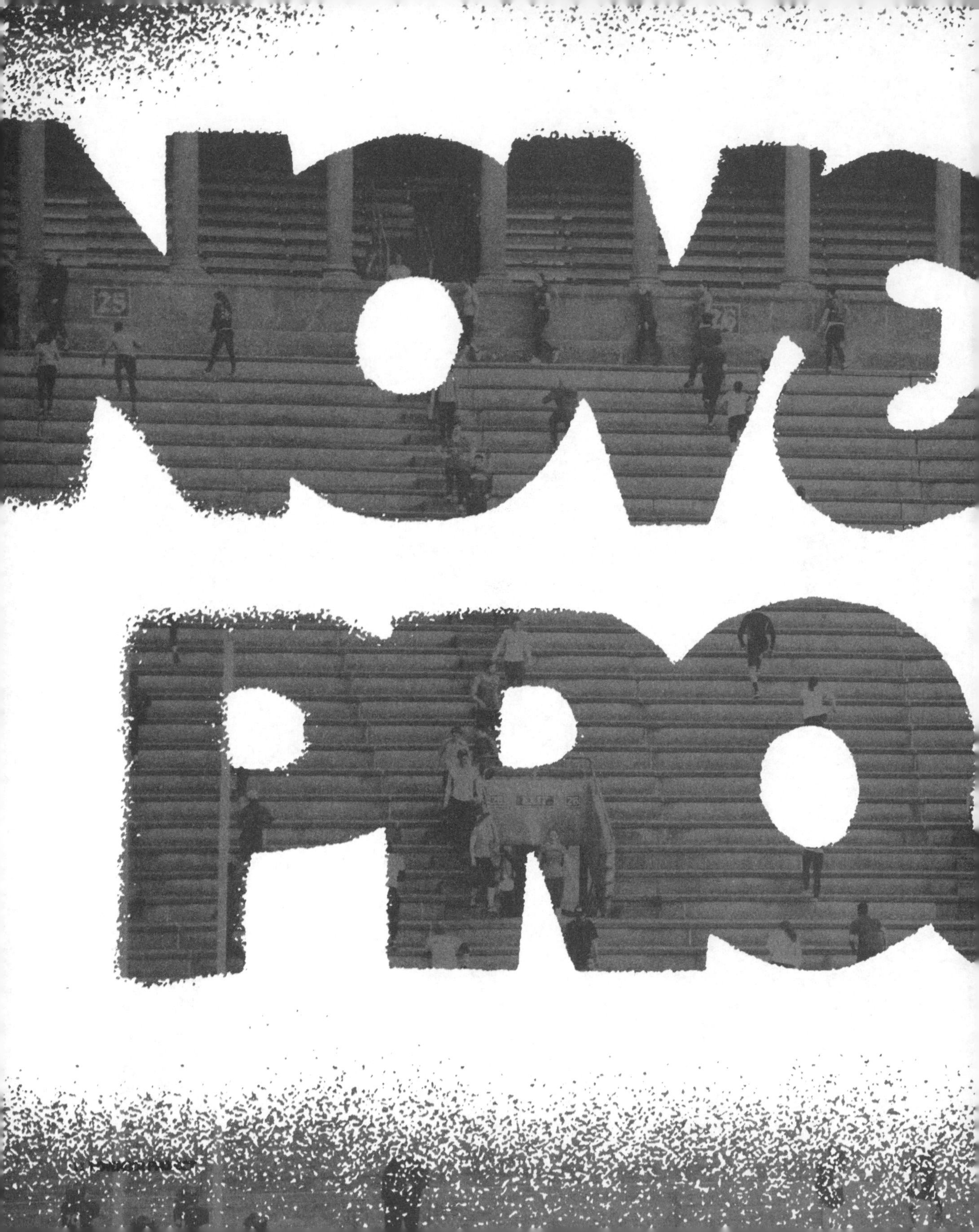

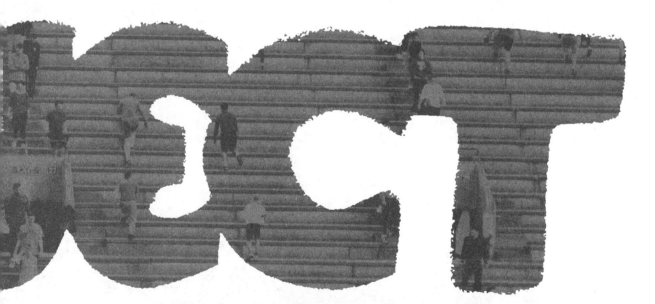

PART 1 **THE MOTHER SHIP**

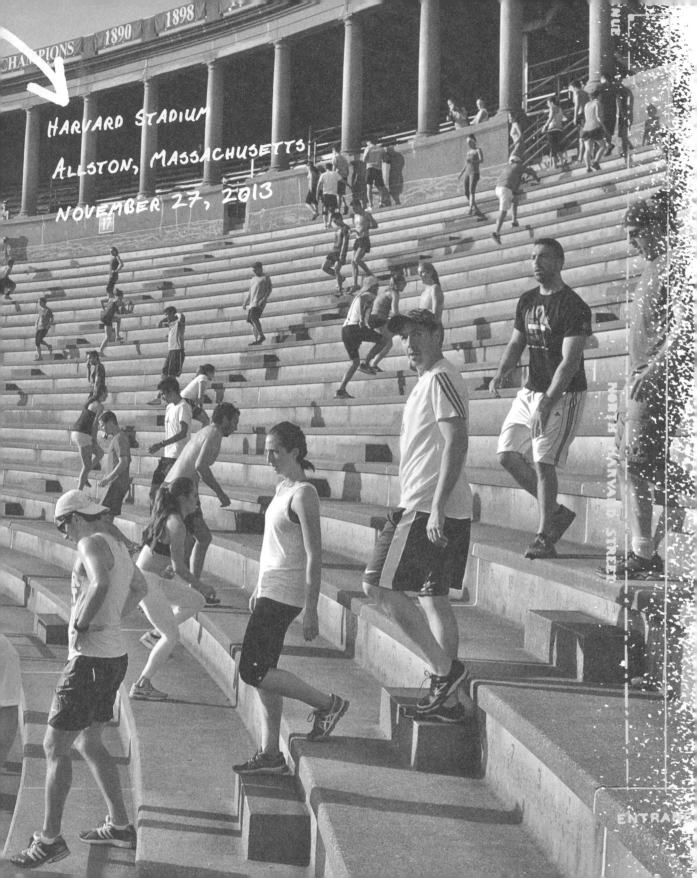

HARVARD STADIUM

ALLSTON, MASSACHUSETTS

NOVEMBER 27, 2013

CHAPTER 1

THE NEWBIES

WISCONSIN NOTES

- NOVEMBER PROJECT TAKES THE STRANGE OUT OF STRANGER

- NOR'EASTER SHMOR'EASTER

- TWO MBTA BUS RIDERS BECOME LIFELONG FRIENDS

- ONE PERSON THROWS UP

- HARVARD'S COLISEUM HELPED SAVE THE SPORT OF FOOTBALL

- NOVEMBER PROJECT'S FIRST RECRUIT RUNS "WILD"

- COUNTLESS BOSTON ROWERS HAVE BEEN BORN AGAIN ON THE STADIUM STAIRS

- A STANLEY CUP CHAMPION ONCE WENT BY "NEWBIE"

- BOJAN GUNS DOWN EXCUSES LIKE THEY'RE STANDING STILL (WHICH THEY ARE)

- WHILE HIS OWN TRIBE WAS HOME WRINKLING LIKE FROZEN PRUNES, BG WAS PICKING SUNSHINE WEDGIES IN SOUTHERN CALIFORNIA. YEAH, FUCK THAT GUY.

Maria Cesca wasn't sure this was such a good idea. Her husband and sons thought she was nuts. Her flight had landed late the night before and she was rolling on 3 hours of sleep. But here she was, at 5:45 a.m., shivering and bleary-eyed in a deserted bus stop at the corner of Harvard Street and Commonwealth Avenue in Allston, a gritty neighborhood in west Boston. A cold rain was lashing the stop signs and the wind swinging the street lights. The 48-year-old Florida warehouse manager was nervous as she peered down the empty boulevard while scanning for the number 66 bus. Not a soul or machine in sight. She bounced from foot to foot, trying to keep warm, no idea what lay ahead.

All because of the big guy.

On a recent trip to Boston from her home in Coral Springs, the Brazilian-born Cesca and her 23-year-old son Pedro, a graduate student at Boston University, had been running the Esplanade along the Charles River. They stopped to take a selfie with the iconic MIT dome across the water in Cambridge as a backdrop, moving the camera this way and that, trying to get the angle just right.

"A big guy stopped running, approached us, and asked if we wanted him to take our picture. I answered yes, thank you. The big guy took the photo and asked us

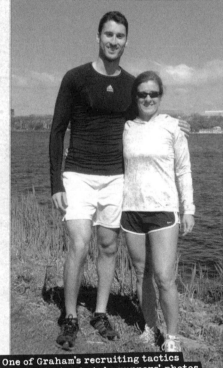

One of Graham's recruiting tactics was offering to take runners' photos along the Charles River.

where we work out, then started telling us about something called November Project. I was so surprised with his kind gesture, taking his time to take our picture and talking with us. In South Florida, people are always in a rush. I went to my son's apartment and looked up November Project at the computer."

Cesca didn't have a chance to check out the curious group during that trip, but found herself in Boston the following Thanksgiving week. She thought about the big guy again and emailed him, asking whether the workout was still on for the next morning despite the monsoon beating down on the city. Within minutes came the reply.

"We always train. The weather is only an excuse for those who decide to NOT show up. Also, the early morning is harsh on the well-rested and the sleep-deprived. ½ the world is 'tired.' Pop out of bed and go intro yourself to Bojan tomorrow. I'm training with our November Project group in San Diego tomorrow morning. The tribe is strong. BG."

Finally, Cesca spotted headlights sweeping the lacquered asphalt, the beams clouded by mist and sliced by furious lines of rain. The bus stopped and the doors hissed open, water dripping off the hinges. She climbed aboard and paid the fare. It was just her, the driver, and two men sitting in different rows. As she stepped forward, she noticed the men were dressed in striped leggings, fluorescent wind jackets, and running caps. Cesca

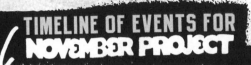

TIMELINE OF EVENTS FOR NOVEMBER PROJECT

SUNDAY, 11:37 P.M., OCTOBER 30, 2011— THE POUR HOUSE BAR, BOSTON

With beer-scented breath, Brogan Graham and Bojan Mandaric give each other what would become November Project's first "verbal."

MONDAY, 8:12 A.M., OCTOBER 31, 2011

Both men wake up hungover, with the naked form of accountability lying beside their throbbing heads.

TUESDAY, 6:30 A.M., NOVEMBER 1, 2011

Bojan and BG meet on the stairs of Harvard Stadium, the site of countless grueling Northeastern rowing workouts. They complete all 37 sections, a.k.a. a full tour.

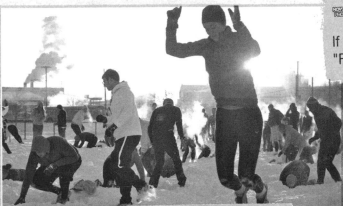

After perfecting her community-growing craft with the Boston tribe, Rakel Eva Sævarsdóttir, seen here, is now leading November Project Iceland.

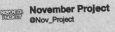

November Project
@Nov_Project

⚙ +≗ Follow

If the voices in your head aren't saying, "Fuck Yeah" let NP fix that. Join for #Frogust

wondered if they were headed to the stadium, too. She took a seat, making note of the storefronts out the window, paying attention to the route.

One of those men was 46-year-old Nicolas Flattes, a sales associate at True Runner, which had just opened a store in Newton. A technical rep from New Balance named Sara Wild had recently visited the staff and told them about a local social-fitness group, that it represented a fresh direction in running, and was even the subject of a *Runner's World* cover story. Flattes thought it sounded weird and crazy, but interesting. He knew Wild was a sub-3:05 marathoner and a one-time professional soccer player, so "my first impression was that the group might only be for ultra and elite athletes. I thought I'd have no place there."

But he also thought that some quad work might speed up his recovery from a calf muscle tear he'd suffered while training for his second half-marathon. The leg injury, however, was the least of his pain. The previous year, his 11-year marriage had collapsed and it was still raw to the touch.

"The relationship went up in smoke as if it never happened. We had two children, a six-year-old daughter and a one-and-a-half-year-old son. She told me to move out and get my own place. It was a complete shock. Our marriage had been rocky and we had moved from Boston to Vancouver in the hopes that things would get better, but they only got worse."

After his ex-wife gained full custody of their children, Flattes found himself shut out, even by one-time friends. Numerous attempts to see his kids failed. Exhausted and worn down, he went home to Boston to regroup with family and figure out his next move. Five months later, he was nervously jostling on a city bus on his way to a strange stadium at the world's most prestigious university. "I had no idea what was going to happen," he said.

The bus whined to a stop across the road from an iron-gated athletic compound, across the river from Harvard's main campus in Cambridge. Flattes followed a short, tanned woman and the other man down the steps and back into the wet blackness. All of them headed in the same direction. They smiled shyly at each other and walked between two brick columns. Were they even allowed to be here? Through the rain, Cesca and Flattes could make out points of light bobbing a few hundred yards away, headlamps of runners going up and down.

"It was a magical image," Cesca recalls. "It looked like the lights were flying. Everything was new. The rain getting in my eyes was so cold. I could hear some voices but I couldn't see the people yet, only the lights."

THURSDAY, NOVEMBER 10, 2011

As rowers, they tracked and quantified everything. Naturally, they created a shared Google Doc for their new fitness endeavor. Titled "The November Project," they filled it with miles run, times for tours at Harvard Stadium, flipped decks of cards, and dumps taken behind construction fences.

 WHEN YOU GOTTA GO, YOU GOTTA GO.

MONDAY, NOVEMBER 7, 2011

Just to keep it weird, the boys hit the road with a deck of cards in their pocket. After running to a mutually agreed-upon spot, they drop down and knock out pushups and sit-ups based on the value and suits of flipped cards.

WEDNESDAY, NOVEMBER 2, 2011

Bojan runs 3 miles to BG's apartment. BG then runs Bojan back home. They christen this workout the "Door to Door."

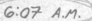

They passed the end zone of the football field and rounded the corner of the gray concrete stadium. They found an open archway that led into the lower cavern. A number of bikes were chained to the wrought-iron fencing, rain-beaded helmets dangling from the handlebars. Flattes could make out concrete columns and staircases leading up to a square of bruised sky. He was chilled and glad to be out of the rain. "I made my way up the back stairs to the top of section 37 and put my bag in the driest place I could find. Then I saw a guy run up at top speed, stagger behind the wooden bleachers, and throw up. I thought, this must be the place."

Nervous, Flattes then made his way down to the group gathering at the bottom, all arms and heads, writhing on a metal landing that overlooked the northern end zone. It looked like 100 people at least. He was impressed. Clouds of breath rose here and there, mingling, vanishing. A shirtless Asian dude was wearing a swim cap, goggles, and Hawaiian board shorts. An older man was barefoot. People were chatting and laughing and hugging; others kept their heads down against the pelting rain. Flattes looked across the artificial turf, emblazoned with a red H in the middle, toward the goal posts and scoreboards. He scanned the red Ivy League championship banners that rung the stadium's upper portico. The most recent national title was dated 1919. This place was old, he thought.

Built in 1903 and shaped like a horseshoe, Harvard Stadium was designed to conjure a classical Athenian coliseum, complete with an upper colonnade and gated archways. Inside, the 37 seating sections are each terraced with 30 rows of concrete benching. At ground level, gates give way to the field. You can almost picture lions being released to eat the Christians or hapless professors denied tenure. One writer described the arena as "the aristocrat of American sports amphitheaters."

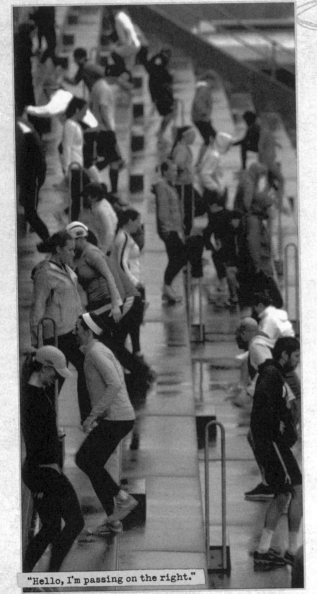

"Hello, I'm passing on the right."

THE NEXT 6 MONTHS

Lather. Rinse. Repeat. By the third month, pangs of boredom start creeping in, even as they are occasionally joined by friends. They talk about inviting random strangers to join them and hopefully race against.

FEBRUARY 2012

Grassroots gear makes its first race appearance at the Super Sunday 5-Miler in Cambridge, Mass. BG comes in 18th place, Bojan in 73rd (33:53). Both men beat their time goal. The race has since become an annual November Project-Boston tradition, with huge tribe turnout.

november-project.com/super-sunday-5-miler/

WEDNESDAY, MAY 2, 2012

For shits and giggles, Bojan creates a November Project website. Not to be one-upped, BG immediately starts a Twitter account.

HTTP://NOVEMBER-PROJECT.COM

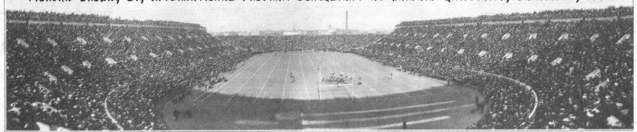

"HARVARD STADIUM'S AN HISTORIC VENUE FOR SURE, AND NOT JUST FOR THE YALE-HARVARD GAME. IKE AND TINA TURNER PLAYED HERE. BOB MARLEY PLAYED HERE. JANIS JOPLIN'S LAST CONCERT WAS HELD HERE. BUT THEY WERE ALL JUST THE UNDERCARDS."

—MORGAN BROWN, 31, INTERNATIONAL PROGRAM CONSULTANT AT HARVARD UNIVERSITY, CAMBRIDGE, MASS.

When it rains, the stadium smells earthy, like history, and, fittingly, it has a claim on several firsts. It was the first stadium built for U.S. college athletics and was the first permanent—and largest—reinforced concrete structure of its time. But perhaps the arena's most famous first was as midwife to football's forward pass, a development that not only saved the game, but pretty much shaped the NFL we know today.

In the late 1800s and early 1900s, football was a hot running and kicking game on college campuses. But it had morphed into a blood sport, a mash-up of rugby and bar brawling, with punches, eye gouging, throttling, pig-piling. And death. At the end of the 1905 college football season, 18 fatalities were reported across the country, along with dozens of disabling injuries. Harvard's president demanded rule changes or he would scrap the program. And if the sport were killed at Harvard, many feared it was all but doomed at the national level.

So U.S. president (and Harvard alum) Teddy Roosevelt stepped in. He organized the Intercollegiate Football Conference—a collection of 28 colleges and universities and the forerunner of the NCAA—which came up with 19 rules to make football safer. Among them, no tackling out of bounds or below the knee, and no striking the ball carrier in the face. It shortened games from 70 minutes to an hour and instituted a mandatory 10-minute rest between halves. There was a push to widen the playing field, too, but Harvard Stadium wasn't built to budge and school officials nixed the idea. As an alternative, they adopted the forward pass, one of the first programs to do so. And, in 1906, the Crimson's first pigskin sailed through the Boston breeze. The forward pass helped popularize the radical changes to the game, and along with it came the rise of the star quarterback and entirely new playbooks.

"It's hard to tell what's sweat and what's rain," a voice laughed behind Flattes.

It was Sara Wild from New Balance. Her wet hair, slicked back and ponytailed, was plastered against her neck. "Glad you made it," she said. Wild had just finished up with the 5:30 group. "It's darker, so it's easier to hide," she smiled. The early squad was born as a way for Graham and Mandaric to get their own tours in before leading the 6:30 workout. But that secret didn't hold, and at last count, the early group had swelled to nearly 100 racers all chasing the long-legged Graham in the dark.

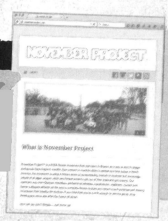

WEDNESDAY, MAY 2, 2012

The first tweet from the NP handle arrives in the cybersphere: "Come one, come all #novemberproject is in full swing. Next meeting @ Harvard Stadium 05/09 @6:30am." A pal at Marathon Sports retweets.

November Project
@Nov_Project
Building a worldwide community by empowering humans of all fitness levels through fierce, free, weekly workouts.
WARNING: We roll 21 cities deep.
#21HumpBeat

November Project @Nov_Project · 20h
Just show up, 6:30AM this WED at the bottom of section 37, Harvard Stadium & u can join us for a wrkout
👤 Nov_Project

"All right!" a robust voice from a few rows above suddenly cut through the chatter. "Listen up, listen up . . . Let's get going. I'm pausing now for dramatic effect . . . Okay, let's get a little bounce."

Flattes couldn't make out more than a pair of broad shoulders and a hooded face rising up against the rain. Like a swell at sea, hoods and caps began bobbing all around him, an energy lifting and crashing against itself, the metal floor of the overlook shaking.

"Okay, slow turn to the right. Look at the people around you. Give them your best murder eyes. Keep bouncing." Eyes widened, brows narrowed, a few people laughed. "Okay, for all my OCD friends, let's go ahead and make a slow turn to the left." They bounced and they bounced and—"Stop! Good morning!"

"Good morning!" a chorus barked back.

"Y'all good?"

Like cannon fire, "Fuck yeah!" ricocheted across the field and back again, the syllables hammering down like massive exclamation points. Flattes felt them in his chest.

"Raise your hand if today is your first day."

Flattes, Cesca, and some 10 other tentative arms went up, all of them greeted with thunderous clapping and hooting.

"Fuck yeah, welcome," Mandaric said, pacing back and forth like a rapper stalking the stage.

Typically, the thunder-voiced Graham, with his manic enthusiasm and spontaneously absurd wit, rallies the troops for the Bounce. But on this morning, Mandaric, often seen as the serious and quiet one, despite his dancing and rapid-fire slang, was in command. The Serbian got off on dismantling perceptions. He'd been doing it his whole life. And Cesca, for one, felt his vibe, the energy from the crowd, like it had fingers and arms, lifting her off her feet. November Project "was already unlike any workout I'd ever been to."

"Okay, today is PR day," Mandaric continued, "so most of you know what to do—race your asses off. Forty minutes on the clock. If you brought a shirt to be tagged, take it up to section 36. Evan's gonna start the big kids in waves of 10. Newbies, follow me out this exit for a little pow-wow."

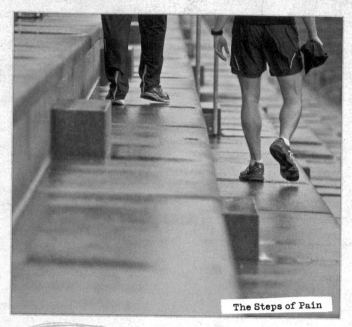

The Steps of Pain

Flattes, Cesca, and the other first-timers gathered at the lower concourse, nervously-curiously-excitedly looking up at Mandaric as he shifted from foot to foot, long thick legs disappearing beneath a black windbreaker. He pushed back his hood, revealing the beads of rain running down his bare temples. Even to Flattes, who stands 6 feet 5, the Serbian was imposing and no-nonsense.

"Okay, bring it in. Closer. You should be touching the person next to you. Body heat is good, especially this morning. Here's the deal: November Project is a free, grassroots fitness movement, started by me and my college rowing buddy Brogan Graham, who's in sunny Southern California right now dancing with the sunbeams. You can give him shit when he gets back.

"This all started as a way for me and him to stay fit in the Boston winter. Then after 6 months, we got bored racing each other at the stadium and sent out a tweet to see if anyone would join us. And the next day, one person showed up. We were fuckin' ecstatic. Her name was Sara Wild and she still owns the fastest female time for a full tour. She took a chance on us just like you're taking a chance this morning instead of hitting your snooze bar. We believe that chance will not only pay off physically and mentally, but will help you make this world a better place."

Flattes stood wide-eyed. He'd read the *Runner's World* piece, but had no idea that Wild was November Project's very first member, that she'd been coming for all 18 months. She was so mild-mannered and unassuming. He was finding the whole thing captivating, even though he'd been involved with meditation and yoga centers where group encounters and personal contact were part of the experience. He'd also survived boot camp in the U.S. Navy. But here at Harvard Stadium of all places, he felt something different, something raw, open, exuberant, vital.

"One thing we never do in our daily lives is look each other in the eye," Mandaric continued. "We avoid contact with other human beings. November Project is about changing that. So turn to three people in your area, give them a hug, look them in the eye, and find out where they're from and one more thing about them. Because without them, and without you, these workouts wouldn't happen."

A cacophonous babble reverberated around the concourse: town names, book titles, movies, sports teams, college names. Mandaric was jostling about the fray, too, hugging and chatting. After 60 seconds, he stepped back.

"Alright, alright. Now for today's workout. On your first day, we suggest shooting for a half tour, which is running up the big steps and down the little crimson ones until you get to section 19. You may think, 'section 19? Fuck that, I'm a marathoner or a varsity rugby player, watch me eat this whole damn stadium.' Well, if you can do that your first time out, in under 40 minutes, you'll have my respect. But after 10 sections, you're gonna find that these stairs are no fuckin' joke."

Indeed. The stone benches at Harvard Stadium are almost 2 feet tall, which for the average runner means stepping up at a near-90 degree angle, your thigh almost parallel to the ground. And at 3 feet deep, the foot tends to land at the front-to-middle of the next row, requiring significant lift to keep going up and forward. That's

"I FIRST LEARNED ABOUT NP ON TWITTER. ABOUT TWO YEARS AGO. I SAW A TWEET THAT IF YOU CAME TO NINE WORKOUTS IN A MONTH, THEY'D GIVE YOU A BRAND NEW PAIR OF NEW BALANCE. I'D JUST STARTED RUNNING AND I NEEDED A PAIR OF SHOES. I'VE BEEN COMING EVER SINCE. I'VE BEEN TAGGING SHIRTS ALMOST AS LONG."

—XANDER MILLER, 21, PHARMACY STUDENT AT NORTHEASTERN UNIVERSITY

31 high lunges per section, including the very top step, which is more of a lip. ("Skip that top row, you end up robbing yourself of an entire section," Graham says.) Multiply that by 37 and you're talking 1,147 upward lunges. With 40 minutes on the clock, those arms are swinging. Cue the jellied quads and urgent conversations with God.

Most of the high school and college crews assembled in Boston over the past 5 decades are intimately familiar with the "Steps of Death." In the 1960s, Harvard's legendary rowing coach Harry Parker took a page from the books of West Coast Olympians who used stadium running as part of their training. Parker considered the steep, solid steps at Harvard Stadium perfect conditioning for the leg portion of the rowing motion, offering his oarsmen a unique combination of cardiovascular and muscular intensity. He took his teams to the arena no matter the weather, shoveling snow to make way for winter workouts. With scores of national and Olympic medals to Parker's credit, other area squads soon followed his regimen. "[Rowing] is not quite fun the way other sports are, like kicking and maneuvering in soccer," he once said. "It's not a game. Basically, it's hard work."

6:39 A.M.

Cesca, Flattes, and the others followed Mandaric as he jogged up the access stairs, back into the rain, and down to the bottom of section 37. Dawn had broken and the campus clock tower was shrouded in mist. The faster runners were already closing in on section 19, little

"I DISLIKE TOUCHING PEOPLE, AND BEING TOUCHED, AND I ESPECIALLY DON'T WANT TO HUG STRANGERS—ESPECIALLY NOT SWEATY STRANGERS—THAT'S DISGUSTING. WHEN I WENT TO MY FIRST NP SOMETHING PERCEPTIBLY SHIFTED INSIDE OF ME. I ACTUALLY FELT IT SHIFT. I CAN'T EXPLAIN IT VERY WELL, BUT SOMEHOW IT JUST FELT RIGHT TO BE THERE. NP IS SOMEHOW MORE THAN JUST NP. IT IS PART OF MY LIFE, PART OF WHO I AM. I FEEL SUCH GRATITUDE TO BROGAN AND BOJAN FOR CREATING THIS SUPPORTIVE, LOVING, WEIRD COMMUNITY."

—MARY ANNA YRAM, 50, RESEARCH COMPLIANCE COORDINATOR AT HARVARD'S STEM CELL AND REGENERATIVE BIOLOGY DEPARTMENT

smeared bits of color streaking down the faraway steps. Mandaric lined Cesca, Flattes, and the other newbies in a row. "Okay, left foot up. Get ready. Go!" A wave of abilities and body sizes splashed up the steps, some nervous and tentative, others going out too fast, with something to prove.

After two sections, not only were Cesca's lungs standing at attention, but so was her entire body, her entire being. A young woman fell in and introduced herself. "Her name was Alex and she asked if I was a newbie. She was very kind and explained the workouts and began running with me," Cesca said.

From the top of section 36, the smell of Krylon spray paint wafted from the upper bleachers, the rattle and hiss of cans hard at work. Dozens of colored shirts were draped across the wooden benches. A lithe dude, face masked in a construction-style breathing mask and shod in a walking-boot, limped about with blackened "November" and "Project" stencils in his hand. His partner, wearing a bandanna, bank-robber style, and a headlamp, was pulling more clothes from a pile and flattening them out. At the end of one row, a Jeep tire cover.

Mandaric sauntered toward section 1, ignoring the rain splashing off the stone benches. He high-fived runners coming down the small steps ("Nice work, friends") and cheered others to the top. He spied a few folks clustered at the bottom, catching their breath, fiddling with their watches, and rallied them onward. "Turn and go. That's it, Michaela. You got this. All the way to the top. Keep moving. Turn and burn."

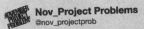

Nov_Project Problems
@nov_projectprob

⚙   +⚫ Follow

Who pooped at section 10? Not cool #PRpoop #novemberprojectproblems @Nov_Project 💩

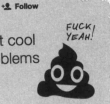
FUCK! YEAH!

By section 30, his seventh section, Flattes's shoes were sopped and his quads torched. He dialed back his pace. The steps were so dark and wet, almost like black ice, that he could see his reflection in them. He stopped to take a few pictures on his phone, the lights of Cambridge and Harvard campus greased on the horizon. A couple sections ahead, the air was being parted by a series of hearty call-and-responses.

"When I say 'November,' you say?" a female voice sang out, boot-camp style.

"PROJECT!"

"When I say, 'Wake up,' you say?"

"SHOW UP!"

At section 19, a dude starting belting out a Bon Jovi tune: "Halfway there, oh whoa, livin' on a prayer." At least a dozen voices joined in. Flattes smiled and had to remind himself that it wasn't even 7 a.m. and he was at an Ivy League playing field, not a hair metal show.

Laura Ingalls, aka DJ Phoenix: Mornin' Brogan! Question for you . . . so I've been backing off on my NP workouts as I'm gearing up for my marathon, but I'd really like to come cheer everyone on tomorrow morning. Then I got to thinking . . . It's the day before Halloween . . . do you think it'd be fun if I brought my DJ equipment in and played some tunes on my big speakers for the workout? Toss in a few halloween songs etc?

BG: FUCKING FUCK! That's an amazing idea!!!! Can you do both groups? FUCK! That's such a great idea!!!! FUCK! So cool.

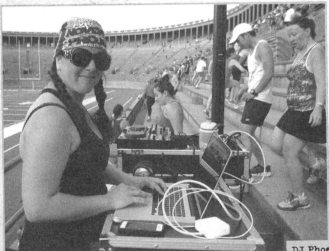

DJ Phoenix: Spinning stadium tunes every month since 2013

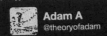

Adam A
@theoryofadam

⚙ +≗ Follow

Wondered why my calf muscles were screaming this AM. Oh yeah, #HarvardStadium @nov_projectprob

Erica Holt
@Erocksawesome

⚙ +≗ Follow

@nov_projectprob Being covered in 18 different peoples sweat after the post workout hug sesh. #worthit

7:20 A.M.

6:58 A.M.

At sections 3 and 2, the faster finishers were leaning over the upper concourse wall, some shirtless, beaded chests cinched with heart rate monitors, some in soaked November Project shirts, cheering the oncoming runners, by name, by outfit, pumping out that finish-line vibe. A boisterous crowd had gathered at the top of section 1, with some forming a human tunnel up the final 10 steps into which soaked bodies disappeared. Grimaces morphed to smiles, legs moved a few degrees faster, hidden reserves were tapped, and hand after hand slapped that magical red box with the white number 1 painted in it. Home base. Then they staggered to the upper concourse, grabbing the railing with both hands to pull themselves forward. Hair flattened and parted by the rain, eyeglasses fogged over, the newly finished joined the other walking wounded. Some sat on the cement, hugging their knees, chests heaving, eyes staring off, coming to, coming back. The air itself seeming to gasp for breath.

Meanwhile, Cesca and Alex had stopped at section 22 to take a picture together. The Brazilian was so amazed by all the smiles and positive vibes that she hardly felt the rain. It was as if weather never existed. "Alex told me about a Brazilian restaurant in Waltham and said if I stopped by, to call her. I was so happy to have a new friend and we decided to do five more sections. I was hooked. I loved every minute of it."

Flattes, who ran by himself, put away 16 sections when time was called. Even though he heard it was raining too hard for the group photo, he saw people gathering at section 1, bubbling, heaving, laughing, lingering in the rain, filling in the rows by the time he reached them on jack-hammered legs. He squeezed in next to Cesca and Alex, still catching his breath. "I don't know how to describe what just happened," he said, grinning. "I'm walking like Pinocchio, but I feel great." He and Cesca exchanged phone numbers and they took a couple wide-smiling selfies. Over the next couple of minutes, the Creature of Section 1 slowly disassembled, its pieces scattering down the stairs and out exits, mounting bikes, heading for running paths, for cars, for homes, for showers, for jobs. The rest of Boston was just waking up, cussing the weather and all the shit that meant for their morning commute.

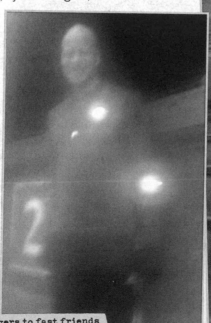

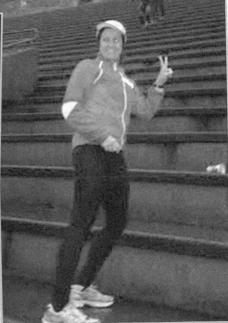

RENEWED FOCUS: From wet strangers to fast friends

Twas the Morning Before Thanksgiving and YEG Was Talking to the Hand

🕐 27th November 2013   👤 bojan   📁 Blog   💬 1 Comment

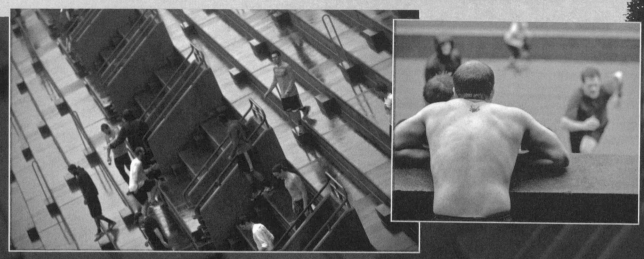

"It's raining" . . . so what? It's water, not nails.

"This storm is gonna create a major clusterfuck down East Coast for holiday travelers" . . . oh well, at least we're not living in Edmonton (Oooohhh no he didn't).

"My photo didn't make it into the facebook album" . . . sit in the front row of the group shot and it will. Unless it's raining in which case camera stays at home and you can take a selfie.

"BG went to left coast to rub neon spandex with people whose 6:30am comes 3 hours later than yours" . . . Fuck that guy and his long legs that make him run fast.

The point that I'm trying to make here by gunning down everything that moves is that excuses are lame statements that your brain is trying to fabricate when you're facing adversity. So kick that excuse in its figurative balls and remember no matter how shitty you think that your particular situation is, it could always be worse.

So be thankful for having an amazing group of friends that even though they're injured will bike in the rain just to spray-paint your shirt. Be thankful for all those fools that will stand around in freezing temperatures while their nose hairs are turning into icicles just so they can cheer you on while you're finishing the last few sections of the stadium. Be thankful for Edmonton tribe that will always make you feel like shit for bitching about the weather. Be thankful for all the amazing humans that will go out of their way to help you find a job, a place to stay, invite you to a social gathering, or ask you out on a date. Be thankful for YOUR TRIBE as they are the only reason that you don't make excuses. I know I am.

Happy Thanksgiving, ya'll! I'll see you on Friday!

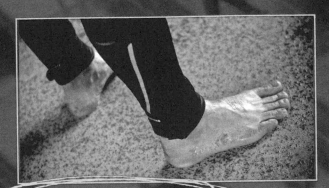

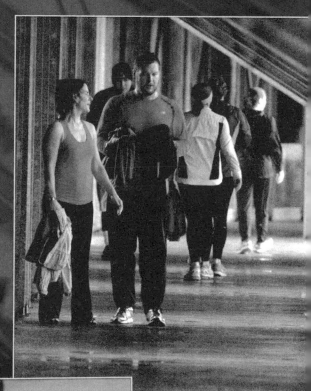

"See, I always say bad weather makes for an amazing workout!"
—Elin Flashman, 42, network and systems engineer, Medford, Mass.

ONE YEAR LATER

"Those few pictures that I took on my first day are symbolic to me now. They were blurry, vague, and fuzzy. A metaphor for what my life was like at the time. I had no idea where my life was headed or where my involvement with the November Project was going. But time passed by quickly. One week blended into another and the months flew by. I got stronger and faster. I met more people. November Project has completely transformed my life."

—Nicolas Flattes, 49,
Sales Associate at the North Face,
Roxbury, Mass.

"The way we start the workouts is very important for me. The hugs, looking in the other person's eyes. Meeting new people is amazing. Where I live, money, status, speed, competition are very important factors. I think NP just got me back to the real me. In our society, we need to come back to the essential social skills. The hugs, the warmth, the acceptance of all ability levels, ages, and status. The energy and vibe at November Project is so positive and fun that it's addicting and contagious. You don't find that inside a gym or club."

—Maria Cesca, 50,
former warehouse manager, running coach,
Coral Springs, Florida

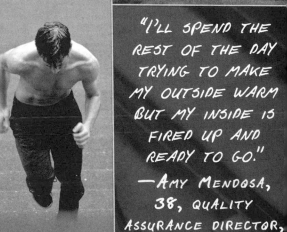

"I'll spend the rest of the day trying to make my outside warm but my inside is fired up and ready to go."

—Amy Mendosa, 38, quality assurance director, Medford, Mass.

NOVEMBER PROJECT'S
HARVARD STADIUM WORKOUTS

BY BROGAN GRAHAM

FROGMAN1

Fifty sections in 40 minutes. Start at section 37 and run to section 13, repeat 13, and run back to 37. This workout was named after a hiker I met on the Appalachian Trail who went by the name Frogman1 (he made sure to let me know that the "1" wasn't spelled out, that it was the actual number at the end of his name). Originally, we'd called this workout "the hiking trip" because the pace was less running and more power hiking. But Frogman1 just seemed to make sense.

Repeating section 13 and heading back into the oncoming fray means everyone mixes together, with the fastest and slowest side by side at some point. And even if it's nonverbal, there's an interaction happening, and that can be pretty powerful.

FIRE DRILL

Forty sections in 40 minutes (full tour, with section 1 repeated three times), sprinkled with squats and pushups. I'll bang a cowbell at random times and runners have to drop for either 5 to 10 pushups or 20 squats (given the screaming quads, most opt for pushups). The idea is to not let people zone out in a robotic groove. It breaks up the

Bill Fallon
@billfallon89
⚙ 👤 Follow

@nov_projectprob got fire-drilled right next to the poop in section 15(ish) @Nov_Project

rhythm. Interrupting the forward progress means people have to push that much harder to finish before the buzzer. The value of the 40-minute cutoff is that everyone can show how far they've traveled in the same block of time, giving the group a mutual feeling of accomplishment and a measurement to beat the next time. Also, the alarm sounds for the entire group at the same time and quittin' time is something that we can all feel good about!

ROBOTMAN3

This workout uses the stadium's top level. Runners start at section 37 and when they get to section 19, they head to the upper concourse, where they run back to section 37 to begin again. A full Robotman3 ends up being 57 sections, with short runs connecting each of the three half-tours. It's a mind game. It seems easy when you start, but most don't finish under an hour. Robotman3 was named by Joey "Big20" Kile and his right-hand man, Steve Christensen, now coleader of November Project DC. They loved the name and the idea of this kind of workout. The amount of shared space, passing, and mixing that goes on when you cram the whole tribe between 37 and 19 . . . I can only say that this thing is awesome, fucking awesome.

BACK TO THE FUTURE

A full tour, with members going back to the previous section whenever they hear a randomly struck cow bell. This simulates race-day conditions, in which you must con-

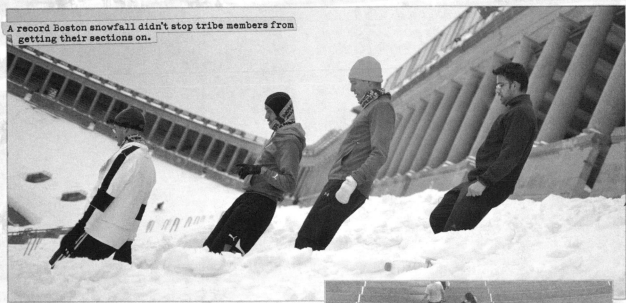

A record Boston snowfall didn't stop tribe members from getting their sections on.

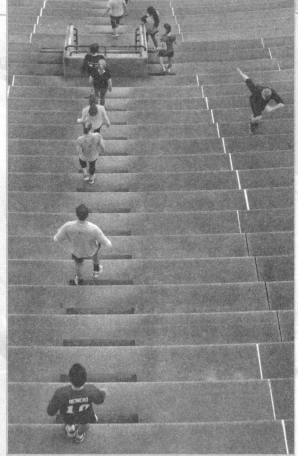

tend with a setback and then be forced to pick up the pace to meet your goal time. It's a mental game that drives positive vibes. People hate this one. Straight up. There are few who don't groan when they hear the bell go off. It makes me laugh because people don't groan when they have to hit the deck for Fire Drills. Maybe we should combine these two just to see who's actually happy to be here and who's here to get a date . . .

PR DAY

Self-explanatory: 37 sections as fast as you fuckin' can.

We used to give away frozen pizzas to the fastest men and women, then New Balance running shoes. From spring through fall, we have a PR pig named Phoebe; a black pot-belly cutie that belongs to married core members Jake and Martica Otto, who first met at NP. If you PR'd, you got to have your picture taken with Phoebe at section 1. You'd see a shit-ton of profile pics change on PR Wednesday when Phoebe was at the stadium. We also tag shirts on PR day and usually have a DJ. We make it festive while introducing racing to new athletes, supporting improving athletes, and celebrating seasoned athletes. Everyone likes PR'ing.

THE TRIBE IS...

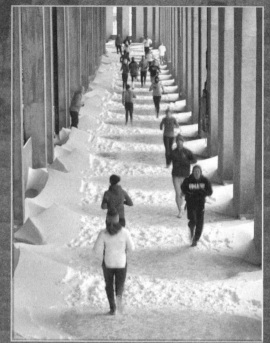

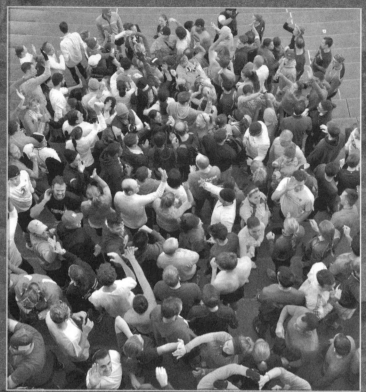

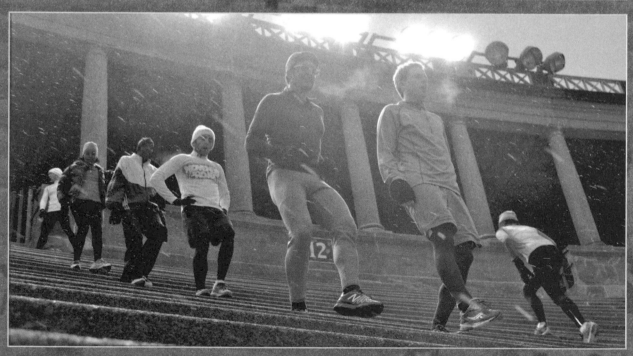

THE TRIBE IS STRONG.

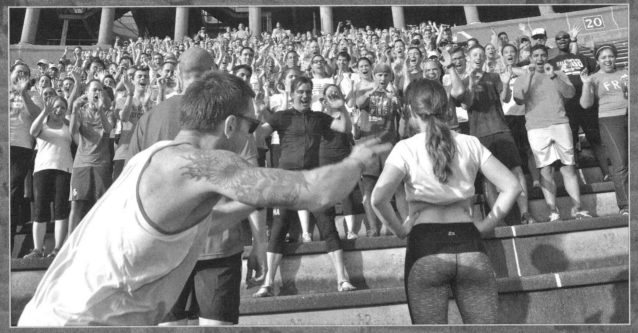

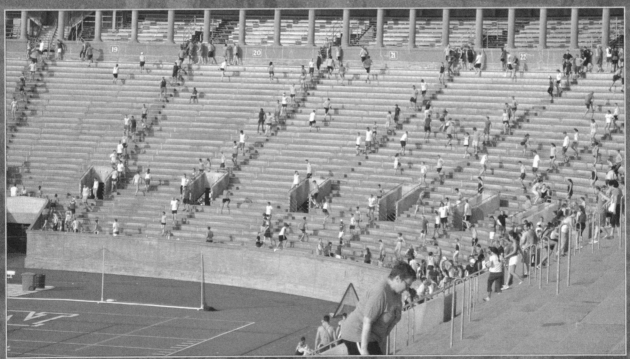

SARA WILD: Newbie Zero

Sara Wild, a 3:04 marathoner, holds the distinction of being November Project's first recruit. The Portland, Oregon, native is humble, quick to laugh, and quietly bangs out blistering stadium tours while openly resisting the over-the-top weirdness that runs through the veins of many tribe members. But being the lone person to answer November Project's first open invitation, the soft-spoken 26-year-old holds a special place in NP lore, having paved the way for every tribe member since. She's also indirectly responsible for the creation of the "We Missed You" page on the NP website, which playfully shames members who break their "verbals," the NP term for telling someone you'll be at the next workout. We caught up with Wild one winter morning at a Starbucks in Brighton near the New Balance office where she works as a product manager.

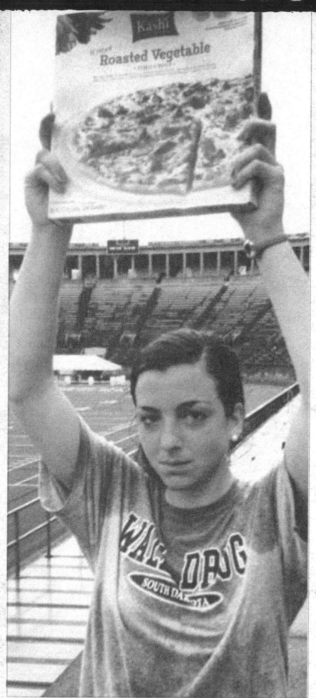

"When I told my dad I was going to meet some guys I met on Twitter, he didn't really like that."

CD: *What's your athletic background? I heard you played some pro soccer.*

SW: Well, sort of. I played in a women's pro league in Sweden after college. I played all through school. Soccer was my sport and I ran because I had to, not because I liked to. I did track in high school and college, just to stay fit. After moving to Boston, I decided to run more, and the New Balance people encouraged me, forced me, to run a marathon.

What were you doing at True Runner when you met Nick Flattes?

I was a field rep with New Balance. I'd put on clinics. You educate stores about your product, your brand, lead group runs, test runs. True Runner was one of my favorite stores in Boston. We were there for their opening and I did a New Balance clinic. November Project was a piece of my spiel about running in Boston, the community run aspect. What we try and talk about a lot is building your community, and New Balance is really part of the running community. I encouraged True Runner to come for a workout. I also saw it as a great way to get to know the associates. A lot of them had just moved to Boston. NP is always a great place to come when you're new in town. You get to meet 300 people right away.

Being the first-ever newbie, you're kind of NP famous. Do you think about that distinction?

Someone was going to show up. I'll take it. It's just fun to work out really hard with a bunch of people really early and be done for the day.

And it all started with a tweet?

Yeah, so a friend of mine from New Balance, we went to the stadium three or four times after work and tried to do the stadium. We were doing the little stairs and thinking, "Someday, we'll do the big stairs, and wouldn't it be cool if we got more people from work to do this with us?" But that kind of fizzled out. Then I saw a tweet from Marathon Sports. They had retweeted some November Project tweet about working out at Harvard, something like, "Join us tomorrow for some stairs." So I replied, "Really? Will you be there tomorrow?" And they were like, "Come on join us." I wanted to work out anyway. I wanted to try the big stairs anyway. They were going to be there, but I really didn't know who or what they were.

Seems ballsy-borderline-foolish to meet up with two strange dudes you'd only met online.

When I told my dad I was going to meet some guys I met on Twitter, he didn't really like that. But it ended up being okay. I mean it's 6:30 a.m. in a public space. Nothing really bad's going to happen. It was to work out and if no one was there, I was still going to do it. It was convenient with my schedule and close to work. And fortunately it turned out to be pretty awesome.

Did you research what November Project was?

Oh, no [laughs]. I didn't really get it. I don't think I really got what November Project was until maybe a month later when Brogan and Bojan started talking about working out together in November and needing to stay in shape after college.

Take me through your first day and your impression of the guys.

Well, obviously everyone's first impression is, "Holy shit, these guys are huge." I walked into the stadium and saw a couple guys standing there and we kind of looked at each other. I asked, "Are you . . . is this . . . are you guys the November Project?"

Were they surprised to see you?

I was more nervous and a little uncomfortable, so I didn't notice their reaction as much. One of them said, "If it's your first time, take it easy, just do half." I was like, "Come on. I can't be the girl that shows up and only does half of their workout."

You took it as an insult?

Totally. I'm always trying to prove people wrong and accept a challenge. "Take it easy," basically means "step it up." I definitely tried to stick with Bojan as much as I could, but I know at the end I was sucking wind. But I did the full tour. I don't think I've ever not done the full workout, because it's like "the challenge of the day" and you can't not do it when you're there with everyone else and all that excitement. Bojan and Brogan are aggressive, not yelling but cheering. Like anyone knows, their personalities are so huge that when you're there, you really get into it.

Are you surprised at what it's become?

I don't know, because every week it got bigger. There was never a time where you thought, "Well, this is going to end." Every week, new people were showing up. It seemed like such a consistent progression. Maybe the whole 17-cities thing's a little surprising because Boston is such a perfect place for something like this. A small city, easy to get around. It's got that recreation vibe. You can wear sneakers going out on Friday. It has more of a workout feel than, say, New York. That it has spread across the country, including New York, that's the most surprising part. But then again, when people meet Brogan and Bojan and find out what they're all about, it's hard not to think it wouldn't work anywhere.

What kept you coming back every Wednesday?

The killer workout that I could never do on my own. That feeling of blood in your throat and your muscles shaking, and all day you feel that workout. I try and take the stairs at work but after the stadium workout you're sucking wind on that first flight. It's a great feeling, completely destroying your body for a half an hour or 45 minutes. That's all it took. Knowing that I would never do something like that on my own, knowing that it's the people around you, pushing you.

BG said it was the PR pizzas that hooked you.

Haha, that was pretty fun. I don't think I ever ended up eating one of those pizzas, because I would bring it to work and leave it there in the freezer.

When did they start that?

They started talking about PRs right away. They said, "If you get a PR, let us know and we'll get you a pizza next week." I didn't really believe it, but I made sure to let them know when I got a PR, and then they went and got me a pizza. Then they started doing PR pizza day through Stone Hearth Pizza, which is near the stadium. The lower your PR, the less you paid for a pizza straight from the oven. It was like, wow, this *is* about community. This pizza place is supporting these workouts.

What is your PR for a full tour?

I don't know, under 25 minutes. I think it's listed somewhere. But I'm sure there are girls who have taken it down by now.

 Marathon Sports @Marathon_Sports · 1 May 2012
Call it a tweetup. Meet @Brogan_Graham 6:30am tomorrow, Harvard Stadium, 37 sections of 31 stairs. Up the big, down the small. Repeat.

 Brogan C. Graham @Brogan_Graham · 1 May 2012
Be clear @Marathon_Sports - the AM fitness/ninjas who meets up in various locations in Camb, Bos, & All/Brigh are the #novemberproject

 Brogan C. Graham @Brogan_Graham · 1 May 2012
Tons of beasts trying to get fit before dawn @BostonDotCom @marathon_sports @timjohnsoncx @BostInnovation ALL ARE WELCOME!!! 6:30AM start.

Brogan C. Graham @Brogan_Graham · 1 May 2012
Anyone who wants to join us tomorrow at 6:30 AM at Harvard Stadium shoe up. #novemberproject lives on.

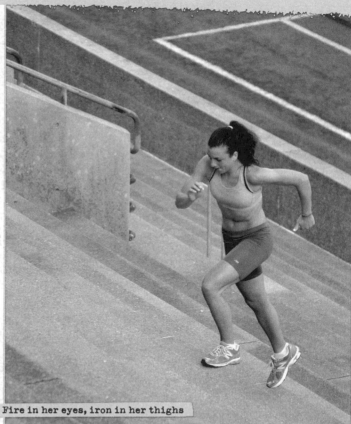

Fire in her eyes, iron in her thighs

(EDITOR'S NOTE: WILD'S PR IS 23:27, WHICH STOOD FOR THREE YEARS.)

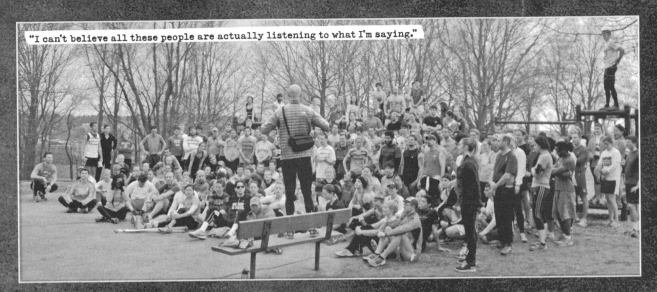

"I can't believe all these people are actually listening to what I'm saying."

We missed you this morning, Ali

🕐 16th May 2012   👤 bojan   📁 We Missed You   💬 0 Comments

Inspired by last minute workout no-shows we're creating the "We Missed You" section. This part of our website will be featuring all those friends that told you that they'll meet you for a workout only to bail last minute for various reasons including but not limited to: "feeling tired", "it's too cold/hot outside", "it's raining/snowing", "the sun is too strong", "it's too humid my hair will frizz out", "I'm sore from yesterday's workout", "I forgot I have to be at work early" while staying in bed, or any other awesome excuse that we all used or someone else used on us.

This morning we really missed our friend Ali that was suppose to make her first time appearance with the November Project gang. Ali canceled on her friend Sara (Wild) at 5:45am via text message after deciding that staying in bed is much better than working out, meeting cool new people, and having fun. Ali, we hope that your sleeping time was enjoyable but we also hope that next week you'll choose November Project instead.

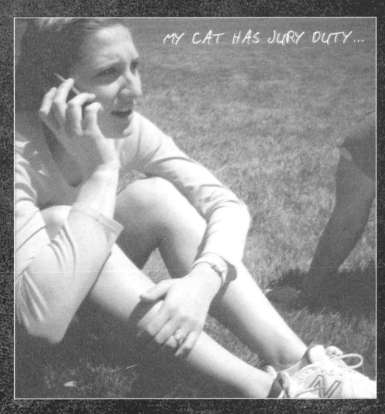

MY CAT HAS JURY DUTY....

We Missed You This Morning, Daniel

🕐 19th November 2012   👤 bojan   📁 We Missed You   💬 2 Comments

Let me tell you a little story about our dear friend, and a family member, Daniel Kirk Graham. Aside from being known among his closest friends, as "Dan the Soccer Player," having a Lacoste chest tattoo (very classy), he is also in great physical shape (just recently ran 50 mile race), and is better looking of the two Graham brothers (the younger one being our Co-Founder, Brogan Full-of-Himself Graham).

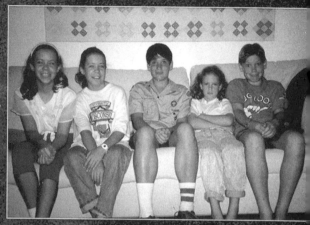

From the early days, Daniel, assured his physical dominance over his brother Brogan by constantly kicking his ass, which led to Brogan's commitment to hard-core training, thinking that one day he'll dethrone his older brother. Despite Brogan's 15 hour/day training regiment, that day has yet to come.

But on the morning of Monday, November 19th, Daniel showed his weakness. While in Boston for his brother's birthday celebration, Daniel committed to coming to one of the November Project™ workouts. The #DestinationDeck location was little over one mile away from where Daniel was staying and he still decided not to show up. Why?

Details are remain unclear at this time. Is it possible that proximity to the Atlantic Ocean negatively impacted Daniel's body so used to harsh conditions of Wisconsin tundra? Should we assume that Dan (is it okay if we call you Dan?), lost his contact lenses, had trouble finding his workout gear in the dark, didn't want to wake up the people that he was staying with by turning on the lights, finally gathered himself but then dropped his toothbrush in the toilet, and stubbed his toe on a bathroom doorstep? These are all just assumptions; The real reason of why Dan missed this rare opportunity to workout with the tribe will never be known. The only thing that we do know is that if his mother can make it to the NP workouts (Hills Session just days before) so can you – We Missed You, Dan!

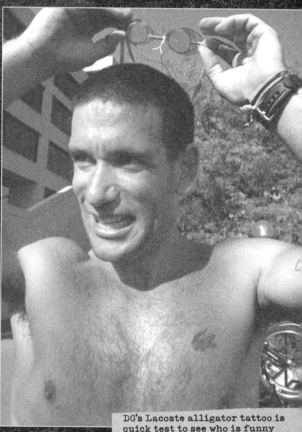

DG's Lacoste alligator tattoo is quick test to see who is funny and who to avoid.

We Missed You This Morning, Chris Marshall

🕐 12th July 2013　👤 bojan　📁 We Missed You　💬 0 Comments

Chris Marshall is a badass marathon runner, the only tribe member that recruited the whole Division I basketball team to join in on a #DestinationDeck, and the guy that's been lobbying for runners safety on Summit ave so hard that we named revolutionary no-parking-on-the-hill-during-the-workout-rule after him. But this morning Chris Marshall made a horrible mistake – he bailed on his verbal. In the efforts to recruit more racers he sent this tweet to @mochnaczmonster "Friday am. You, me, a hill, and @Nov_Project"

Inspiring tweet no doubt. Hell, if I got that tweet I would be so worked up for the workout that I would have to watch Rocky 4, Rudy, and the Hoosiers back to back to back because I wouldn't be able to fall asleep from all the excitement. But Chris Marshall didn't have to stay up all night watching inspiring 90's movies. He slept well in the comfort of his bed. He slept so well that he tried to cover his sleepy tracks with this lame tweet blaming foot problems for the missed workout.

Dear Chris Marshall let me tell you something about foot problems... I know a guy whose toes are so infected that they might fall off but he was there this morning cheering people on. I know a girl that has stress fractures in her foot sidelining her from running for few weeks but she was there this morning doing #InjuryDeck. I know a girl that's training for a half ironman but can't run because the walking boot and crutches will be messing up her stride for the next 6 weeks – but she was also there this morning cheering on her tribe. See the pattern here?

So please, next time you're bail on your verbal just say that you slept in, don't blame it on injury because there are a lot of injured people out there that still come out because they said they would. We love you, Chris Marshall, we hope that your foot heals soon, but most of all We Missed You this morning.

Chris Marshall @goNUchris　　　　　　　10 Jul
@mochnaczmonster Friday am. You, me, a hill, and @Nov_Project
↩ Reply　↻ Retweet　★ Favorite　••• More

11:26 AM - 10 Jul 13 · Details

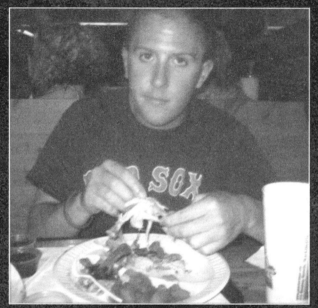

Chris Marshall @MayorOfBeacon · 12 Jul 2013
Foot banged up again. Had to miss @Nov_Project
Hope y'all had a great workout

7:32 AM - 12 Jul 2013 · Details

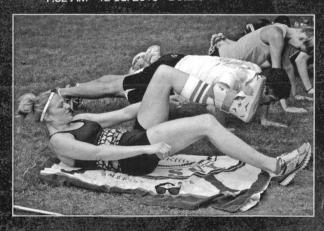

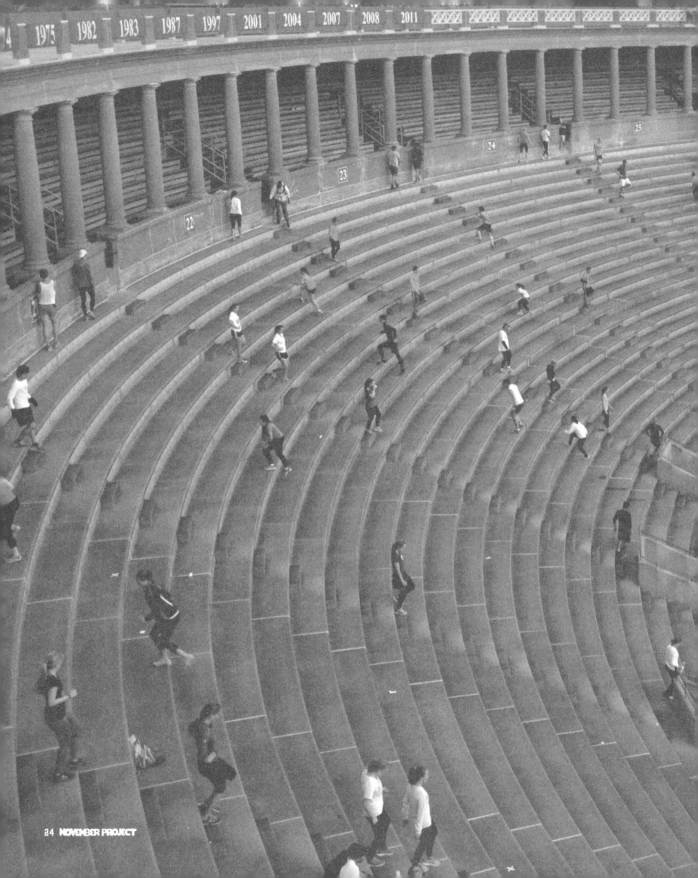

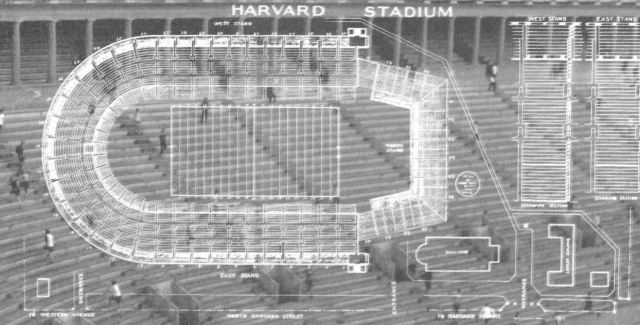

HARVARD STADIUM BY THE NUMBERS

4.5: Months to build

250,000: Cubic feet of concrete

1906: Harvard became one of the first college teams to employ the forward pass

22,000: Original seating capacity

30,323: Seating capacity

848: Football wins

383: Losses

50: Ties

4: National football championships since 1903

1919: Last year Harvard won a national title

1: Number of times Bob Marley played the stadium

1970: Janis Joplin performed her last concert on August 12

548: Calories burnt by a 160-pound athlete running a full tour

#GrassrootsGear

🕐 2nd August 2012   👤 bojan   📁 Blog   💬 2 Comments

The time has come for November Project family to start rocking official NP gear and represent the tribe that has proved that you don't need to drop insane amount of dollar bills to be fit. How are we going to do that? #Grassroots style! We're turning down perfectly printed shirts that are already flooding our closets and racks at local GoodWill to something way cooler and more badass—#GrassrootsGear.

On Wednesday 8/8/12 we're having a Bring Your Own T-shirt (B.Y.O.T.) day at November Project. From a simple v-neck cotton T to a lightweight racing tank, bring any kind of white or light blue shirt. It MUST be plain, solid, white OR light blue without writing/prints/logos. This will be your ONLY opportunity to have 1st edition of November Project shirt design as the stencil will be retired into a framed memorabilia after the event and will never be used again. Don't miss out on the chance to own a piece of fitness revolution history.

Your shirt will be created by the uber creative November Project staff during your workout next Wednesday. Please label your shirt tag or mark your collar with a sharpie so we can keep that many shirts straight. It goes without saying that next week we'll have a pretty rad group photo and we hope you and your shirt can make it.

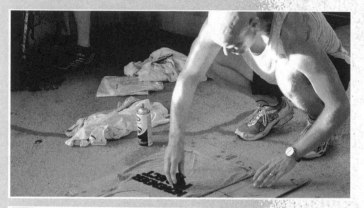

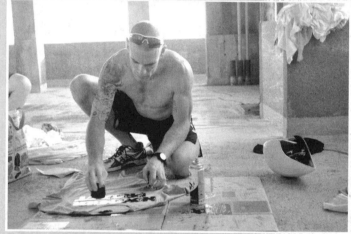

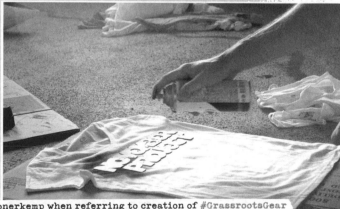

#Grassrooting: Term coined by NYC leader John Honerkemp when referring to creation of #GrassrootsGear

Positivity Award @Nov_Project

🕐 18th September 2012   👤 brogan   📁 Blog   💬 2 Comments

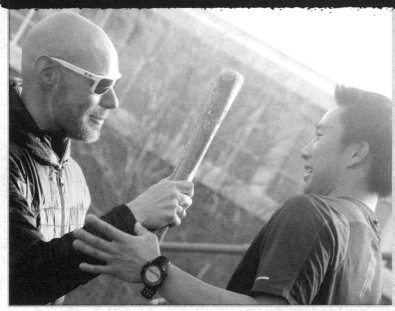

The team vibe that we've all created at November Project is key for rough workouts, harsh weather, and when we're feeling like we could have used those extra hours of sleep. We need to continue to boost one another with positive comments, high5's, and sometimes a simple pat on the back.

You may see a wooden oar handle floating around the tribe at many of the workouts. If you get a chance to get closer to that handle you'll see the words "NOVEMBER PROJECT" and your city branded up and down the sides. This is our **November Project Positivity Award**. We're awarding it after almost every workout to one member who bounced out of bed with an extra spring in his/her step and brought the rest of us to a new level. You may nominate someone for an outside event or for helping you through a workout. This award will never have to do with speed or strength but will always go to the person who shows the best attitude. This can be displayed in the form of fun, encouragement to others around them, putting the tribe first, recruiting more racers, and generally being an awesome person to train near. With many of our core values of account-

ability, racing, team bonding, and training in all conditions coming from the sport of rowing, we thought that the award was pretty much perfect.

If you end up with the award, you'll be asked to bring it along to the next NP session so it can be awarded to someone else. In the day or two that you own it you'll be encouraged to carry it with you (all the time). Keep building your tribe by showing up ready to race and build community. One day you'll have this handle in your hands and you'll be posting your photos in awesome/odd places around town for all to see . . . and that day, my friend, you'll completely understand. This is the #PositivityAward.

We hope you have a great day and we'll see you shortly after your alarm clock goes off. Stay positive.

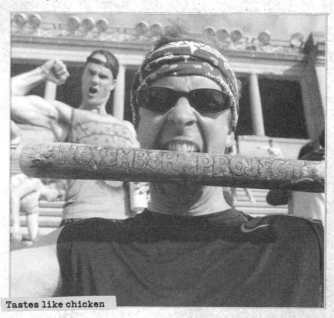

Tastes like chicken

ANDREW FERENCE,
Captain, Edmonton Oilers

"November Project is exactly like Fight Club, except with hugging."

NHL defenseman Andrew Ference is the former alternate captain of the Boston Bruins (2007–13) and the current captain of the Edmonton Oilers. After helping the Bruins win the Stanley Cup in 2011, Ference staged a grassroots victory parade through Boston, where he towed the trophy behind his bike and posed with fans, tweeting along the way. The 37-year-old father of two is a seasoned stair runner, active on social media, and coated in tats. It was just a matter of time before the energetic Canadian and November Project happily crashed into each other.

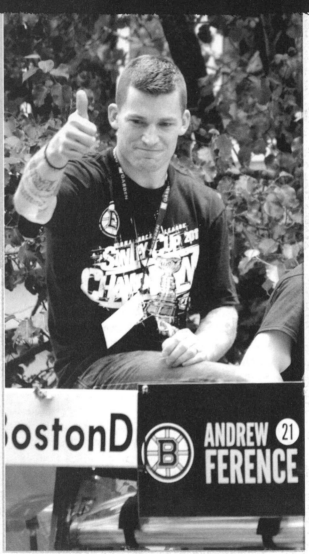

CD: *How did you first learn about November Project?*

AF: I was running stairs on my own at Harvard. The Harvard rink was one of the rinks we could skate at during the lockout [2012–13], so I incorporated the stairs into my workout day. I threw it out there [on social media] that I was doing the stadium if people wanted to join me. I had about five or six people come and do it. So I was kinda doing an NP-like thing before I even knew of NP. Then, literally within a week, I went into Landry's Bicycles and the owner and I were talking about some of the workouts I was doing to stay in shape during the lockout. I mentioned the stadium and he pointed me in the direction of November Project. He said, "Check these guys out, they go pretty early, they go hard, and they're pretty fit." The reason I had put it out there on Twitter for people to come join me is because I was bored. Running stairs on your own sucks. It's so easy to bail out, to do five less sets. No one's watching. I was actively looking for that accountability. Even if they're not faster than you, at least you know they're watching you and you have to push it a little harder than you would on your own. The timing was perfect. I checked them out the very next Wednesday.

I know you went to the newbie meeting. As a professional athlete with plenty of stair experience, weren't you tempted to skip and just get going?

I was just following rules. Hockey players do well following the rules. We're used to schedules and being told what to do, when to show up. Even though I'd been running the stairs, I figured I should do what I'm told. I'm definitely glad I did. I would have no doubt been called out if I thought I was too good for the newbie meeting.

What was your reaction to all the hugging?

The guy at Landry's didn't really tell me anything about the hugging or the yelling or the vibe. I didn't know what to expect. I was just trying to figure it all out. That early in the morning you just go with the flow. Just take it all in. I didn't know it was an every time thing. It was cool. I'm pretty open to that sort of stuff. You look around and there are a lot of girls who looked real fit and dudes with their shirts off looking jacked. I thought, *okay, this is a good group. If you gotta high-five and hug a few people, there's nothing wrong with that.*

What was your initial impression of BG?

It probably took me a few times before I got a good impression, but right off the bat, he's loud and fast and pretty energetic. There's just certain people who walk into a room and the room gets quiet and people just listen. He's got a presence, which is great for what he's doing. He's a super-fit loud dude who seems to be very friendly. He's not the bad stereotypical jock dude who's like a rooster puffing up his feathers.

And Bojan?

The brains behind the operation. The safety department. The dude isn't as loud but he's the one who's in the background taking it all in and making sure things are happening the way they're supposed to be.
If I need to get something done or need info, Bojan's definitely the one I'll go to. BG is busy riffing all over the place. When I'm in the mood to throw ideas around and brainstorm, BG's perfect for that. We'll go back and forth for a half hour and we've probably talked about a million things and think we have it all figured out.
They're both from my world. Super-fit jock dudes. But

something I don't like so much about my world is everybody jockeying for the alpha male position and not being themselves. Those two guys are open and talk like normal friends. You can call them up and talk about marriage, your kids, your dreams. You don't have to be a full-on dude all the time. It's nice to have friends who are super-athletic and macho when they need to be but have that element that makes for a great friend. They have been a great addition to my life.

Together, they're a perfect storm of fitness positivity.

They're perfect for what they're doing. I couldn't understand it at first. They were putting so much effort into it and it doesn't cost anything. I didn't get it. But they're just made for it. They have the type of personalities—boisterous, very energizing. I mean they're not simply patting people on the back. They're motivating, making sure you get the most out of it. You wake up that early, you want to get the most out of being there. They're rallying the troops, but once people are there, they're definitely helping people get to another level, not allowing you to slack off and give a half-ass effort. That's pretty cool. And think about the diversity of people that they've been able to bring together under this secret little fight club. I mean, that's kind of how I view it. I think I told Brogan once, "You guys are exactly like Fight Club. I mean, you don't punch each other. There's more hugging." You feel pretty cool to be part of that group. You're surrounded by a whole bunch of people just like you. We all kind of like the same thing, but we're all different in our own ways. It's pretty neat what they've been able to build.

How did the workouts impact your training?

It was a great supplement for sure. I'd do the stadium in the morning, go home, and get the kids to school. Then go back into the gym at 9 or 10 for some more hockey-specific stuff on my own. That supplement is amazing. It gets me woken up in the morning and gets me dialed into my workout for the day. That later workout is so much better after NP. I'm fired up and ready to go. I have this conversation with my hockey trainers all the time. They're old-school guys with these book workouts where this is the perfect way to move your muscles for hockey, this is how hockey works. I always come at them from the side of mental workouts. Where are those workouts that push you to the next level, where they hurt, where your muscles are burning so much more than they would in hockey? I call them my "brain buster" workouts. That's where NP has helped me. You're maxed out at the stadium and keep pushing yourself. That's a mental workout. To push your body past that and keep up with the fast group and not slow your pace down, that, to me, is the most powerful part of those NP workouts. It's definitely paid dividends. In hockey, I will never reach that point of pain or exhaustion in a game. It just doesn't happen. I've been in triple-overtime in the Stanley Cup Playoffs and you're tired, sure, but mentally, it's nothing. I've been here, I got this. As long as you have your hydration and nutrition. I've always looked for those kinds of workouts.

You're now one of the coleaders of the Edmonton Tribe, the third to come on board after Boston. When you were trading your Bruins uniform for the Oilers, you told me you thought it'd be too cold to start a tribe up there. What changed your mind?

We were able to drive the numbers up during the summer, but then we had to have the conversation: what do we do when it gets to minus 40? Is it okay to be working out? We honestly didn't know. Was it stupid? I mean, when you promote that anyone can show up, what happens if someone shows up and is underdressed, not being smart? That could be dangerous. And what if someone does get hypothermia, do we know what to do? So we had to go through those questions and what's the smart thing to do here? I can't say we ever really answered them. We just kept going and we educated our tribe. We had a night where our version of The North Face gave a talk on layering and how to properly dress and we pumped that through our social media channels. At least we could say, we told you so.
As we started hitting some of those cold days, then it became this badge of honor when people did show up, bragging rights. We did a new stencil, but it's so hard to spray paint in the winter. So we did a badge you can sew on, like a Boy Scout badge. That became our thing. I think we've given out a couple hundred. And you only get it once. We actually have to reorder because we're all out.

You're known for being community- and environmentally minded, very much in line with the NP vibe. Did those two things feed off each other?

One hundred percent on the community stuff. As for the environment, I always assume people who get outside and enjoy it are usually more dialed into it. But definitely the community stuff. Everybody's welcome. For Pride Week, we were the official place for the Pride Run and Walk, for the LGBT community. Poor, rich, whatever color skin, I just love bringing everybody together. When it does become the community and not just talk, that's where it's awesome. We've had so many people who are new to the city and NP is their group of friends. This is their family. You start seeing them doing stuff on the side. They're going on camping trips together, taking trips to run marathons, and it has nothing to do with us as leaders. The feedback we get isn't about the fitness

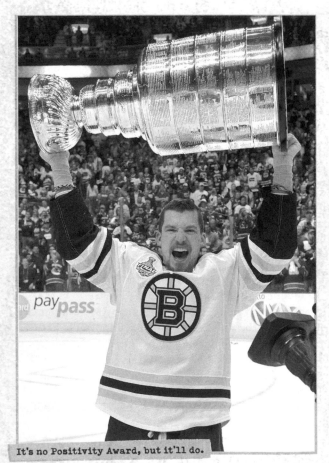

It's no Positivity Award, but it'll do.

as much as it is for making people feel part of something.

My favorite recruit to this day is this drag queen from the Pride Parade last year. I said, "You gotta show up and come work out with us." She showed up and it was awesome. She still comes except for the really cold days. For anybody to feel comfortable, that's a real source of pride for our group. There's no backstory on you. Everyone starts at the same level. You're sweating it out, hurting just as much as the guy next to you. It brings everyone down to the same level. It's just great.

How would you describe NP in one word?

Interesting. It baffles people. It still baffles me. What are we doing?

Weirdest thing about NP?

I find it weird that more cities aren't doing it. It's weird to stare into people's eyes and tell them something about yourself. That's still a little weird to me.

What's the biggest misconception about NP; what might be keeping people at bay?

I didn't know there were misconceptions. Maybe that it's some kind of scheme, that it's just free. Where's the hook? But everybody who comes out stays. That's the cool thing that I've noticed. I don't think there are a lot of one-timers who come and don't come back.

Where do you see NP going, what's the potential?

Spreading to other cities. It will become kind of normal. All the big cities will just have it.

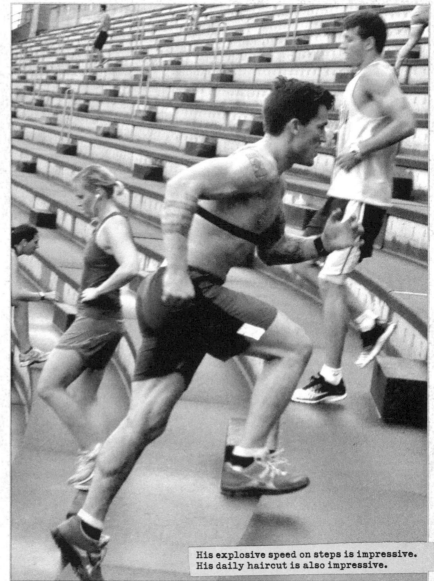

His explosive speed on steps is impressive. His daily haircut is also impressive.

Then there's that source of pride trying to get people on podiums. Everyone's training for something. Everyone has goals. That competiveness at NP workouts where you get those fast groups which are pushing the intensity levels up, you'll see people not just trying to stay fit, not just pushing to run races, but to do really well at races. Hopefully, you'll see more tagged shirts on podiums. Then you'll have inter-city pride and competition between cities. (NP)

The Boston Bombings: The Tribe Is Strong

On Monday, April 15, at 2:49 p.m., two pressure-cooker bombs ripped through the crowds gathered near the finish line of the 2013 Boston Marathon. When the smoke cleared, two young women and an 8-year-old boy were dead, more than a dozen maimed for life, several hundred injured, an entire city traumatized. In the wake of such devastation and mass tragedy, Graham and Mandaric had to decide whether to go forward with the Wednesday workout at Harvard Stadium. In a stroke of terrible timing, the theme for that particular session, hyped the previous week, was "pack day." The idea was to fill backpacks with weights or books for an extra challenge on the stairs. The guys chose to hold the workout, but not take to social media as they typically would in the days prior. With Boston still reeling and the bombers on the loose, they didn't expect much of a turnout, maybe a hundred, probably less. Almost 500 souls showed up that morning, all of them seeking solace and communion. —CD

Harvard Stadium
April 17, 2013

"I needed that human contact. I needed to touch another person, to talk to another person who'd ran the marathon that day, to get someone's else reaction. I needed to see people wearing their jackets. I needed them to show me their medals because we never got ours. We all had stories and we wanted to share, so you don't feel like you're the only one it happened to. People were crying, I think we all shed a tear. We were all there to get our sweat on, our hugs on, our fuck yeahs, and it was just awesome to see so many people alive and doing something they enjoyed without the fear. You could sense that feeling of security. Nobody's going to hurt us here. I think if I missed that workout, the recovery process would have been a lot worse. For me, NP was a life saver."

—Rosa Evora, 48,
Housing Advocate, Brockton, Mass.

"At the end, a whole group of us met at section 25 or 26, because a lot of people got stopped at mile 25 and 26. There was an eerie kind of silence. I don't even think we took a group photo that day. It was a solemn vibe. I felt I should say something. My usual role is, 'Fuck and shit and the crowd goes wild.' But that's not going to work. It was also not right to say, 'Let's move on and get beyond,' because the dude was still marching around the neighborhood. It wasn't the right vibe to be, 'Let's be upbeat and just smile this off.' But I'm also never from the school of 'Let's just hang our heads and cry,' but that's not exactly right; even be-kind-to-strangers wasn't right. I was also connected to a lot of people who were really stirred up. For the first time in my life, my usual I'll-figure-this-out wasn't cutting it."

—Brogan Graham

"NP WAS AN ANCHOR FOR ME IN THE DAYS AFTER THE BOMBING. I HAVE A SYMBOLIC PICTURE OF THE 26TH SECTION THAT I TOOK. I THINK I CRIED FOR A GOOD PART OF THE TOUR."

—KATHLEEN MEEHAN, 27, REGISTERED DIETICIAN AND NUTRITIONIST, BOSTON

"MY VERY FIRST NP WORKOUT WAS THE WEDNESDAY AFTER THE ATTACK. I WAS AT THE FINISH LINE WHEN THE BOMBS WENT OFF AND I WASN'T QUITE SURE HOW TO DEAL WITH THE EMOTIONS I WAS HAVING. I WENT TO NP THAT MORNING, NOT NECESSARILY FOR THE WORKOUT, BUT TO BE SURROUNDED BY PEOPLE WHO WERE MOST LIKELY TO UNDERSTAND WHAT I WAS GOING THROUGH. I'M NOT SURE IF IT WAS THE ATMOSPHERE OF THE CITY AT THAT MOMENT, BUT EVERYONE WAS SO WELCOMING AND I NEVER FELT LIKE A NEWBIE. I WENT FOR THE HUGS AND I LEFT WITH SO MUCH MORE. I'VE BEEN GOING EVER SINCE."

—MEAGAN KELLY BUFANO, 38, INFECTIOUS DISEASE RESEARCH SCIENTIST, BOSTON

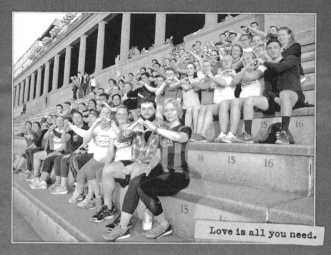

Love is all you need.

"I REMEMBER WHAT I WORE. I REMEMBER WHO I TALKED TO. I REMEMBER THE VIBE. BUT I DON'T REMEMBER THE WORKOUT, WHO DID THE BLOG POST RECAP. IT ALL KIND OF JUST FLEW BY . . . BUT IT BECAME MUCH MORE OBVIOUS WHAT NP WAS TO OTHER PEOPLE ASIDE FROM 'THE SHOW,' THE IMPACT IT HAD ON PEOPLE'S LIVES."

—BOJAN MANDARIC

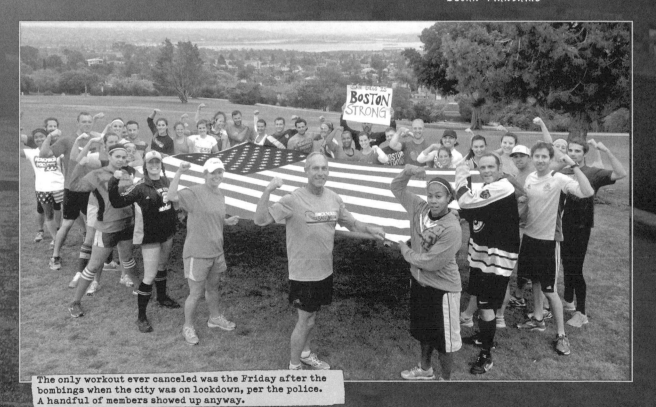

The only workout ever canceled was the Friday after the bombings when the city was on lockdown, per the police. A handful of members showed up anyway.

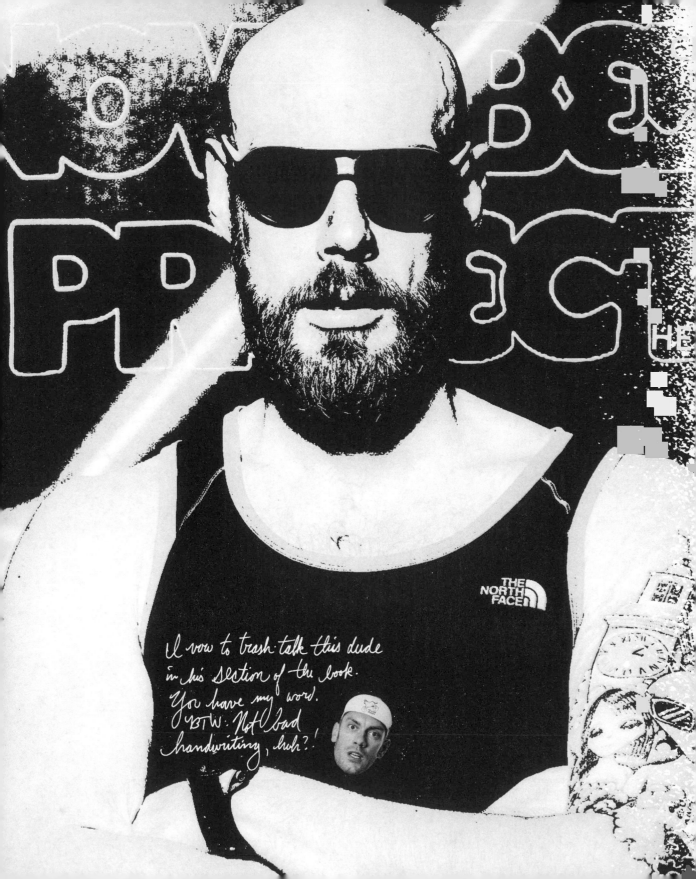

CHAPTER 2

BOJAN THE SERBIAN

BY BOJAN MANDARIC

WISCONSIN NOTES

- THE DAY BEFORE THANKSGIVING BROUGHT RAIN, COLD, AND SOME FIERCE RACING

- THE TRIBE IS #WEATHERPROOF BUT MY CAMERA IS NOT, SO ENJOY SOME MEDIOCRE iPHONE PHOTOS

- PR DAY WAS A HUGE SUCCESS

- EDMONTON STILL REMAINS THE COLDEST PLACE ON EARTH!

- AXL ROSE IS A MUSICAL GENIUS

One of the 20 preset alarms on my phone went off at 4:30 a.m. I'd been setting this one every Tuesday night for 2 years now and had lovingly named it "#RiseAnd-Shine, You Bitch!" The all-too-familiar melody that some Apple software developer named "Piano Riff" looped once before I punched in my code to make it stop. As I lie in bed a few moments, I imagined blues pianist Fats Domino getting up at 4:30 a.m., and that being the chord he'd play to start his day:

Da-na-na-na-na . . . I woke up this morning at zero-fuck-early . . .

Da-na-na-na-na . . . My lady was still in bed thinking I was crazy . . .

Da-na-na-na-na . . . Fumbling through the darkness I stubbed my toe on a door jamb . . .

Da-na-na-na-na . . . I should just go back to bed and sleep 'til the weekend.

That morning, I was going to be running the show on my own. BG was away for Thanksgiving at his almost-wife's family thing in Southern California. It was late November 2013, the last Wednesday of the month, which meant we were racing 37 sections for time. PR Day. The plan was to do my workout with the 5:30 a.m. squad, change into something warm and dry (extra pair of socks and underwear for the second part of the workout makes all the difference), and then lead and motivate the 6:30 a.m. group.

I snuck out of the bed, leaving my wife, Emilie, behind. Emilie had been amazingly supportive of my "extracurricular #FREE fitness activities" that, by this point, had turned into a second full-time job. Just a few weeks earlier we discussed an idea that BG and I were throwing around—flying the leaders from the seven cities we were in at the time to Edmonton, Canada, for a November Project meeting of the minds. We still hadn't met half of them face-to-face. While social media was a big part of our ability to spread the word and further this community, we knew a virtual relationship among the leaders wouldn't cut it.

Emilie knows first-hand the impact of November Project. Her athletic background consisted of a high school cross-country team that she joined just because all her friends were on it; they ran until the group got far enough away into the woods to safely stop and socialize. Now, she was putting away 50 sections of Harvard Stadium before work and hitting a yoga class in the afternoon, all in preparation for her first half-marathon.

"Yeah, dropping thousands of dollars out of our pockets to fly people to the coldest place on earth in December to talk about free fitness makes perfect sense," she said. "It's not like we're saving up cash for a down-payment on our first house or anything."

Damn it. I hate when she uses sarcasm against me. That's *my* move!

"But none of this makes sense," she continued, now seriously. "You two clowns have been defying logic from day one, so why stop now? Just make sure you come back with one of those warm Canadian toques."

I rolled up to the stadium at 5:20. The early group was small, maybe 25 to 30 hunched-over bodies trying to protect their hands from the wet chill by pulling jacket sleeves down over knuckles. Most of them had to be at work early; others wanted to get a workout in before their holiday travels, but they were all ready to start moving. I led a short, warm-up Bounce, explained the workout, and took off with the first wave of runners. Less than 25 minutes later, I slapped the top of section 1. Not a PR but a decent showing considering the nasty conditions. I stood at the top for a few minutes, gathering my wits while my lungs and heart started talking to each other again. I tried to decipher the shadows that were streaking up the last few dark sections like ghosts.

THURSDAY, MAY 3, 2012

First recruit, Sara Wild, shows up at Harvard Stadium. She not only keeps up, but posts a blazing full tour time of 28:30, just a few minutes behind Bojan and BG. The promise of a large frozen pizza the following week for her accomplishment buys her future attendance.

SATURDAY, MAY 5, 2012—THE FIRST NORTH FACE ENDURANCE CHALLENGE

BG takes off in the middle of the night to drive to Bear Mountain, New York, to race the marathon relay with his childhood friend, Nick Van Sicklen. They win and receive medals from ultrarunner star Dean Karnazes. Racing becomes a core NP ethos and is buttressed by the new hashtag #raceeverything. november-project.com/cinco-de-redtube/

I had to go with Nick over Bojan, Boj just wasn't ready yet. He was still #RACE SomeTHINGS

"That's it, buddy, turn and go!" I yelled at the silhouette, no idea who I was talking to. "Two more sections . . . don't leave anything in the tank."

As the figure got to the top of section 2, I recognized Andy Ullman, a 5:30 a.m. regular from Cambridge. His thick lumberjack beard must have sponged up an extra pound of rain water. "Yeah, brother, you got it, that's it! The last one!"

I don't know if my cheering helped or he had paced himself correctly, but Andy flew up the last section like he'd just started the workout. But at the top, all the gracefulness and ease of movement from moments before vanished as his back curved, his hands dropped down to his knees, his head hung between his shoulders, and his dried-out mouth squeezed out an eerie, animal sound.

"Aaaaahhh!!!" he groaned, his lungs struggling to support his words. "Fuck! . . . Fuck! . . . Man, this . . . never . . . gets easier . . ."

"No, it doesn't," I replied. "PR?"

Andy looked away from his feet, his face fur hiding a smile. "By 15 seconds!"

"Fuck yeah, dude!" I raised my right hand and we high-fived. "All right, I got to get ready for a 6:30 group. Nice job today!"

A lot of people ask how November Project is different from other fitness groups. The clearest answer is in the Bounce. I don't even remember when we started doing it, but the idea is to get everyone dialed into the workout. Back in our college rowing days, before we got on the water, we'd huddle over various items to focus on during the practice. It allowed the coach to set the tone for the

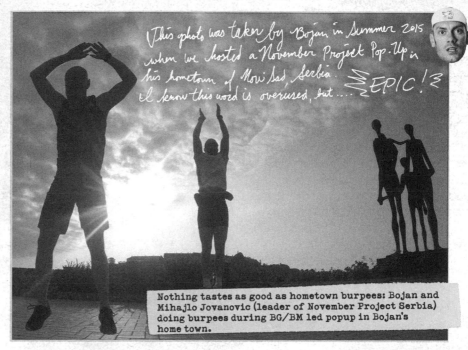

This photo was taken by Bojan in Summer 2015 when we hosted a November Project Pop-Up in his hometown of Novi Sad, Serbia. I know this word is overused, but . . . ≋EPIC!≋

Nothing tastes as good as hometown burpees: Bojan and Mihajlo Jovanovic (leader of November Project Serbia) doing burpees during BG/BM led popup in Bojan's home town.

workout and put everyone on the same page. With a few hundred people looking to us three times a week, our attention wasn't about explaining the technique of running stairs or hills, because that's easy to pick up. For us, it was more important to establish the energy for the next 60 minutes. And the NP vibe is anything but serious. When a newbie finally shows up, they're usually still intimidated and anxious, but all that crumbles away after a few silly chants, some strategically placed F-bombs, and a round of full-body bear hugs.

I was stoked to be the hype master that morning. Normally, I didn't "hold the mic," the term BG and I use for the person making announcements and getting the group fired up. Not because I wasn't comfortable or didn't think I could do it well. When I had the opportunity, I was all over it. But I always passed the mic to the giant tattooed guy standing next to me because, simply put, he's the best I've ever seen.

THURSDAY, MAY 31, 2012

Repeats on a monster hill in well-to-do Brookline are announced for a Friday morning workout. Conflict between the athletes and the residents ensues.

november-project.com/the-summit-ave/

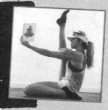

THURSDAY, JUNE 14, 2012

Local yoga instructor Goldie Kaufenberg becomes the sixth member of November Project when she shows up with a bunch of her dedicated yogis. Despite the sudden swell in numbers, BG and Goldie only have eyes for each other. Since this day, NP Boston has a majority of women over men.

So, BG in one word: LOUD. I'm talking caps-lock-turned-on, this-one-goes-up-to-17 LOUD. We met in 2002 and then spent 4 action-packed years as teammates rowing for Northeastern University. We lived together on three separate occasions, and for a few years we battled as crew coaches, him at our alma mater, and me at Syracuse. On his wedding day he'd ask me to stand next to him and his older brother as he was trying to get through his vows without choking on tears and blowing snot bubbles.

As a teammate he was an incredibly hard worker. He never hid his lack of a rowing background, but he compensated for it with a relentless work ethic and amazing strength. He was always down for an extra workout, a game of pick-up basketball, or a stadium tour on our day off. But it's not his height or his physical presence that's so impressive. It's the way that he talks to strangers, like he's known them his whole life. It's the way he weaves a silly sense of humor into the most serious conversations without coming across as disrespectful. It's his constant need to pull stunts like spending a night under the Mass Ave Bridge on a pylon that can only be reached by boat, just so he can say that he did something that hadn't been done before.

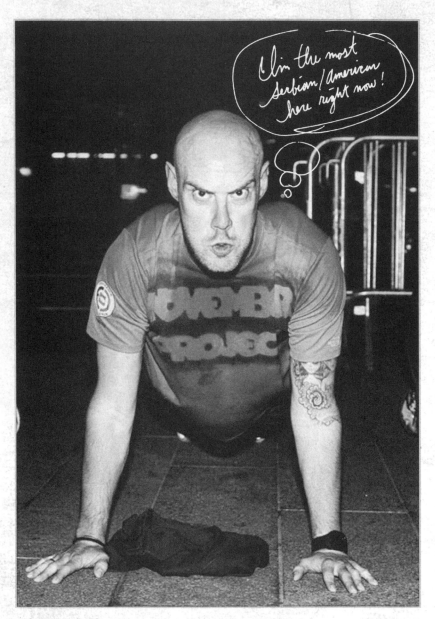

I'm the most Serbian/American here right now!

SATURDAY, JUNE 23, 2012—BIG MAN RUN, SOMERVILLE, MASSACHUSETTS

BG and Bojan are asked, "Are you the November Project dudes?" by a complete stranger. Ecstasy ensues. Total Twitter following at the time is roughly 20. BG wins the 5-mile race with a time of 27:53.
november-project.com/big-man-run-2012/

WEDNESDAY, JUNE 27, 2012

November Project starts taking group photos after the workout "November Project Style." The straight face, straight back, old school cowboy feel to go hand in hand with #grassroots #community movement that's been spreading around Boston like a wildfire. november-project.com/tradition/

When you share the stage with a guy like that, you just put your ego aside and give him room to shine.

Typically, my role during the Bounce, after BG was finished bringing the hype, was to feed him information to announce: workout descriptions, scalable-option reminders, safety announcements, social events. It was a great symbiotic relationship that we called The Flow. Each workout, like a story, had to have a beginning, middle, and end, and we each had our roles to play to keep The Flow going throughout. It didn't matter who was saying what, who was holding the mic longer, or who was getting credit for all the jokes at the end of the day. If our tribe walked away feeling energized, inspired, healthier, and happier, then we'd done our job.

And as I stood a few steps above the crowd that late-November morning, with hundreds of bodies huddled against the rain, anxiously awaiting my signal, I thought, *I'm not sure I'll ever get used to this insanity*. It's absolutely pissing rain, and yet these people are standing around, waiting for me to tell a few mediocre jokes and send them out to run up some giant concrete stairs. Just a few years ago, all BG and I wanted was to race each other, and then find some other fast fuckers to race. And now, at this same moment, in seven cities around North America, people were getting ready to bounce, hug, and drop F-bombs because of our gangly asses. This had definitely become much bigger than we ever anticipated, which reminds me, I need to book a fuckin' van for Edmonton when I get home . . . Okay . . .

"Let's get a little BOUNCE!"

Even though I was wet and cold, after the workout ended I took a slow bike ride home, enjoying the rain pouring down my face and singing a Guns N' Roses classic I knew all the words to before I could even speak English, *"'Cause nothin' lasts forever, even cold November rain . . ."*

I've never done any drugs (not even weed), but I'd imagine the feeling I get after the workout is over—that moment after I take the group photo, tell the crowd, "Have a great day!" and recognize the fact that hundreds of people just ran concrete stairs in the rain because of something that my college friend and I decided to do after a few cold Pabst Blue Ribbons in a frosted mug with lemon (to classy it up), and that a motherless kid from the former East Bloc was breaking new ground in America—has to be what being high feels like. I don't need drugs. I have my tribe.

NOVI SAD, SERBIA: SIXTEEN YEARS EARLIER

It was an unseasonably warm January afternoon. I got home from rowing practice with two of my teammates. My father, teary eyed, greeted me at the door. He told my friends it wasn't a good time and showed them out. Two police officers sat at our dining room table, looking like they just got caught with their hands in the cookie jar. For all my years on this beautiful planet, I never saw cops look this way. Their expression did not resemble THE STARE that I expected to see from a uniformed officer. You know THE STARE, the one perfected by cops and customs officers that makes you stutter, sweat bullets, and feel like you're smuggling drugs for no apparent reason? I knew THE STARE all too well.

My father had been on the force for decades. He was one of those guys who climbed the ranks fast. He graduated from the police academy at the top of his class. After logging time with the Special Forces, he became Unit Commander. A decade later, he was the commanding officer for Novi Sad's entire city police department. Every cop knew his name, which automatically made me somewhat of a celebrity in police circles, and not in a good way.

(handwritten margin note:) We still do the PBR's w/lemon. Must have started back at Northeastern

SUNDAY, JULY 1, 2012

November Project becomes known around Boston as "the Fight Club of Running Clubs"* because of the odd way NP is promoted or uncoached or FREE or all of the above. BG and Bojan continue to keep the workouts, vibes, and stories of NP weird and hard to follow (for normal people).

* NHL hockey player Andrew Ference claims he coined this term. Anybody want to argue with him?

MONDAY, JULY 9, 2012

Monday workouts added. Each week is a new destination in the city in which the group meets to do pushups and sit-ups based on flipped decks of cards. This is called the #DestinationDeck and continues to make Bostonians who train with NP discover parts of the city and shake up their usual run routine. november-project.com/monday-workouts/

THE FIRST TWO RULES OF NOVEMBER PROJECT ARE THAT YOU MUST TALK ABOUT NOVEMBER PROJECT.

You know how hard it is to be a teenager in a town of 350,000 where every cop knows your dad? It sucks! Many of our high school parties that were broken up by the cops, my dad knew about before I even got home. Every time I got pulled over for a random traffic checkup (pretty common in Serbia to prevent drinking and driving) the word made it to "Mandara," my dad's nickname, stemming from our family name, Mandaric.

"License and registration, please. Oh, you're Mandara's kid, eh? Does your old man know you're getting in trouble?"

"I'm not getting myself in trouble, sir. I'm on my way to practice."

"Yeah, yeah, don't let me tell your pop you're riding that moped like a punk."

"Yes, sir! I won't do it again, sir!"

For the record, I never acted like a punk, as I knew that any asshat moves would make it back to my dad. Yet no matter how innocent I was, every time I talked to a cop in a uniform I felt like their look was tattooing giant "GUILTY" letters on my forehead. I hated THE STARE, but for some reason not seeing it on the face of the two officers in my dining room scared the shit out of me. Something was very wrong here.

My dad put his shovel-like hand on my shoulder and guided me onto the couch in the living room. That scared me even more. We never showed physical affection to each other, not since I can remember. When Serbians greet each other, they shake hands and kiss three times on the cheek. Depending on the occasion, this can mean welcome, farewell, happy birthday, or congratulations, among other things. Serbians are also very big on hugs, especially if the alcohol is flowing. And the alcohol is always flowing. It's not uncommon to see people starting their day with a shot of rakija—fruit-flavored brandy with an alcohol content slightly lower than rubbing alcohol. But no matter how many liters of rakija had been put away, my father and I never really hugged, or kissed, or even high-fived for that matter. He grew up in Communist Yugoslavia and carried the tightness, the rigid obedience to rules and order, with him after the country broke apart

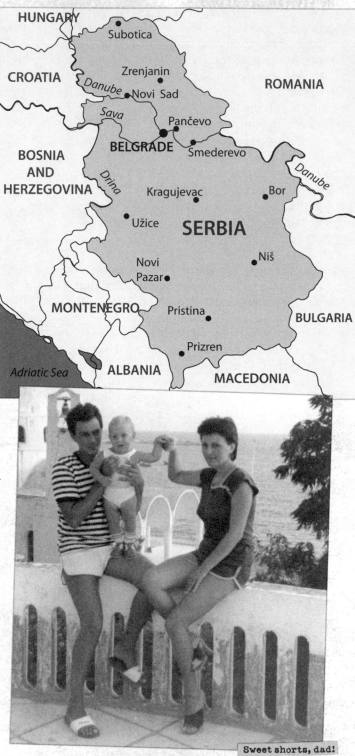

Sweet shorts, dad!

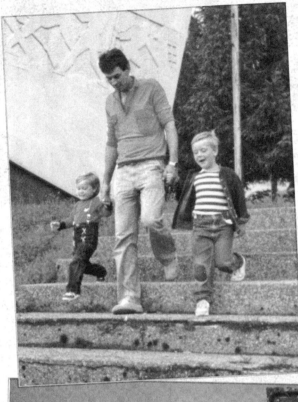

in 1991. Even though we were now Serbians, free to evolve and explore, he remained a Yugoslav. And we remained distant.

Early on, though, there was plenty of physical contact, just not of the tender variety. He exclusively initiated these interactions, and the medium of expression was dependent on the situation. Service-issued leather belt, fly swatter, wooden spoon, and open fists were some of the popular items that ended up marking my glutes, and sometimes lower back, depending on how good his aim was, every time I "misbehaved." And I apparently misbehaved a lot. My father would moderate arguments with my younger sister, Olivera, by whipping my ass so hard that I had to eat dinner standing up, weighing in that as an older brother and more mature individual I should know better. As I got older, the whippings stopped, but my dad and I remained physically distant and neither of us tried too hard to bridge the gap.

So when he put his hand on my shoulder, my heart dropped.

We sat down on the opposite ends of the L-shaped couch, his shoulders pointing upward as he placed elbows on his knees. His proud 6-foot-2-inch frame, which, at 16, I was closing in on, all of a sudden appeared tiny and insignificant. He took a long drag from a cigarette. Usually, I would snark about second-hand smoke, but it didn't seem like an appropriate moment. I don't remember his words or how he delivered the news. I just remember having millions of questions flying through my head. I wanted to say something, but nothing seemed right. So I finally just asked, "When is the funeral?"

To this day, I still don't know the actual cause of my mother's death, nor do I have any intention to find out more. That morning she came back from the night shift at the hospital, where she worked as a delivery room nurse, picked up around the house, cooked lunch, and went into the bedroom to take a nap. My dad came home and found her lying in the bedroom, motionless. Rigor mortis had already set in. He called the emergency line. But because health care resources were so scarce at the time, ambulances would only go out for a real emergency. And since the death had already occurred, there was no rush. A few of my dad's cop buddies were the first to show up. Olivera told me that the autopsy report said something about her heart, but I didn't want to read it.

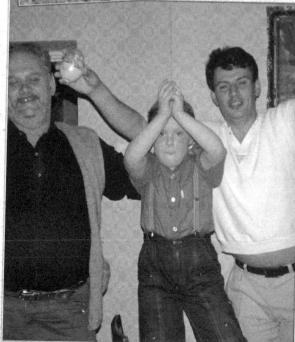

Bojan has been running steps and chilling out in high-waisted pants his entire life.

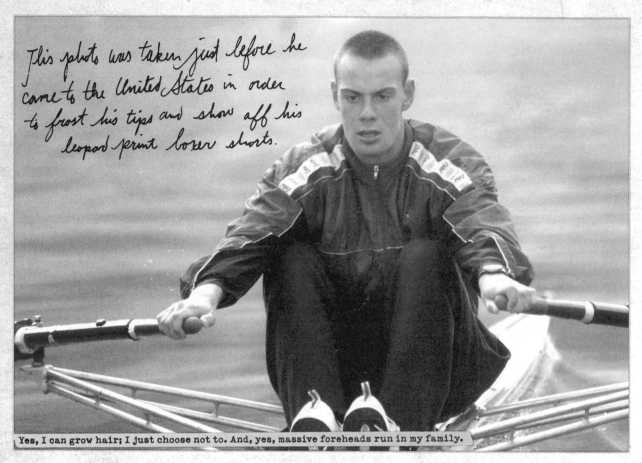

This photo was taken just before he came to the United States in order to frost his tips and show off his leopard print boxer shorts.

Yes, I can grow hair; I just choose not to. And, yes, massive foreheads run in my family.

At the funeral, I didn't want to look inside the open casket. I didn't want her motionless body to be my last memory of the beautiful woman who had taught me loyalty, patience, and humility.

I'd started rowing about a year before my mother passed away, but I was never too serious about it. My hometown rowing club, Danubius 1885 (River Danube in Latin), had a long history of successful oarsmen who represented Yugoslavia at many a prestigious regatta and at the Olympic Games. But after the breakup of Yugoslavia and the economic and political turmoil that engulfed the whole region, rowing fell into oblivion despite a handful of oarsmen on the international rowing scene. None of those guys, however, trained or competed in Yugoslavia during the season. They all rowed for major colleges around the United States. Only during the summer would they come home to compete for the National Team.

The state of local rowing clubs, especially the one in my hometown during the late nineties, was dismal at best. The boats and the equipment were severely outdated. Resources for high-level training were minimal, yet to me rowing seemed increasingly like something that I would really enjoy. It's an outdoor sport. It's on the water. No skills are required. You get to move while sitting down! And the yearly membership was really cheap. Check, check, check, and check. My mom gave her blessing as long as my grades didn't suffer. My dad didn't care as long as I wasn't out getting arrested. So in April of 1996, at age 15, I took my first rowing stroke.

Shortly after I learned the basics, I started competing. And I sucked. A lot. The first time I got into a single scull, I flipped and fell in the water, flailing and clutching on to the boat, kicking my legs, but unable to get back on board. My coach suggested I keep flipping on purpose to get the fear out of the way and figure my way back into the boat. This was a skill that became very useful a few years later during a chilly February workout that involved a collision with a submerged log. Let's just say that doing burpees in a steaming shower room is a good way to prevent pneumonia.

The great thing about rowing is that it's truly one of the few sports where talent is not important. It's all about the effort. Some of the best rowers in the world are pretty clumsy and uncoordinated. However, their training ethic and dedication is so unwavering that they've conditioned themselves into excellence just by working really fuckin' hard. Initially, I wasn't that serious. I was happy with the new friends I was making and the occasional race that I competed in. Out of 12 workouts per month, I'd go to maybe seven or eight—just enough for the coach to put me in the racing lineup.

But once my mom wasn't around anymore, I was looking for any excuse not to engage in my father's awk-ward attempts at parenting. I just needed to be out of the house. My dad tried, he really did, but all those clumsy attempts would soon be engulfed in flames when he started dating again. Less than 6 months after my mom's passing, I noticed that he started dressing up to go out. At first he tried to keep it secret, but then one day I got home to both apartment door locks being bolted (something we did only when we went away on vacation), and I walked in to find my dad with a woman I had never seen before, hanging out in the living room. I said a super-awkward hello and went straight to my room. Neither of us said anything to each other that day, but it became pretty obvious that our strained relation-ship just got significantly weaker. I didn't know what the appropriate number of months, or years, or days were to start dating after you lose your spouse, but for 16-year-old me, it was too soon.

CHCK!

When a carbon fiber oar hits the water at the optimal angle, it makes the most beautiful *CHCK!* sound—the result of air being pushed out of the puddle that an axe-shaped oar blade creates at the beginning of every stroke. It's called the catch. Anyone who's ever experi-enced the perfect catch has also felt the boat suddenly become more responsive, lighter, and easier to control. When I heard that *CHCK* for the first time, I was hooked. I felt free, like the training wheels had been taken off the bike, and all I wanted to do was hear it over and over again. But accomplishing a perfect catch 200-plus times in a row during a 2,000-meter race is not an easy feat. Oarsmen at the highest level are able to accomplish it, but they've spent thousands of hours achieving balance, relaxation, calmness, all while moving up and down the slide tracks at 34 to 36 strokes per minute as their bod-ies are fighting fatigue caused by the lactic acid buildup in every single skeletal muscle.

Since my rowing club held two workouts per day to accommodate kids with different school schedules, I made it my mission to get to both just so I didn't have to be at home. My deteriorating relationship with my dad consisted of daily fights over the stupidest things, like not putting the dishes away after washing them or "walk-ing around loudly" while he was resting from a night

NS SPORT PLUS
MESEČNI MAGAZIN SPORTISTA NOVOG SADA
Godina VIII • Novi Sad, Avgust 2001 • Cena 10 dinara

MEĐUNARODNI SPORTSKI SUSRETI NOVI SAD DORTMUND AMIJENS 2001

BOJAN MANDARIĆ

No fucking way!! The cover of "NS SPORT MAG"!? Did you tell the writer to "Put me on the fucking cover"!?
#ROWING NERD #SUPEREURO

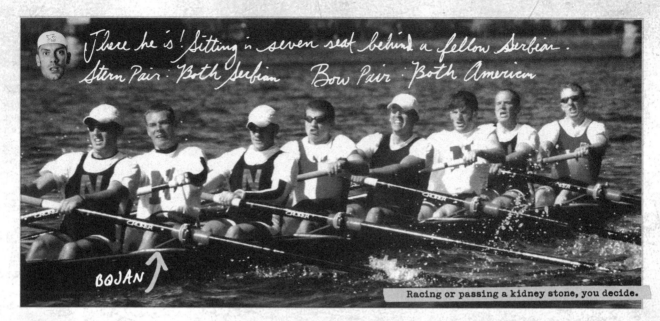

There he is! Sitting in seven seat behind a fellow Serbian. Stern Pair: Both Serbian   Bow Pair: Both American

BOJAN ↑

Racing or passing a kidney stone, you decide.

shift. But at the boathouse, things couldn't have been better. Two-a-day workouts proved fruitful in helping me get super comfortable in a rowing shell. The *CHCK* sound became something I was hearing more and more, and as a result I started crossing the finish line in front of most of the guys from my rowing club, half of them several years older than me.

My first try for a national team berth was in double-scull at the Junior Balkan Rowing Championships in Belgrade. I was 17 years old and got paired with Emil Jakovljevic, a five-foot-ten 18-year-old, who looked more like an NFL fullback, and who been rowing since he was 12. Only the winning boat from the national team trials, out of a dozen entries from around the country, would make the team. We were confident that we would make the cut, but after a slow start and a few snags in the final race, we crossed the finish line less than a second behind the winning crew from Red Star Rowing Club. We were devastated. But while loading our boat on the trailer, the coach told us that as a host country, Yugoslavia might get a second entry if one country didn't send a crew for the field of seven boats. Two days later, we got the news: Albania was out. We were in! The only downside was that as a "B" boat we weren't eligible for medals, so even if we placed we'd get skipped on the podium. Emil and I didn't care. We were just stoked that we had a chance to represent our country, and both

agreed that we HAD to beat the Yugoslavia "A" boat.

The race was in the early afternoon on a sunny September day. The crosswind was blowing warm air from the starboard side, creating small, annoying waves that can disrupt the balance of a less-experienced crew. Emil and I were used to the choppy Danube water, unpredictable currents, and the occasional whirlpool that would sometimes spin smaller boats 90 degrees without warning. A little crosswind on Ada Ciganlia, a man-made lake a few miles west from downtown Belgrade that was often used by locals to cool down during hot and humid summers, was no big shakes. We pointed our bow a few degrees away from the center of the racing lane in anticipation of the wind that was going to push at us during the first few strokes.

"All hands down," said the voice from the tower. "Attention . . . GO!"

Yugoslavia "A" had a decent start and was immediately going back and forth with Greece and Romania, fighting for the first three spots. Emil and I were about a half-length back, tussling with Bulgaria for the fourth spot. Turkey was another half-length behind. Our plan was to stay calm for the first 700 meters and not get reactive.

At the 500-meter mark, all the crews had settled into their rhythms and were strategizing their next move. Greece, rowing at a long 34 strokes per minute, was pulling away, leaving Romania in second place and Yugoslavia "A" in third. Emil, who was stroking at a collected 32 or 33, glanced over to his right shoulder and, seeing that Yugoslavia "A" was within the reach, signaled, "HOP!" This was the sign that our 10-stroke move was coming on the next catch. A little confused about his strategy to attack at only a quarter into the race, but without time to argue, I went for it. And just like that, in 10 strokes we were even with Yugoslavia "A." Emil signaled another "HOP," followed by, "Let's pull away." *You don't have to tell me twice, Bud*, I thought.

Yugoslavia "A" tried to respond with a move of their own, but we kept inching farther and farther ahead, taking over third place. Then Romania, still in second place, took off. Greece noticed Romania attacking, but didn't bite, and continued their long strokes, waiting patiently for the move to end. With 750 meters to go, Romania attacked again, causing Greece to respond. Emil and I found ourselves in a no-man's land between two crews battling for gold and a crew we set out to beat fading to a length behind. Crossing into the last 500 meters, we wanted to make a statement: Beat the "A" boat with as wide a margin as possible and show the national team coach who the real "A" boat was.

Emil bumped up the rate from 36 strokes per minute to 40 in two strokes, and in another two strokes we were at 43, a crazy pace, just about red-lining. With 250

meters to go, Romania, in lane four, entered our peripheral vision. Completely delirious trying to follow Emil's violent cadence, I somehow mustered, "Romanians are right there." In Emil's head, that translated to "Go apeshit!" I don't remember much of those last few strokes. Our coach told us that with 100 meters to go, he clocked us at 48 strokes per minute. That was also the point where we passed Romania and started closing in on Greece. Spectators watching from the grandstands said that we had so much speed that if the course was 50 meters longer we would have won. But we didn't. We came in 1.4 seconds behind the Greek crew. But still, we were excited out of our minds. We destroyed the "A" boat by a few lengths of open water, and even though our legs and shoulders were screaming from the built-up lactic acid and our throats were scratched raw from a jacked-up breathing rate to the point where we could only use signs to communicate, we thought that the day couldn't get any better. That is, until we got off the water and our coach told us that the crew that had beaten us had just won a silver medal at the Junior World Championships a few weeks before, and that the Romanian crew that we overtook in the final strokes finished fifth in the grand final. Not too shabby.

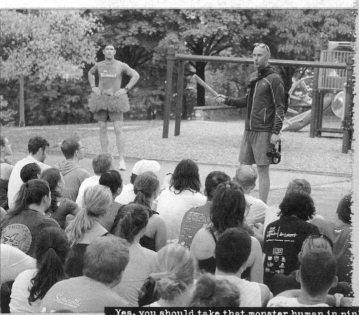

PROPER WAYS TO MISPRONOUNCE BOJAN'S NAME

- Boy Ann
- Boyanton
- Boyancé
- Boj-Anne
- Bojan (like Trojan)
- Bohan (Spanish)
- Bojane (French)
- Bouillon (Cajun)

Fun Fact: I change the way I say his name every... single... time. Each is different, like snowflakes.

Yes, you should take that monster human in pink tutu behind me seriously.

↑ *Look at him go!? He's dressed like everyone's most responsible uncle. Uncle Bojan! Seen in this photo, Uncle Bojan rolls out the #Positivity Awards on Friday in Boston.*

After that race, I went on to represent my country for 6 years, competing in numerous international regattas, World Rowing Championships, and Collegiate Championships. I won more than 100 medals, but hands-down my most memorable race to this date is the one I wasn't supposed to be in and didn't get a medal for. Now this is the part where I can drop a cheesy line about how "It was all about the love of the game"; or that "Leaving a part of yourself out there on the water is the true driving force." To a certain extent both are true, but for me those are lines for motivational posters. My strongest driving force is turning what others see as super-challenging and sometimes impossible into reality. I guess that could be a motivational poster, too. I'll take the royalties if anyone wants to print it up.

HUSKIES

I'd never heard of Northeastern University (NU). The only things I knew about Boston were the Celtics and Larry Bird. As an 18-year-old living in the Balkans, everything I knew about America came from heavy-metal song lyrics, late-night broadcasts of NBA games, and badly dubbed movies like *Caddyshack* and *Animal House*. I'd studied English in high school for a few years, but what I learned was more like British English and it never felt right in my mouth or my brain, didn't climb from the lungs and throat the way Serbian did. English words seemed all crunched and chewed up and pushed out through pursed lips. And then the spelling . . . In Serbian, everything is spelled phonetically, so even the 50-character words aren't hard to spell. But English, man oh man . . . the confusion between *fairy* and *ferry* gets me in trouble on Twitter even today.

I first learned of Northeastern through a 6-foot-7 human mountain named Veljko Culafic. Veljko rowed at Partizan Rowing Club in Belgrade before going to high school in Florida to complete his senior year. Being a strong dude and a super-skillful rower, he was heavily recruited to row in the United States. He chose NU, where he was coached by highly regarded Buzz Congram. After his junior year at NU, Veljko decided to spend his summer trying out for the national team. We met at the rowing camp in Belgrade, where guys from rowing clubs from around the country competed for positions in the four-man boat that would go to the World Championships in Linz, Austria.

I clicked with Veljko right away. After our first workout, he asked if I'd ever considered applying to a college in the United States. After realizing that rowing could be a way to get an amazing education outside of Yugoslavia, I knew I had to pursue the opportunity. But I had to get a scholarship. At the time, my dad was making around $300 per month, which was considered a decent salary for a police commander. But to pay for a single four-credit class in the US, he'd need to work for more than a year without paying any bills. It had to be a full-ride scholarship or nothing.

By this time, Buzz had decided to retire, passing the reins to his assistant, John Pojednic. John was a lightweight rower who came to Henderson Boathouse from Boston College, a few miles downriver. At age 26, he was the youngest coach in the Intercollegiate Rowing Association, the league that administers the U.S. Collegiate National Championships. John was put in a unique,

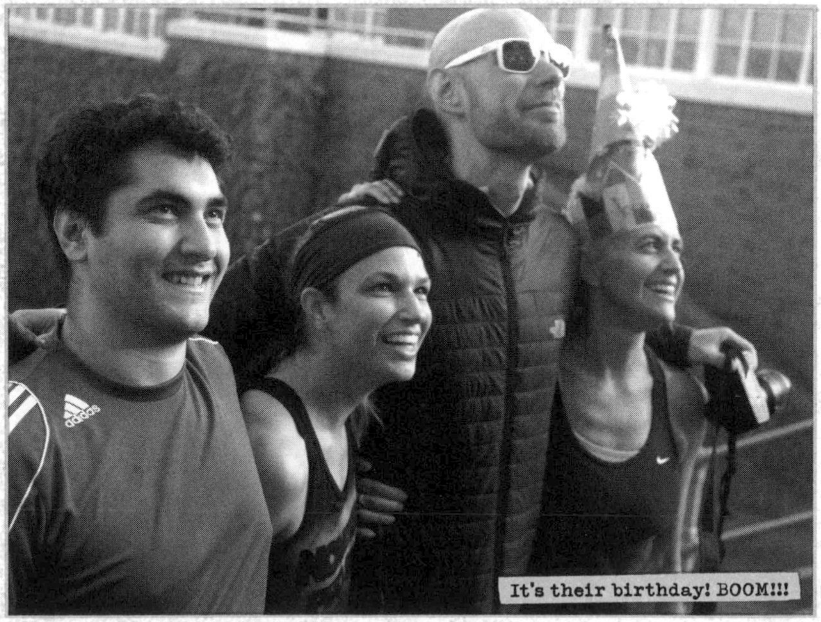

It's their birthday! BOOM!!!

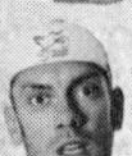

FunFact #110: Bojan and Lil usually miss at least one ferry each time we're in SF visiting our family in Oakland @the North Face

and I would imagine very stressful, situation where he had to sustain the success and excellence that Buzz had brought to the program while coaching guys only a few years his junior. But he did it, and he did it well. His dry sense of humor, no-bullshit attitude, and way of maintaining coach-athlete boundaries helped continue the sterling legacy of the Northeastern Huskies crew.

Veljko suggested that I get in touch with Coach Pojednic. As soon as I got back to the computer that afternoon, I fired off an introduction email. Meanwhile, later that summer, I made the Yugoslavia national team boat and went on to win a bronze medal at Worlds. Pojo was impressed with my results and, bolstered by a great recommendation from one of his best guys, he offered me a full athletic scholarship.

Since I'd already enrolled in the first year of university in my hometown, Coach Pojednic saw the opportunity to transfer some of the credits I had accrued and enroll me as a sophomore at NU. That meant that I was eligible to row in the varsity boat, which under NCAA rules at the time had to consist entirely of upperclassmen. Freshmen, on the other hand, had to spend their first year of eligibility racing other freshmen before they could move up the ranks.

The first time I touched the US soil was on March 22, 2002. I had $200 in my wallet and two duffel bags full of clothes. As my plane broke through the layer of clouds approaching East Boston, all I could see was a dark gray ocean. I swam in many seas around Europe, but I hadn't yet been in the ocean. I kept thinking, I can't wait to dip my toes in that salt water. At Logan Airport, I was met by an NU alum who gave me a plane ticket to Atlanta. He told me I was heading to a training camp at the site of the 1996 Summer Olympics, where the whole team had already started their spring training.

I shared a room with Justin, a senior coxswain from Florida, and Petar, a Croatian national team oarsman who came to Northeastern a few months before I did. Even though less than a decade earlier the Croats and Serbs had viciously battled each other for territory back home, I was glad to have, through Petar, some connection to the old country. The door to our room was propped open as guys kept coming in to introduce themselves. One dude walked in wearing only beach shorts, towering a few inches over my 6-foot-4 frame, showing off what appeared like 18-pack abs and shoulders that

resembled a bookshelf. He had a square jaw and a buzz cut, and looked very much what I'd always imagined Americans to look like. He had perfect posture. A mountain man just like Veljko.

"What's up, man, I'm Brogan," he said, shifting his weight from leg to leg, like he just got off a 20-hour flight and was trying to get the blood flowing again.

"Hi, I'm Bojan."

"What is it? Boy . . .?"

"It's Bojan, spelled B-O-J-A-N, but that 'J' you pronounce as 'Y.' So, it's Bojan."

"Cool," he responded sizing me up, still shifting about. "We've all heard about you. Serbia, huh. So you rowing with freshmen or varsity?"

"Varsity. At least that's what Coach told me."

For a split second, Brogan looked like he didn't understand what this Serbian fellow was saying. A storm cloud passed across his face as his expression morphed from friendly to dead serious. And then he belted out a long, gorilla-loud "FUUUUUUUUUCK!!" and stormed out of the room.

I turned to Justin and Petar.

"He thought you'd be rowing in the freshmen boat," Justin said. "They need one guy to make that lineup really fast. You would have been perfect."

I stared at them for a second and then at the empty space between the door jamb that had been almost entirely blocked out by Brogan's body moments earlier. The only thing that kept going through my mind was, "Holy shit, that human monster is just a freshman?!"

THE SECTION I DIDN'T WANT TO WRITE

When two heartless pricks detonated bombs near the finish line of the 2013 Boston Marathon, my reaction was different from my wife, Emilie's, from my friends', from most of Boston. I wasn't shocked. My world wasn't instantly turned upside down. I was sad that this kind of shit still happens. I was sad for my American friends. But, unfortunately, it wasn't the first time I saw devastation, heard the boom of explosions, tasted smoke in my mouth.

If you were watching CNN in the 1990s, you remember the implosion of my homeland, Yugoslavia, after the collapse of the Soviet Union. You probably recall names like Bosnia and Herzegovina, Croatia, Slovenia, Serbia, and Kosovo. When I was 9, the country where I was born

Jumping ahead 13 years and Justin stops #PaulLeak* on the street in New York City when he sees Paul's #GrassRootsGear. They meet, hug, shoot and send a selfie video to Bojan, and go on their way. * Paul Leak is the Co-Leader of November Project NYC

and raised, among the most liberal of the satellite nations within the Eastern Bloc, fractured pretty quickly. Even provinces within republics were splitting apart, everyone declaring independence, old tensions rising and turning violent. I'm sure it was really confusing to you. It was pretty confusing to a teenage me, too.

But of all the fights and struggles in Yugoslavia in the late eighties and early-to-mid-nineties, it was the two upheavals in Kosovo—10 years apart—that rocked my world the most.

First, a little history lesson. Kosovo is the southernmost of Serbia's two provinces, bordering Albania, and is deeply entwined in Serbian heritage. In the 14th century, the Serbs fought a crucial war in Kosovo against the Ottoman Empire in which the Empire's leader, Sultan Murad I, was killed. Even though the Ottomans eventually overtook that area, historians argue that if it weren't for that battle, Europe would look very different today.

In the early nineteen hundreds, Serbia was very prosperous. After WWII, as part of Yugoslavia's fairly moderate socialist regime, it became an attractive destination for Albanians who were fleeing from a more severe form of Communism back home. By the late 1970s, the traditionally Christian Serbian population had become the minority. But under the imposed atheism of Communism, religious and ethnic differences were kept at bay, and everyone, more or less, was living harmoniously. We were Yugoslavians first.

After the Eastern Bloc began wobbling in the late eighties, the majority Albanians in Kosovo began demanding independence from Serbia, and with that demand came violence. Police stations, government buildings, and homes were attacked. Police officers from other parts of Serbia, including my dad, were sent in to quell what was seen as an internal flare-up. He did two 6-month tours, but things didn't get better. Casualties on both sides were mounting. Then my mom, a nurse, was called to Kosovo to help out in local hospitals. When one of my parents was gone, the other one would stay at home. But they still had to work, including night shifts. Sometimes, my grandparents stayed with my sister and me. Other times, it was just the two of us for long stretches of the day and night. I was 8 and Olivera was 6. We learned early on how to take care of ourselves.

Eventually, diplomacy got the leaders of both sides to the negotiating table and things calmed down for a while. But the first Kosovo conflict was just a preview for the rest of the country. Slovenia and Croatia were the first republics to declare independence from Yugoslavia, doing so on the same date in June 1991. Bosnia followed 8 months later. Bloody conflicts were soon raging in most parts of what used to be one country. "The Brotherhood and Unity," a term coined by the socialist party to describe a melting pot of nationalities, cultures, and religions, had turned into 5 years of senseless fighting, burned-down homes, hundreds of thousands of refugees, and economic sanctions. The life that I knew for the first decade of my life—new clothes, well-stocked store shelves, safe streets, vacations in Greece and Croatia—had come to an end.

When I was almost 17, tensions in Kosovo flared up again, this time multiplied by 50. It was 1998. And this time, diplomacy didn't win out. A heavy, sustained NATO bombing campaign was launched in the spring of 1999 to halt the violence. The Serbs were seen as the aggressors and our assets were targeted in retaliation, including many in Novi Sad, my hometown, the second-largest city in Serbia after Belgrade.

I remember watching BBC and seeing jet fighters take off from Aviano Air Base in Italy, and then maybe 10 minutes later, there was a boom. The windows just shattered from the impact. The first bomb that fell on Serbian soil made impact 500 yards from my house. I was scared shitless. My dad was at work. My sister and I were the only ones at home. It was fucking insane. So, my dad calls right away. He's like, "You know where all the guns are"—since the day I was born, he had taught me how to use them—"Get all the guns, pack a light bag, and start walking toward me, but don't take any main roads. Take the side roads."

Life went on that way for 2 months. During those 60 days, they hit everything we needed to sustain a normal existence. The oil refinery, just outside of the city, was shelled to fucking rubble. I saw all the burning smoke from my window. You would see airplanes flying around and anti-aircraft tracer rounds lighting up the sky. A few moments later, you'd see an explosion somewhere in the vicinity of a bridge or the TV station.

But Serbians are fucking strange people. When something is going really bad, people rally behind it. "Oh fuck that," Serbs will say. "We're going to show everybody the middle finger. Fuck the world. You're going to bomb us? You're going to knock down our bridges? We're going to create a human shield on the bridge. All right, knock us down now!"

Usually, shit would go down at night, so during the day we'd go about business as usual. And for me, that business was still all about rowing.

There was a naval base on the Danube River. Serbia doesn't have a sea, but it does have a bunch of rivers. At the time, we had a couple of ships and a few cannons—nothing that we could go to war with—but they were enough to shoot down some airplanes. And they were located maybe one kilometer from my rowing club. So we'd row by the base, clenching our butt cheeks. Eventually, the NATO bombers knocked down all our bridges, cutting us off from the rest of Serbia. So when we launched onto the water, we'd end up rowing between the broken halves of bridges that had collapsed into the river. But for the team, we were more pissed because our practices constantly got interrupted. Five kilometers into the workout, you'd have the air raid sirens go off and have to turn around and go back to safety.

Arrangements were made for us to train in Hungary. Since we were all 16, 17, and 18, we had to get special permission from the military to leave the country during a time of war. I remember at customs, the guy would look at us three times and he'd be judging the shit out of us. Anyway, we were in Hungary, rowing twice a day. It was awesome. I was crushing the competition. But off the water, we spent the bulk of our time glued to the TV, watching CNN and BBC, trying to figure out what the fuck was going on back home. Professionally, it was a great time, but personally, it was one the worst periods of my life.

Initially, I didn't want to get into any of this political-military stuff in this book. I'm only including this because

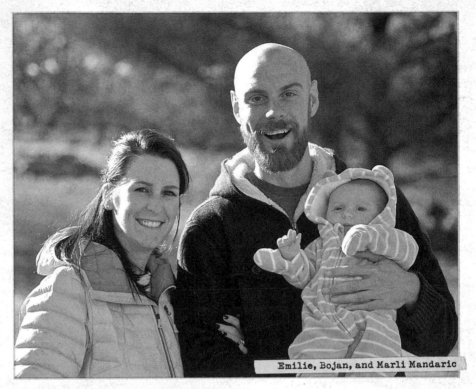

Emilie, Bojan, and Marli Mandaric

Caleb, aka Bookman (he'll explain that one later), thought it would give the reader some additional insight into why I can come across as a serious and intense dude. I guess Serbia gave me my game face, and the shaved head and tats don't help, but I digress . . .

I don't have beefs with anyone; my heart is open. At Northeastern, one of my closest friends was Petar, a Croatian fellow. In the boathouse, we were all one unit, no divisions, no Croats, Serbians, Canadians, Americans. We were all—and will remain—Northeastern Huskies. At November Project, one of my favorite dudes, and a hardcore NPer, is Kosta, the Albanian. That's what NP is all about: community—all backgrounds, all levels, all ages, all persuasions. That's why when BG and I talk about a world takeover, we're not kidding. We're using positivity, high-octane vibes, and weird antics as our weapons. I've seen what violence and hatred does. As I write this, my wife Emilie is 8 months pregnant with our first child. And I'm going to bust my ass to make sure our daughter comes into a world built on love and community, respect and understanding. An army of fit, positive fuckers. Yeah, that's what I'm trying to help build every day.

"crushing!"??

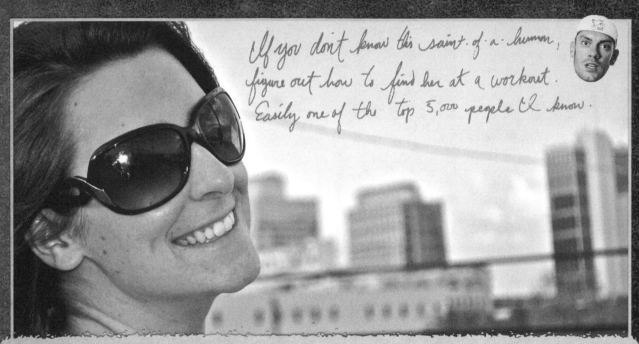

If you don't know this saint of a human, figure out how to find her at a workout. Easily one of the top 5,000 people I know.

I HATE NOVEMBER PROJECT, I LOVE NOVEMBER PROJECT by Emilie Mandaric

🕐 7th December 2013   👤 brogan   📁 Blog   💬 7 Comments

One of the best people I've known in my life, Emilie Mandaric, is today's guest blogger. I've watched her over the last few years start as a skeptic, transform into an athlete, and grow from negative to neutral to full supporter of our movement. She and I went for a 1.5 mile run two years ago and we were forced to stop and take many rest breaks before we were done. Fast forward two years and Emilie has found her way to the finish of countless 10Ks, #Frog-Man1s, and even a few half marathons. Her progress as a runner is an entire story in itself and I couldn't be more proud to have watched from the sidelines. I am also very happy to see that we're actually getting this post up and live *without* her husband and my dude (Bojan) knowing about it. This is the annoying/awesome November Project seen through the eyes of Emilie Mandaric:

Brogan asked me to write a guest post for NP and keep it a secret from Bojan. As I rarely get the opportunity to surprise Bojan, I said yes. I sat down and typed out my thoughts, then erased them, then re-typed them, and then walked away and tried again. Finally, this logorrhea (<—the true "medical" term for "word vomit") dialogue was born . . .

At this point, I think we all know what November Project means to a lot of the tribespeople. It means hugs, friends, kick-ass workouts, race PRs, and, let's be honest; looking better naked . . . and maybe sharing that with someone. What November Project means to me, as the wife of one of the co-founders, is many things. This has evolved over the past two years from hatred and intimidation to love and pride.

So, keeping it real, let's talk about how regularly I said "I HATE NOVEMBER PROJECT" in the beginning. It's true. November Project was an unstoppable force, figuratively barreling through my household, and my life.

1. **WE USED TO TAKE VACATIONS.** We now take November Project vacations. This means we travel to places that have current or prospective NP locations, and/or travel to places with killer stairs that we can crush, at 6:30am . . . on vacation . . .

2. **We used to have a normal amount of clothing.** We have earned so much free #grassrootsgear that it doesn't fit in our dresser drawers anymore . . . seriously, we need a third dresser just to hold our (awesome) tagged gear.

3. **I used to have socially appropriate boundaries.** I want to hug EVERYONE now. I was on a job interview last week, and when it was over I had to remind myself I shouldn't hug my interviewer. It's instinct now to stick my hand out and high-five every runner I see running by. It's like I shit rainbows now. This is what NP has done to me.

4. **I used to have free time.** We have met so many great people from all walks of life, and have endless opportunities to immerse ourselves in fun activities. Now our calendar is full; filled to the top.

5. **I used to participate in "normal" social activities.** I can run now . . . and do a full stadium . . . and do crow pose. Prior to NP I couldn't complete six sections or run a mile. I am now expected to participate in 5Ks, 10Ks, even half marathons without much notice because I am an athlete now. Who have my friends become?

6. **We used to have dinner dates.** My concept of romantic gestures is now all screwed up; it's gone from a surprise candlelit dinner, my LBD (men: that's code for little black dress), and designer pumps to an early morning #weatherproof half marathon in Hyannis in February and having my husband run the entire race next to me, cheering me on with soaking wet feet.

At this point in time, two years later, with seven cities and hundreds, perhaps thousands of people waking up to meet at 6:30am to sweat, love, and hug, November Project is still that unstoppable force barreling through my household and life, but it's a welcome one. I have to tell you the phrase "**I hate November Project**" has been eliminated from my vocabulary. I've replaced it with "I am so proud of my husband and Brogan; and all of us might be a bit crazy, **but I fucking love November Project.**" If you invest one month, one day, one week, or even one hour with NP, getting to see what Bojan and Brogan have started, I think you too will drink the Kool Aid, hug it out, and proudly say "**I Love November Project**" ("f-word" optional, but highly encouraged).

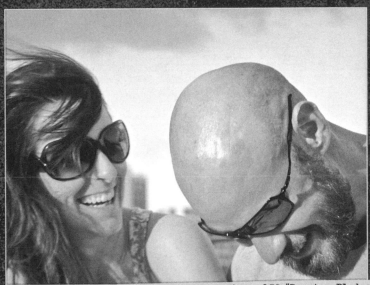

Photo by @Brogan_Graham of IG #Dooster_Pledge

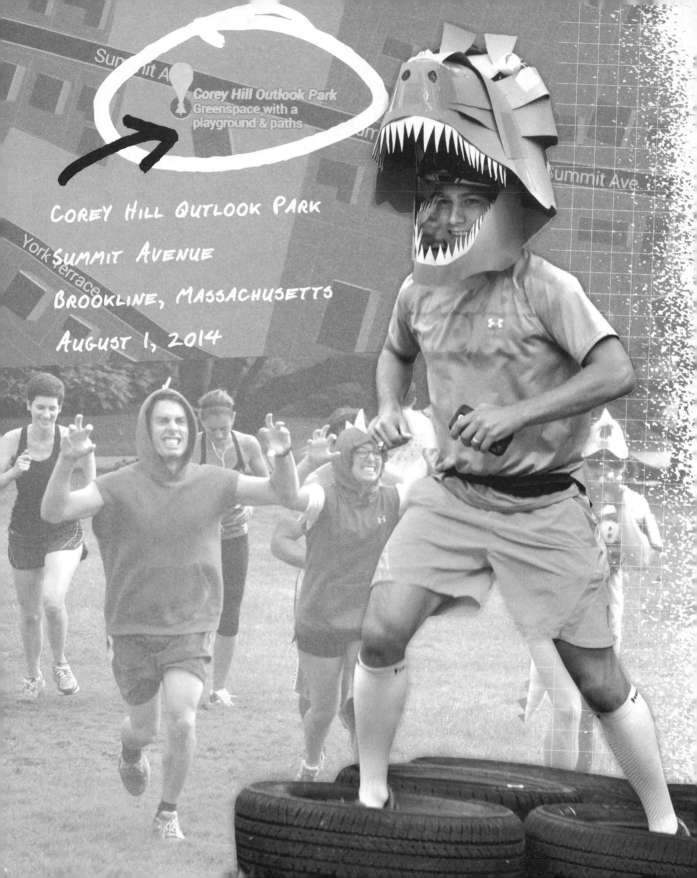

Corey Hill Outlook Park

Summit Avenue

Brookline, Massachusetts

August 1, 2014

CHAPTER 3

#DinoPoolParty

Wisconsin Notes

- BG scales a barbed-wire fence

- Sometimes it rains tires

- Full frontals with extra helpings of cross country spice

- Hold on, is a Chinese dragon technically a dinosaur?

- We do our little turn on the catwalk, yeah, on the catwalk

- The tribe can swim

- Two kids fall asleep with memories to last a lifetime

- Tribe member John Vining tap-dances his way out of a sticky situation

- Never steal, kids; and always return what you borrow

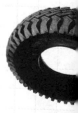

John Vining: Dude, what's the address of that shop with the tires?

Brogan Graham: The corner of Thor Terrace and Cambridge Street in Allston. I'll meet you tomorrow at 5:15 a.m.

JV: 5:15 it is.

BG: Grand.

Early the next morning, John Vining, an architectural designer from Woburn, pulled up in front of a small auto body shop in his Dodge pickup. It was dark, the streets quiet. Graham had asked for help hauling some tires for the Summit Avenue workout. Vining waited 10 minutes or so, killing time by scanning the radio. Then out of the gloom across the way, a large figure materialized wearing a dark singlet, yellow bicycle cap, red shorts, and a backpack. No matter how many times he'd laid eyes on Graham, he was always awed by his solid size and fluid movements—even though Vining himself stands 6 feet 3 and, at 47, could still dunk a basketball on a regulation rim. Graham looked almost out of proportion against the store doorways, NO PARKING signs, and overflowing garbage cans. He spotted Vining in his silver quad cab and waved, but kept moving.

"I thought, where the hell is he going?" Vining said. "I wait some more and all of sudden, he comes around the corner from another building, as if he had just looped around the block. Then he disappears again. I'm like, what the fuck?"

Finally, a few minutes later, Graham appeared at the driver's side door.

"I can't find the tires," he said. "I rode my bike past here the other day and there was a stack, but I don't see them anymore. Let's jump in the truck and look around."

So Vining and Graham prowled the gritty neighborhood, looping down dimly lit

side streets and alleys, past several auto body yards. They turned another corner onto a dark, narrow lane.

"There!" Graham exclaimed.

All Vining could see was a 10-foot-tall fence with barbed wire on the top and padlocked chains across the gates. Then through the chain links, he spotted several stacks of large used tires. "I'm like, 'Dude.'"

But before Vining could say another word, Graham was climbing the fence, then pulling himself onto an adjacent tree that had grown over the top, providing clearance over the barbed wire. From there, Graham swung down and dropped to the cracked asphalt work yard. Distant wisps of light were starting to peel the sky. Vining wondered what he had gotten himself into. Here he was, a married, 40-something-year-old father of two teenagers. Even his kids wouldn't be caught pulling a stunt like this.

"I'm standing there and the thought occurs to me: Channel 7 News. Think of the footage if there were security cameras anywhere. Two guys wearing neon November Project shirts, one jumping the fence. Then I'm thinking, *How the hell are we going to get those tires?*"

All of a sudden, one flies over the fence. And another. Graham is focused like some kind of Looney Tunes discus thrower, heaving one skyward while reaching for another, his long tattooed arms a blur of color and motion. Sixteen tosses in all.

"I can't keep up with him," Vining said. "I get one in the truck and here comes the next one and there's a third and now one's rolling down the street, another bouncing off in a different direction. I'm like, man, we're gonna get in big trouble."

Graham scrambled back over the fence, helped Vining corral the stragglers, and they hopped back into the cab like the Duke boys after outgunning Sheriff Rosco P. Coltrane. They then hightailed it to Summit Avenue, just a pair of smoke tracks in their wake.

Meanwhile, on the second floor of the blue house near the park at the top of the hill, 4-year-old Grace L'Esperance-Chouinard and her little brother, Micah, were pulling on their costumes. Today was the day. They'd been buzzing with Christmas-like anticipation all week. Grace wriggled into a forest green T. rex onesie with a white-spiked hood

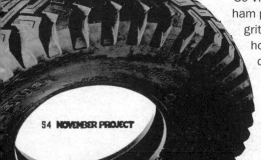

while checking the view through her little brother's bedroom window, which looked out onto the street. Micah stood in a lime green outfit with a marsupial pouch, yellow spikes running down the back, and a tail. Their inflatable dinosaurs were downstairs waiting by the front door.

Ever since that morning last spring when she and her family were pulling out of their driveway and the brightly colored runners stopped and waved at her and her little brother in the backseat, Grace had been fascinated by them. Every Friday morning, she dashed to Micah's room to watch the people running up and down their big hill. She loved their colors. In winter, she could see them in the park through the bare trees, running and rolling and jumping up and down. Sometimes her mom, Jordanna, brought them outside to watch. They once set up a water station at the end of their driveway and drew up posters, just like a race. Many runners stopped by to say hello and slap Grace's outstretched hand. They knew her name. She especially liked the big giant with the colored shoulders. He crouched down to give her a high five whenever he saw her, her tiny hand disappearing against the expanse of his palm. He carried a curious old stick with him and sometimes let her hold it.

Jordanna L'Esperance-Chouinard, a public school psychologist in neighboring Newton, had also been won over by Graham's charm, dislodging her initial assumption that he was some kind of jock asshole. "But he wasn't. He's super kind and gentle and funny. Plus, you're nice to my kids and you're in." With summer winding down, she told Graham and Mandaric they were wel-

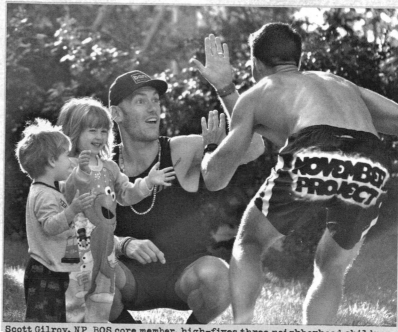

Scott Gilroy, NP_BOS core member, high-fives three neighborhood children.

come to incorporate their backyard swimming pool into one of NP's workouts. Graham's face lit up like a kid's. He had an idea. "What are Micah and Grace's favorite animals?" he asked.

At 236 feet above sea level, Corey Hill Outlook Park is the highest point in greater Boston outside of the Blue Hills. The green space is divided by the aptly named Summit Avenue, with the oaks and maples lining both sides of the road providing a sense of continuity. The park's southern parcel contains a tidy, low-gated playground with a scalloped, cast-iron water fountain, while the northern section is open, with a handful of benches, a sundial, and a large sloped lawn that provides bruising views of Boston and Cambridge.

JULY 2012

November Project starts attendance incentives like $50 credits at Marathon Sports and FREE memberships to Hubway, Boston's then-new bicycle share system.

WEDNESDAY, JULY 25, 2012

"PR Pizzas" become a regular thing. Local pizzeria Stone Hearth becomes the official "go-fast" award. Your time is how much you pay for pizza. Thirty-seven sections in 34:00 minutes (and a PR) got you a 12" pizza of your choice for $3.40.
november-project.com/pr-pizza-day-by-stone_hearth/

WEDNESDAY, AUGUST 15, 2012

"If we ever get more than 300 members in a single workout on a Wednesday morning, we'll get November Project tattoos," BG and Bojan tell a mob of 100 members at Harvard Stadium.
november-project.com/tatsfor300/

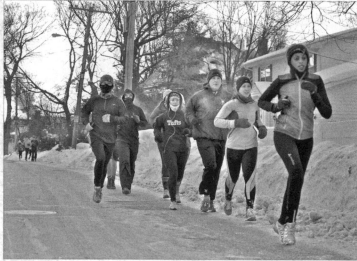

To reach the park under your own steam from either direction is no walk in the park (see what I did there), but especially from the eastern, Brookline side, where the road ascends almost a half mile, starting at an 8-percent grade and peaking at 17 percent in the final quarter. Underneath their slacks and skirts, longtime residents are bona fide Quadzillas. As one of the few steep inclines in the area, the hill is popular with cross-country teams, cyclists, and ROTC units from local colleges. The Boston Marathon's famed Heartbreak Hill, in neighboring Newton, is a mere mound by comparison. Summit Ave is more like Rip-Your-Heart-Out-And-Stuff-It-Back-Down-Your-Throat Hill.

"Our coach at Northeastern, after a Saturday river workout, instead of going home, he took us to the hills," Graham said. "It was really rough, a scarring workout. We did maybe four or five hills. You have 30 or 40 very competitive guys standing next to each other, who are constantly in racing mode, and it was all-out sprinting for as long as you could [go]. People were definitely throwing up. That's how we trained back in the day."

When Graham and Mandaric added the Friday workout to the November Project menu in the fall of 2012, things didn't start off so smoothly with the residents in this upper-middle-class hilltop enclave. The vibe at an empty, predawn Harvard Stadium was unbridled exuberance powered by Fuck Yeah! thunderclouds, a collective button-ripping superhero-logo reveal. But that shit wasn't going to play in sleepy Brookline.

Graham and Mandaric already had been reminded more than once about the noise ordinance, which was in effect until 7 a.m., and been on the receiving end of at least one police citation. Even Jordanna and her husband, Adam, were aggravated in the beginning when they couldn't back out of their driveway because of the unrelenting foot traffic. They found Graham and complained.

He listened. And the following week, the boys com-posed a letter of apology, made a hundred copies, and slid one through the mail slot of every door on Summit Avenue. They turned the volume down on the Bounce, from 11.9 to 3 or 4 (though whenever Mandaric was out of town, Graham snuck it back up to 6 or 7). Speaking in a "murder whisper," Graham reminded tribe members to be quiet for the first half hour, to run on the sidewalks, and always stop to let cars pass through. For the most part, from 6:30 to 7:00 the strange and colorful horde moved on mute, save for some low murmurs and the golf-like applause of several hundred running shoes slapping the pavement.

So that first day of August, as the sun was starting to wash over the rooftops and slant across the asphalt, gaggles of silent, running-shoe-clad T. rexes, Stegosauri, and Brontosauri made their way up the hill. Not one, but three multi-person prehistoric creatures, including a Chinese dragon, sidled to the low wall that overlooked the park. At the bottom of the sloping field, Vining and Graham had set up the tires for some football-style high-stepping. Mandaric had meanwhile created four vertical lanes with miniature American flags for hill sprints. This Cross Country Spice would, of course, cap off each pass up the murderous Summit Ave. Never mistake festive for easy at November Project. It tends to be just the opposite. Fun equals fuel.

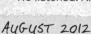

AUGUST 2012

New Balance, headquartered in nearby Brighton, fields anywhere from 3 to 15 employees at workouts. Before long a street-side deal is cut to award NB kicks to any member who trains with the group at least 8 times during the month. Instead of the estimated 75 pairs, New Balance discovers the tribe needs almost 180 pairs.

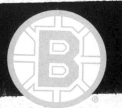

SEPTEMBER 2012

The NHL lockout brings Boston Bruins defenseman and stadium junkie Andrew Ference to the slowly burgeoning movement. His tweets bring a whole new breed of athlete/fan to NP.

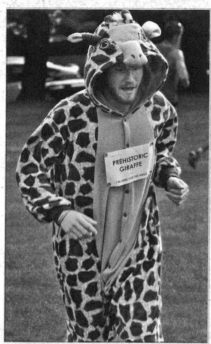

PREHISTORIC GIRAFFE

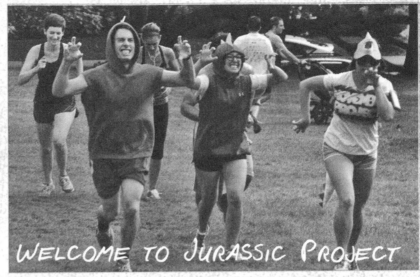

WELCOME TO JURASSIC PROJECT

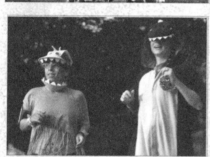

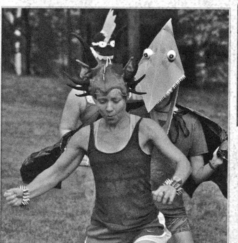

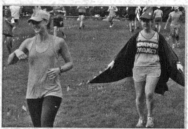

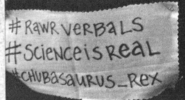

#RAWR.VERBALS
#SCIENCE IS REAL
#CHUBASAURUS_REX

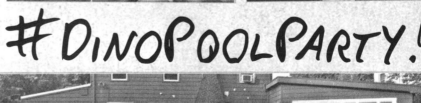

#DinoPoolParty!

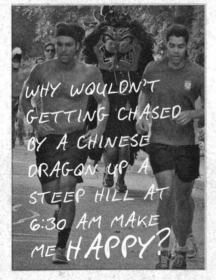

WHY WOULDN'T GETTING CHASED BY A CHINESE DRAGON UP A STEEP HILL AT 6:30 AM MAKE ME HAPPY?

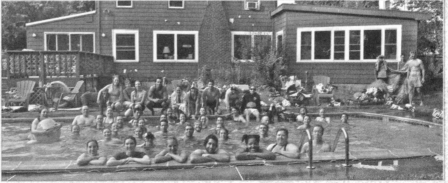

!!!?!??

 Seth Waltz This is the most interesting thing that has happened this summer...in the world...#CNNisstupid #dinosaursrule
August 1, 2014 at 11:17am · Like · 👍 2

 Jim McGowan Dino-flops for breakfast, that's how you kick off a weekend. Epic morning! In for Monday AM.
August 1, 2014 at 11:45am · Like

 Teri Butkiewicz I am really sad that I do not live in Boston to participate in such joy!
August 1, 2014 at 1:12pm · Like · 👍 1

 Mary Anna Dear November Project, I love you. SO MUCH. xoxo Mary Anna ♡
August 1, 2014 at 1:47pm · Like · 👍 4

 Chris R. Payne What Mary Anna said.
August 1, 2014 at 4:39pm · Like · 👍 1

 Amy Ingles I seriously picked the wrong week to go out of town. ☹
August 1, 2014 at 7:35pm · Like

 Jennifer MacCallum O'Meara Happy Happy, Joy Joy all around. What a way to kick off August!
August 1, 2014 at 1:43pm · Like

 ThePositivityAward @PositivityAward · Aug 22
Congratulations Micah and Grace on winning me at @Nov_Project this morning! Thanks for the great pool party! (P.S. I float!)
↩ ♻ ★ 3 ···

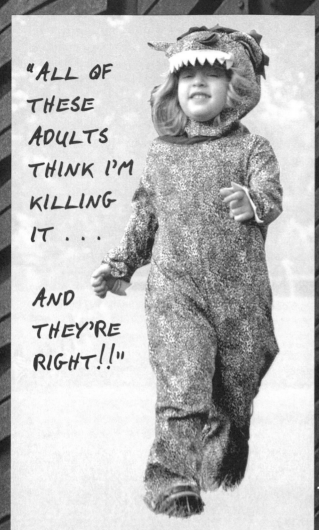

"ALL OF THESE ADULTS THINK I'M KILLING IT . . .

AND THEY'RE RIGHT!!"

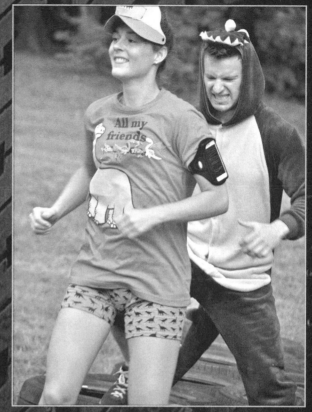

"I LIKED THE TIRES BECAUSE THEY LOOKED LIKE DINOSAUR ROCKS."
—GRACE L'ESPERANCE-CHOUINARD, 4, PRE-SCHOOLER/DINOSAUR, BROOKLINE, MASS.

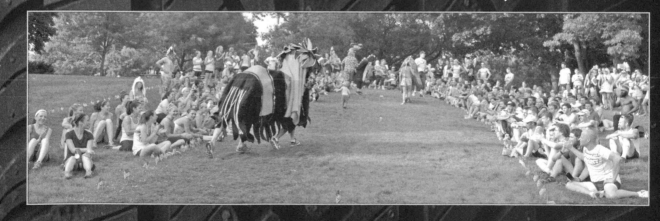

Just before 8 a.m., as many Summit Avenue residents were turning off their coffee makers, plucking car keys from hooks, and shutting their front doors behind them, it was as if nothing had happened. The street was quiet except for a few cars passing through here and there. Birds were chirping. There were no signs that sweaty man or beast had power-roamed the hood for 45 minutes, that a dino runway scene had unfolded at the feet of both a 4-year-old and a 2-year-old judge, that an in-ground pool had bubbled and boiled over with creatures freed from their shells. Just a few wet dinosaur tracks leaving the blue house and headed down the sidewalk remained. Bags had been collected and the flags plucked from the field. Everything as it was.

Except for the tires.

"When we were done," Vining said, "I was like, 'Dude, what are we going to do with these?'"

Graham agreed they should return them. Vining had to get to work, though, so he loaded the tires and took off.

"So now it's eight o'clock," Vining said. "I drive back there and as I pull around the corner, it dawns on me, this place is going to be open for business."

When Vining arrived, the gating and fence were wide open. As he jumped out of his truck cab, a guy walked around the corner from the street and into the yard. In the clear light of morning, Vining saw an old busted-up garage building. He imagined pit bulls, scarred knuckles, thick necks, and short fuses.

"I say, 'Good morning' and I realize he's an employee. He says, 'How ya doin?' and goes into the building. So as fast as I can I'm stacking up tires and I just know the owner is going to come out. So I'm almost done and sure enough, I hear a couple of voices. I'm behind the truck, stacking. He says, 'Excuse me, can I help you?' I said, 'Nope, I'm all set. I'm just returning the tires we borrowed this morning. I work out with this group and we needed tires for a workout.' I tried to talk as fast I could and not stop moving. I'm grabbing the next tire as I'm talking, because I know at any second, he's going to ask, 'How did you get them in the first place?' I'm trying to avoid that at all costs. So he's like, 'Oh, okay.' As I look at his face, I can see he is trying to register what I'm saying, what's going on in front of him. At that moment, I literally pulled the last tire from the truck, stacked it, and got of there as fast as I could. I just know that 10 minutes later he's thinking to himself, *Hold on, how the hell . . . ?*"

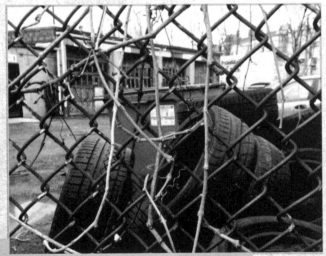

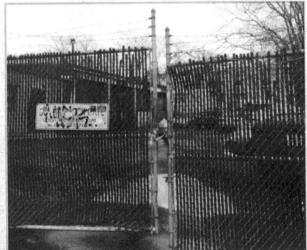

SEPTEMBER 2012

Led by Ference and NHL scout Patrick Burke, NP hosts a stadium workout for the YOU CAN PLAY foundation, which seeks to stop homophobia in sports. Local media is on hand and the atmosphere of inclusiveness surrounding November Project is further projected.

YOU CAN PLAY

WEDNESDAY, SEPTEMBER 12, 2012

November Project breaks 300 members at one workout. "The Tattoo Verbal" video shows the founders getting November Project ink at Pino Bros Ink in Cambridge, Mass. The Hubway bikes used for transportation, the tattoos themselves, and the full production add up to a grand total of $0. Did Bojan or didn't Bojan get a skull tat?

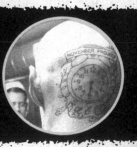

BG: Where did you go?

JV: Dropping off tires and heading to work.

BG: Dude! I was supposed to come with you. Went to grab my bag and you disappeared. Super fucked up man. I mean helpful, I mean fucked up. That's a long-winded way of saying thank you. I can't believe how well this morning worked out. None of those smiles would have been possible without you. When you return the tires and get arrested and get one call from jail, call me.

JV: Yeah man!!!!

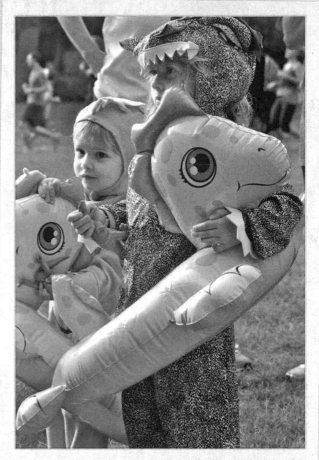

#DinoPoolParty in Boston

🕐 1st August 2014   👤 bojan   📁 Blog

Remember that time when kids asked adults join their pool only if they come dressed as dinosaurs?

Remember when those adults accepted the challenge and in addition to their busy lives, computer jobs, buttoned up shirts, and neckties, took time to carefully craft very intricate T-Rex heads, Stegosaurus back spikes, Velociraptor legs, or Pterodactyl wings?

Remember how a few of the adults took the dinosaur theme to the next level and whipped out a casual Chinese Dragon costume?

Remember how amazed the kids were that whole time?

Remember that time when a guy "borrowed" 18 old tires, dropped them off in his truck an hour before the workout, put the "Yellow Jersey Bike Shop" cycling hat on, and heckled BG's pre-workout talk?

Remember when those old tires and hundreds of small American flags were used to set up the cross-country course?

Remember when a guy showed up with two idiots spray-painted on his shirt?

I still feel like that whole day wasn't real. I feel like I was a part of some strange but unexplainably pleasant dream. If I was dreaming, man that was a fun dream! If that day really happened . . . well I guess nothing is impossible anymore.

On Monday, we'll see you at Sullivan's by Castle Island. Southie people, you have no excuse not to show up! #WeekendEarned

NOVEMBER PROJECT'S HILL WORKOUTS

BY BOJAN MANDARIC

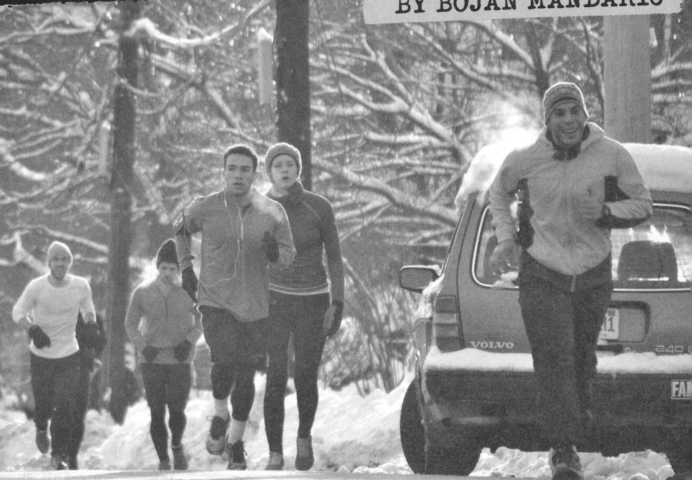

A few months into our existence, people started asking, "When are you going to add more workouts?" At the time, BG and I were still running to and from each other's apartment, popping in on free yoga classes around town, and doing "deck of cards" workouts down by the Charles River. We didn't really NEED to add any more work to our week. However, most of our group was already involved with local running groups and training for road races on weekends, so to help everyone keep the momentum that they'd built on Wednesdays and take it into the weekend, we decided to add a Friday hill-running workout to our repertoire. Here are our regular hill workouts. They're yours for the taking. For just $0.

FULL FRONTALS

Running Full Frontal hills is the least exciting, most boring workout in our repertoire. Yet for some reason, for the first few months that's all we did. And we LOVED IT. The workout originated from BG's and my rowing days at NU, where Coach Pojednic would pile the 40-plus-person roster into university vans, drive up to the hill, and have that same roster race each other all-out up the hill, until he said enough. There was never "we're doing six repeats," or "you have three more to go." The only time we knew we were almost done was when he said, "This is the last one." And even then we weren't 100 percent sure. It was straight-up fucking brutal. Every. Time.

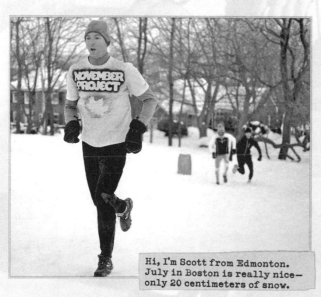

Hi, I'm Scott from Edmonton. July in Boston is really nice— only 20 centimeters of snow.

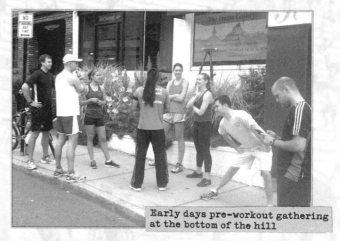

Early days pre-workout gathering at the bottom of the hill

Early on, our newly formed Friday group was pretty small and everyone ran at similar speeds, so you couldn't really hide in the crowd and "take it easy." If you showed up to the hills, you knew that you had to throw it down hard, as everyone else was there to do the same. Whoever dreamed up the acronym K.I.S.S. (Keep It Simple, Stupid) definitely had Full Frontals in mind. All you have to do is run up the hill, turn around at the fire hydrant at the top, come back down, and repeat that five times as fast as you can.

Our meeting spot was at the bottom of Summit Avenue (corner of Summit and Beacon streets) next to the laundromat. Our backpacks littered the flower planter (that at the time didn't contain any flowers), and our start/finish line was the No Parking sign on the corner. We eventually moved the starting line to the top of the hill for two reasons. One: the group was getting too big to meet on the street corner, and the lady from the laundromat was complaining about our shit being all over her flower planters. And two: with the finish line being at the bottom of the hill, in an effort to post some fast times, people would recklessly bomb down the hill with no regard for human life. Lighter runners had a significant advantage doing this, as their weight didn't cause as much stress on their joints as it did on the bigger runners. Both BG and I have a 200-plus-pound frame, and we can report it was an unnecessary strain. So to even out the playing field (and prevent potential injuries), we discouraged reckless down-hilling and instead focused on the uphill push.

UP AND OVERS

Once we brought the starting line to the top of the hill, we realized that there were two sides to this hill. Who knew, a hill with a front side *and* a back side!? Mind-blowing!

Aside from this amazing discovery, we also recognized the fact that our group wasn't getting any smaller. So to keep runners safe, drivers away from vehicular manslaughter charges, and neighbors from complaining, we decided to utilize the full hill (Brookline and Brighton side). This gave us the opportunity to spread out the group, allow runners to enjoy the slightly less intense gradient profile (the back side, though steeper at one point, is much shorter and easier to tackle), and put in longer mileage.

STAIR SPICE

Corey Hill, the site of our Friday workouts, has one large street that goes up and over the hill (Summit Ave) and a bunch of smaller streets that run parallel in an east-west direction. Bisecting the southern side of the hill is a network of pedestrian stairs. We use one of those sets of stairs, named Summit Path, for our Stair Spice.

The path starts by the giant maple tree on Beacon Street and goes all the way to Summit Ave, breaking only a few times to accommodate two side streets that run parallel to Summit. Once we discovered that we could run the full length of the path, we decided to incorporate it as a "spice," or an optional extra credit (that everyone ends up doing anyway). So as the group is coming up the hill, runners have the option to continue to the crossroad at the top and head down the hill for an "Up and Over," or just peel left and down Summit Path for some stair running.

As we got more involved with the trail running (a challenging city activity), we started doing intervals up and down the path. The uneven pace of the stairs, mixed in with some sections of very slight incline across the paved road, mimics trail conditions. I love running Summit Path. It's fun, people are constantly passing each other, and when you get to the top you feel like your lungs are going to burst out of your chest cavity.

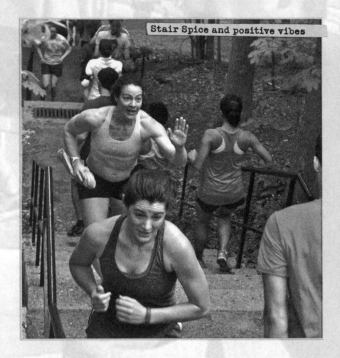
Stair Spice and positive vibes

CROSS COUNTRY SPICE

Cross Country Spice started as an "optional" detour across the grass patch on the north side of the park, just below the stone wall that we use for our morning gathering. Initially, we would place a few cones or backpacks in the corners of the lawn and ask people, as they were coming back down the front side of the hill, to make a little cross-country detour around the cones, enjoy a brief change in scenery, and give us a reason to make them sprint up the grass. But as the group continued to grow, and BG looked for ways to blur the line

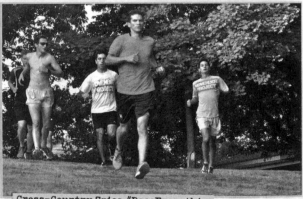
Cross-Country Spice #RaceEverything

between what's fun and what's going to get people severely injured, we started creating obstacle courses using anything from recycling bins, caution tape, miniature flags (hundreds of them to create multiple sprint lanes across the lawn), and, of course, car tires.

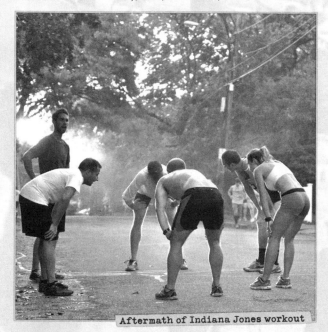
Aftermath of Indiana Jones workout

INDIANA JONES

As I already mentioned, early on we had to race our asses off because the group was so small that you could easily see who was dodging the workout. But we wanted to keep the racing spirit strong as the numbers grew, and one of the ways to do that was to group the runners of similar speeds and have them do Indiana Jones. You may remember a similar torture from middle or high school called Indian Runs.

Indiana Jones forces teams of 5 to 10 people, organized in a straight line, to push each other up the hill. The person in the back of the line sprints to the front, breaking up the long hike up the hill into shorter, higher intensity intervals. Once at the front, that person slows down to a normal running pace. This continues for the entire workout. Because teams are paired up according to speed, every single person is pushing to the limit.

PENALTY BURPEES

You can run up- and downhill only so many ways until you start repeating yourself. So to keep our workouts fresh and creative, we throw in small, quirky elements to break up the monotony, get people to meet new friends, and sometimes even forget about the watch on their wrist that's counting out splits. Hello, burpees, old friend.

Sprinkling in burpees as a penalty for running without a partner during a "No one runs alone" workout was a perfect way to get people to interact with strangers. We would also play various iterations of the game of tag, in which each runner at the top of the hill has to run through the tag area. If touched by a tagger, the runner would have to do five burpees. Some of the smarter runners would calmly run up to the tagger, take their five-burpee penalty, and continue about their workout, while some runners would try whatever they could to escape tagging, as if the tagger was infected with Ebola virus. Most of the time, the chase eventually resulted in tagging, so not only would the tagged runner have to do five burpees, they'd also spend 15 to 20 seconds cutting, juking, and dodging the tagger, getting themselves even more tired than if they were just to do the five burpees. Not a single person involved in this workout ever had a grumpy face. Why? Because we ALL loved playing tag as kids!

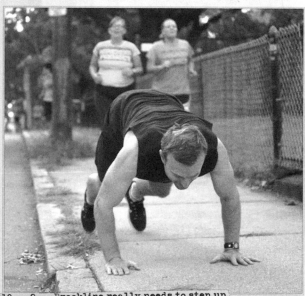
10 ... 9 ... Brookline really needs to step up its weeding game ... 8 ... 7 ...

Ian Nurse
Chiropractor to the B.A.A. Stars

Ian Nurse is a lean, soft-spoken Boston chiropractor. But there's nothing gentle about the good doctor when he straps on his kicks. In 2013, he posted a 2:25.35 at the Boston Marathon, the 44th runner out of 29,000 to hit the finish mats on Boylston Street. Nurse, 37, has been toeing starting lines since his early 20s, claiming the tallest podium step at the Baystate Marathon (Lowell, Massachusetts) in 2003 and the Portland Marathon (Oregon) in 2011. He's lost count of his half-marathon victories—the latest earned at the 2015 Michelob ULTRA Miami Beach 13.1 (1:14.40); his wife, Amanda, came in first for women (1:24.28). November Project has been part of his life since late 2012, with Nurse relishing the Friday hill workout on Summit Ave in particular.

CD: *How did you first cross paths with NP?*

IN: A bunch of my patients had been doing it, so I first heard about the group from them.

Then, randomly, one day, I was running with my wife and some friends in the Newton Hills. I think it was December 2012. Brogan and a few other guys, Joey Kile and Bojan, were on the hill doing their recruiting. You know, they were handing out those little coasters that said November Project and the workout times. They ran up behind and talked to us about NP, and then kept going. When we got to the base of Heartbreak Hill, I could still see them and I was like, "Okay, I want to catch up to these guys." So I went ahead of our group and ended up catching Brogan at the top of the hill. I remember him saying, "We have these great workouts at Summit Ave, and we could get you in really good shape."

Were *you insulted, being a sub-2:30 marathoner?*

Haha, no. I said I'd heard great things. And as a sports chiropractor who deals with a lot of running-related injuries, I thought it'd be a good idea for me to meet the people who were leading this large group. I was already treating a bunch of their runners anyway. I said anytime your people need any type of treatment, or if you want me to talk to your group about preventing injury in the first place, just let me know. Brogan said, "Well, we have a lot of people who offer us that, but they don't ever show up to any of our workouts. If you show up, we can talk about it." So the next Friday I showed up.

Were *you familiar with Summit Avenue?*

I'd been going to Summit for years. It's a really tough hill. But I hadn't done it in a while. It's always a shock to the system no matter the shape you're in. So I was familiar with that type of workout, but I had never seen that many people running the hill at the same time.

What *were your initial impressions of the group?*

I was really hooked. It was a great experience. The whole hugging thing was unique to Boston, so I started going more. Whether they used me as a resource or not, it didn't matter. I just really enjoyed going. The community aspect was totally foreign. It's just not the Boston mentality to hug people, to introduce yourself to strangers, and encourage people. The Northeast is more standoffish. November Project has really changed the demeanor of a lot of people, even myself. Instead of going in for a handshake at NP, I still sometimes have to remind myself to go in for a hug.

And in terms of timing, starting with November Project in late 2012 was really good because I was trying to build my base for Boston 2013. So I incorporated NP's Summit Ave workouts into my first 2 months. And I had a pretty significant PR that year.

You *credit NP with that?*

Definitely. My previous Boston PR was 2:27, so I had an almost a 2-minute drop. To have such a significant improvement in my Boston time was huge.

How would you describe running Summit Avenue to the uninitiated?

It's the biggest hill in Boston. There are a few other big ones, but none as long and steep. Even if you want to take it easy, you are still breathing hard at the top, and it often turns into a shuffle. The first half of the hill is a moderate grade and then you get to this one intersection and it changes a few degrees, and suddenly it's uncomfortable. And coming down, the pounding is tough. It's hard to run slowly even if you want to. It's too steep to keep your balance. You can damage your quads if you're not used to it. I can never convince my [Boston Athletic Association (B.A.A.)] teammates to run Summit Ave. It's just such a demanding hill and the recovery after is pretty intense.

As a longtime marathoner who has logged countless solo miles, what was it like suddenly running with hundreds of people?

Anyone who's ever run Summit Ave by themselves and then gone and run it with November Project [knows that] it's a world of difference. When you're by yourself, you're sucking wind the whole time and it hurts. But there are so many different athletic levels at November Project—you always have someone in front of you to chase down and someone pushing you from behind, and this constant wave of support as you go by, people yelling, "Great job, keep going." Just to have a constant supply of motivation is huge. I've done Summit Ave by myself and am infinitely slower [when I do so].

Any hill workouts that stand out for you?

There was one workout Brogan texted me [about] the night before and said, "I really want you to come tomorrow; we're going to have a crazy hard workout." He said another guy, Owen Kendall [a 2:32 marathoner and a 16:01 5-K runner], would be there. I think Brogan really just wanted to pit the two of us together. I don't think we'd ever run it at the same time, but as two of the better runners, I think BG wanted a little bit of a showdown. The workout was [to do] as many front and back sides as you can in 40 minutes. And in true NP

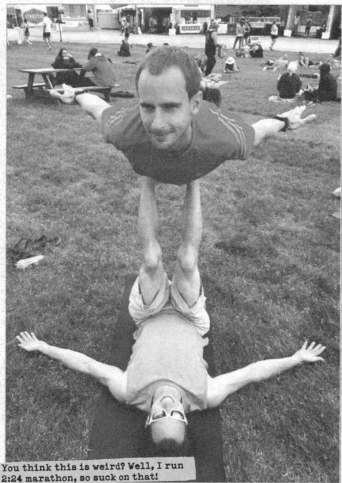

You think this is weird? Well, I run 2:24 marathon, so suck on that!

fashion, Owen and I were competitive but at the same time supportive and pushing each other. He and I were together the entire time except for the last hill, when I pulled away a little, but not by much, and at the end, we gave each other a hug. It was definitely one of the hardest workouts I've ever done. I think we did six hills. It was a lot. My quads were definitely singing the next day. Owen and I have gone on to compete against each other in races, and it's always a friendly encounter.

Describe NP in one word.

The first word that comes to mind is "cult," but I think that has a negative connotation I wouldn't want to associate with NP, so I'll go with "community." Or how about three words? "Positive community cult." Ⓝ

SHARING PUBLIC SPACE: CAN'T WE ALL JUST GET ALONG?

BY BOJAN MANDARIC

Living in a city comes with many perks. One is access to well-maintained lawns, parks, beaches, sculptures, and river paths, all of which can be legally commandeered for any sort of exercise. But sometimes sharing public space presents challenges when a group that relies on verbal motivation and vocal encouragement trains at 6:30 in the morning in a residential neighborhood.

Since most of our workouts were initially held at Harvard Stadium, far from any residential buildings and blissed-out pillow heads, we never even thought about noise. We were built on noise, and we weren't used to getting noise complaints in the early days. How often do you go around thinking about your bones and lungs and nose hairs? Exactly. But when we launched our Friday workout on Summit Avenue in Brookline, and then added the ever-changing rotation of Monday locations, things started to get interesting. Here are a few emails that showed up in the November-project.com inbox.

After a few complaints about running up and down the hill, I and a few NPers who live close to Summit Ave decided to drop off fliers explaining our presence and encouraging residents to join us for a good sweat. It went like this:

NOVEMBER PROJECT

November Project is the workout group that you keep seeing running on Summit Ave every Friday morning. We believe that strong community and motivated members can transform the conventional pay-for-fitness model so we keep our workouts FREE for life. Our tribe of like-minded, forward-thinking people is growing daily, despite the declining temperatures of the late autumn and winter months. As our numbers continue to rise, we realize that our noise levels are following the same pattern. This is creating a disturbance to your Friday morning and we apologize for it.

As a part of the Brookline community we want to continue to use Summit Ave as one of our main workout sites but we don't want to do damage to our relationships with you as a resident of this wonderful street. We will do everything in our power to keep the noise of cheering and coaching to a minimum and would like to ask for your understanding if an occasional, non-intentional slip does happen on future Friday mornings.

Yours truly,
Bojan Mandaric & Brogan Graham
Cofounders of November Project
http://november-project.com

This was one of the first responses:

Summit Ave Resident

To: **November Project**

Name: **Summit Ave Resident**

Email: ▇▇▇▇▇**@earthlink.net**

To the human beings who think it is reasonable to run yelling and screaming through a residential neighborhood at 6:30 AM without any regard for the families who reside there. Guess what? It's really not. Since respect for other people does not come naturally to some folks, there are rules put in place. In the Town of Brookline, we have a Noise Ordinance. You and your 100 plus friends don't get to start screaming on the top of your lungs until 7:01 AM. If you would like to continue to harass my family and my neighbors we can get the police involved for an explanation regarding how rules the work as common courtesy/decency seemingly eludes your group. Why is it that you think that your trendy fitness club entitles you to mistreat middle-class families who are just trying to get some sleep and simply live their lives peacefully? Shame on you for being mind-blowingly insensitive.

Hey Brojan and Brogan

To: **November Project**

Name: **Jerry Casper**

Email: ▇▇▇▇▇**@comcast.net**

Hey Bojan and Brogan,
Thanks for the flyer in my door. I've not complained or even heard you on Friday morns but a bit of advice: if you want to "make nice" by flyer, at least have the balls to leave a contact phone # or email instead of making me look it up, neighbor. Also I assure you that if you wake anybody up, the cops will be called by my neighbors who are more interested in sleep than socializing with a free group when they paid big money to live here.
Thank you for your cooperation and understanding.

And this one. We didn't know that people (and not just robots) actually lived in Kendall Square near MIT, but this is proof that they do. Also, we didn't use a megaphone that morning.

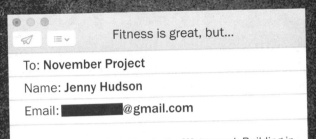

Fitness is great, but...

To: **November Project**

Name: **Jenny Hudson**

Email: ████████@gmail.com

Fitness is great, but I live in the Watermark Building in Kendall, just above where your booming megaphone and yelling participants woke me this morning at 6 a.m. Please keep it down if this is a regular thing or you may have the police there for disturbing the peace. I'm sure you wouldn't want to wake up to a megaphone outside YOUR window. Thank you.

We really did try to take a proactive approach but after a few more angry emails from Summit Ave residents, followed by a police citation for violating the noise ordinance, we knew we had to make some adjustments. So we decided to practice our "safety ninja skills." Tribes around the country (I see you, San Francisco) have since had to sharpen their own Spidey skills and draw up blueprints for good/better relations. Below is what Boston laid down.

Step One: Make sure no member who drives to the Friday workout parks on the street that we're running. Adding large obstacles to an already narrow road increases the difficulty for morning commuters and runners to share the road. So we created the "Chris Marshall Rule," named after a core NP dude who's been running Summit Ave with us since day one. (See Glossary, page 216.)

Step Two: Make sure we remain quiet until the noise ordinance is no longer in effect (7:01 a.m.). That means the Bounce, "Good Morning Cheer," and any sort of coaching and encouraging has to be done in a murder whisper. What's a murder whisper? See the movie *Scream*, or call up your favorite niece or nephew and

shout as soft as you can with some creepy-menace that you're "gonna get them." Or just come to the workout next Friday.

Step Three: Make sure that we're good neighbors and respectful members of the community: always stopping for cars pulling out of driveways; running on the sidewalk instead of the road; sharing the sidewalk with dog walkers and pedestrians; getting to know neighbors and involving them in the workouts and social events.

Fourth and the Final Step: Kill everyone with kindness. Engaging in confrontation never results in a peaceful resolution, so hearing out all the complaints, apologizing for any sort of inconvenience (even if it wasn't caused by our group), and suggesting next steps for a solution creates an environment of trust, respect, and willingness to collaborate.

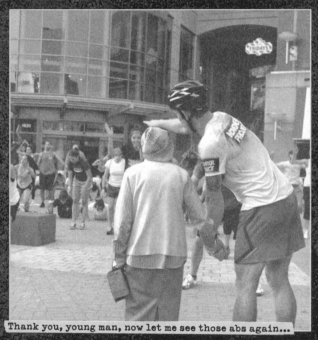

Thank you, young man, now let me see those abs again...

For the most part, our strategy has worked. Despite our significant growth and high-octane vibe, we've established a good relationship with the Brookline Police Department and made some great friends among the neighbors, a few of whom even invite us over for a dip in their pool after our summer workouts. And when I say "us," picture a hundred-plus sweaty bodies splashing, armpit-farting, and displacing so much water that it looks like a kettle of humans being boiled for lunch.

Oh, Brother!

Brookline is a well-heeled town that borders Boston on three sides. It has a population of almost 60,000, and a rich history, including being the birthplace of John F. Kennedy. Other Brookline natives include Conan O'Brien, John Hodgman, and Michael Bloomberg. In recent decades, Brookline has seen an influx of college students, professors, and young professionals. With its stately homes, low crime rate, fine public schools, and ample green space, the community has long been a magnet for celebrities and luminaries, from Saul Bellow, Larry Bird, and Mike Wallace to Jon Krakauer, New England Patriots owner Robert Kraft, and QB Tom Brady and his supermodel wife Gisele Bundchen.

Thanks to generous municipal resources, an ample roster of police officers, and a proactive community relations strategy, crime in Brookline is under control—nothing like neighboring Boston—though city ele-

ments sometimes leak across the borders. Brookline Police Department patrol officer Noah Brother has been patrolling the town, and its dozen or so distinct neighborhoods, for 8 years. For the past 2, he's been assigned to Sector Three, which includes the Corey Hill Park neighborhood. Complaints from the upper-middle-class hilltop enclave tend toward the mild: an overnight vehicle break-in, a car accident, occasional partying in the park, and a group of wild turkeys attacking residents. But for a couple months in late 2012, it became all about a group of wild runners who were attacking the hill. —CD

Officer Noah Brother: In His Own Words

There were a series of complaints from residents on Summit Ave. At first, it didn't seem that big a deal. The November Project was just getting started over there, you know, chanting cadences while people were running. Maybe 30 people at the time. It was more an annoyance. We'd go up there, make our presence known. But within a few weeks, it grew to like a hundred people or more, and progressed to runners running in the streets, that sort of thing.

On our shift, people tend to wake up 6:30 to 7:00, and that's when calls for service start coming in and things start getting busy for us. To deal with people who are just running up Summit Ave, irritating the neighbors, just as you're trying to finish up your paperwork from the previous shift, and getting flooded with all these other calls, it's frustrating.

As the calls kept coming and the group kept growing, I tried to identify the leaders. From what

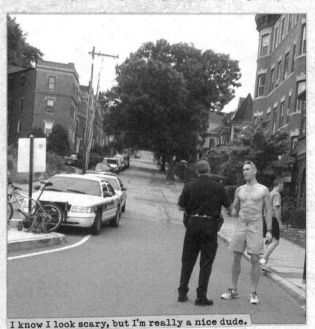
I know I look scary, but I'm really a nice dude.

I understood, it wasn't a business. No one was making money off it. It was just a group of people loosely organized who had decided to get together and run the hills. I identified Brogan Graham as the guru there. I think someone pointed him out to me.

Initially I told him, "Listen we're getting complaints. I appreciate what you're doing, seems like cool idea. But you have to look at it from our perspective. It's a residential neighborhood. You have to make an effort to fit rather than creating conflict with them." He responded favorably. I didn't feel like he was brushing me off. I think he had a desire to fit in with the neighbors. He told me he'd work on it.

The next week or two weeks after, I got called back again. Same time, same place. Now, it's 150 people, and the streets are flooded. There were more runners than I'd ever seen. I'm thinking this is now legitimately an issue. Cars can't traverse the street easily. Even when I'm coming up in my police car, just trying to pull onto Summit Ave was tough.

I went up there, couldn't find Brogan among all the runners. I just parked at the top of Summit Ave and thought, *How am I going to deal with the situation?* I'm not going to write 150 jaywalking tickets for a dollar. It would take me all day. But we do have a nuisance bylaw, which is generally utilized for loud parties, but it doesn't have to be that specific. It's two or more people causing a nuisance inside or on the street, and are loud enough to be heard by neighbors in their own home. It starts with a hundred-dollar fine, then goes to three hundred, and then we take court action after that.

So I sat in my cruiser and I called him on his cell phone—I had his number—and I said, "You need to meet me over here." The ticket was already written and I said, "Here you go." It wasn't meant to be punitive, but more of a wake-up call. "I talked to you last week and you said you'd take care of it and I'm still getting calls, so you didn't take care of it." And Brogan's response was, "Well, I'll just get everyone to donate a dollar and we'll take care of this." I think I said, "That's not the point. It's supposed to be a wake-up call. My intention isn't to penalize you, just to give you a kick in the butt."

Complaints from the upper-middle-class hilltop enclave tend toward the mild: an overnight vehicle break-in, a car accident, occasional partying in the park, and a group of wild turkeys attacking residents. But for a couple months in late 2012, it became all about a group of wild runners who were attacking the hill.

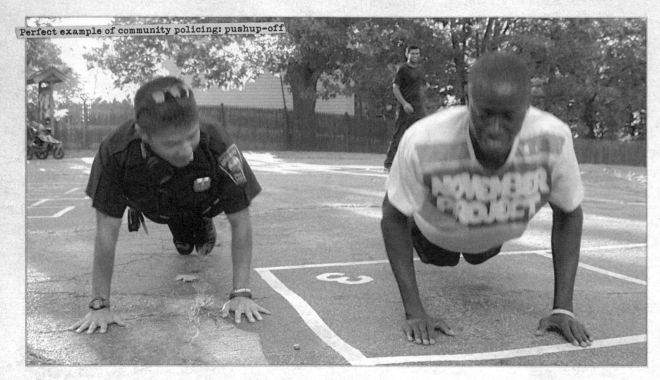

Perfect example of community policing: pushup-off

The next week, I came by and everyone's running on the sidewalk and they started having crossing guards at the intersections so cars could get in and out. From time to time, we'll get a call. You're not going to completely eliminate it, not going to make 100 percent of the people happy 100 percent of the time. For the most part, the complaints are few and far between. I think they did a good job on their own nipping it in the bud.

Shortly after I started interacting with Brogan, and not long after I gave him the citation, I got a call from my cousin, who said, "I just saw you on Facebook. I run with the November Project at Harvard Stadium and they were talking about Officer Brother in Brookline on their blog." I'm like, "Oh my god." But it was a short blurb thanking me. I thought it was cool. I thought back to when I was in the police academy and we were all out running and singing, and I'm sure the neighbors didn't always appreciate that early in the morning. But there's a balance.

Last winter, I came up one day, and we'd had a big snowstorm, a couple feet. I took a swing up there and I see a bunch of November Project people out and they're all up there, shoveling out people's driveways. I'm like, what the heck is going on here? I couldn't believe what I was seeing. Especially since I'm paying a guy a hundred dollars to plow *my* driveway. I hooked up with Brogan and he said they'd been wanting to do something like that for a long time, to give back to the neighborhood. "Things lined up at the right time, so we came out here and shoveled all the driveways." I'm like, "That's amazing. You know how happy I'd be if I woke up and someone shoveled my driveway for me?" It was a nice gesture.

"Someone had taken pics of the shoveling workout and I emailed them to our community relations division and I said, "Hey, Lieutenant, you might be interested in this, a textbook example of a successful community policing project. Initially, it was adversarial and now they're shoveling people's driveways." They reposted it on Twitter and they got a record number of same-day retweets in department history." NP

#ShovelShuffle

BY BOJAN MANDARIC

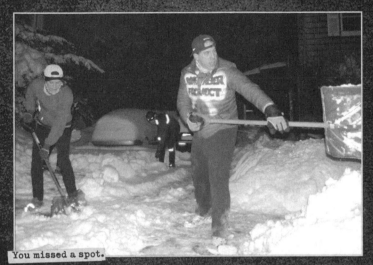
You missed a spot.

Ah, the New England winter. It seems like every year we are genuinely surprised by it. "Oh no, it's January and we're having eight inches of snow! Let's declare the state of emergency, cancel school, and shut down public transportation! We're not ready for it!" Oh, the humanity!!!

Turn on the TV and the situation becomes even more intense: 54 minutes of weather coverage, 2 minutes of Patriots coverage, 2 minutes of weather coverage at Gillette Stadium, and 2 minutes of actual news. Even the commercials get bumped into one of the two screens within the screen while the other one is playing Doppler storm tracker. The bottom line reads "Breaking News" followed by all the school closings on the loop while the weather guy is throwing a pot of boiling water into the wind to illustrate how cold zero degrees is. It's pretty safe to say that if a story during New England winter doesn't involve snow or the wind chill, it's not newsworthy. And that's how we became the news.

Thursday, throughout the day—this was January 2014—BG and I were shooting texts back and forth, trying to figure out what to do for the Friday morning workout. Johnny the Weatherman was preparing us for

another Snowmageddon of epic proportions, calling for a foot of overnight snowfall. Unlike skiers and snowboarders, runners don't get very giddy about the fresh powder. Especially runners in Boston. Being one of the oldest cities in United States, Boston was designed for horse and carriage traffic. A lot of the one- or two-way streets have very narrow sidewalks and don't have the capacity to host plows, cars, pedestrians, runners, and snow banks all on the same stretch of the road. So, usually the smallest ones on that food chain (pedestrians and runners) end up having to use their Spidey sense to avoid getting swept up under the plow, slipping on the ice, or getting run over by a lady in an Audi who thinks that just because her car is all-wheel drive, she should ignore the fact that the road surface is completely slick.

I saw a golden opportunity to make nice with our Summit Ave neighbors: clear some sidewalks and driveways as part of the morning workout. BG was not into the idea.

"We were up Friday morning listening to the sounds of cheering from the group making their last efforts running up Corey Park through the deep snow. My kids and I were watching from the windows and thinking, 'What a crazy group of individuals.' Then I walked outside and saw that the entire driveway was shoveled! What a fantastic Friday morning gift as I was trying to get to work! Keep up the great workouts!"

—Chris, Summit Avenue resident (comment from NP blog)

"Not everyone will bring a shovel. We'll end up wasting people's time. Plus, Brookline issued a state of emergency. No parking anywhere!"

"Dude, do you remember the time we asked people to dress up in capes and feathers?" I asked, reminding him of the costumed workout that we'd held just before Halloween. "All it took was a tweet, and people came! In some epic costumes!" I told him that the worst thing that could happen is that it would be just him, me, and Derrick (one of our core members who lives at the bottom of the hill and rarely misses the workout). "We'll have three shovels, we'll tell some jokes, and we'll go home."

No one loves standing in the circle telling jokes more than BG, so I knew that the idea of three idiots dressed up in puffy jackets, standing on top of the snowed-out hill, and telling jokes with shovels in their hands at 6:30 a.m. would be appealing to him.

"We may even score some points with Summit Ave neighbors," I said. "They'll poop their pants when they wake up and see shoveled-out sidewalks, AND the hill will be clear for running."

So the tweet went out: "Tomorrow 6:30AM at Summit Ave. Bring shovels if you can. Please RT!"

I arrived around 6:15 a.m. with two shovels. There were already four people standing in snow a foot deep, each holding shovels of their own.

"*Yes! I fucking love Twitter!*" I thought, just before

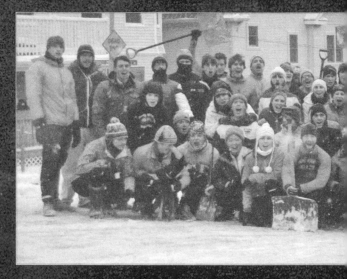

BG's voice interrupted my internal self-high-five.

We took a moment for "The Company Meeting"—a last-minute detail polishing session that we perform a few steps away from the gathering crowd, minutes before every workout.

"All right, what are we doing?" BG said, still a bit doubtful about what was about to go down.

"Not everyone will bring shovels," I said. "So we'll split the group in half—the ones with shovels and the ones without, and we'll team them up. The ones with shovels will pick the section of the sidewalk and start shoveling, while the ones without them will run down and up the front side of the hill. Then they'll switch. Forty minutes total."

And so we went. About 70 members, many unrecognizable under balaclavas and ski goggles, turned what was supposed to be a 40-minute workout into an hour-long run-shovel-run event. When the sidewalks were cleared, driveways were next. Jacket sleeves turned into snowbrushes, and eventually every house on both sides of the street had a clear driveway, sidewalk, and a brushed-off car. Our sentiment after the workout was, this was pretty fun, but I wouldn't put it in the pantheon of amazing adventures. We set out to accomplish two goals: have a good workout, and clear the hill from snow so we can run it again. What we got was amazing local and national media coverage, not to mention tons of brownie points with the neighbors.

Like I said, "I fucking love Twitter!"

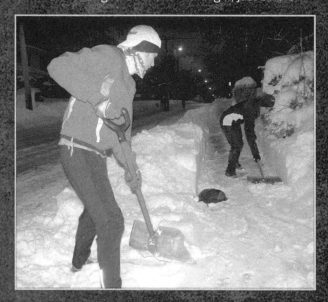

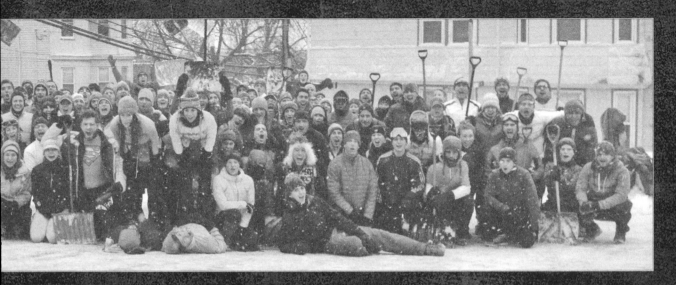

"IN BROOKLINE, YOU GET FINED FOR NOT SHOVELING YOUR SIDEWALK AND FROM WHAT I COULD SEE FROM THE WINDOW, THERE HAD BEEN A SIGNIFICANT AMOUNT OF SNOW, MAYBE 12 INCHES. SO I STARTED PUTTING ON CLOTHES TO GO OUT AND GET BUSY. I LOOKED OUT THE WINDOW AND SAW THE SIDEWALK HAD BEEN SHOVELED. IT WAS A MOMENT OF COGNITIVE DISSONANCE. HOW DID MY SIDEWALK GET SHOVELED? I'VE BEEN SLEEPING. I TURNED MY HEAD ONE WAY AND THEN THE OTHER. THE SIDEWALK HAD BEEN SHOVELED AS FAR AS I COULD SEE. AND JUST AS I WAS PONDERING THIS, A COUPLE OF WOMEN SHOWED UP AND SHOVELED OUT MY NEIGHBOR'S CAR. I DON'T KNOW IF THEY KNEW SHE WAS A WIDOW WITH A RECENT HIP REPLACEMENT, BUT THEY MADE QUICK WORK OF IT. THEN I REALIZED, THESE ARE THE FRIDAY PEOPLE. NOT ONLY DID THEY DO ALL THE WALKWAYS, BUT THEY STILL MANAGED TO DO THEIR WORKOUT, TOO. WE TALKED ABOUT IT AFTER AMONG THE NEIGHBORS. EVERYONE WAS JUST DELIGHTED."

—MARK LECCESE, EMERSON JOURNALISM PROFESSOR AND SUMMIT AVENUE RESIDENT

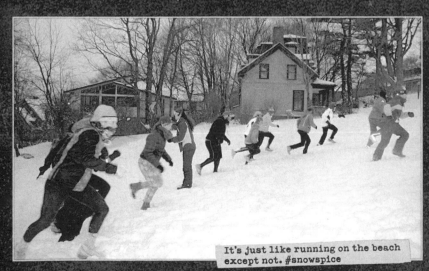

It's just like running on the beach except not. #snowspice

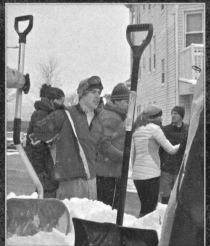

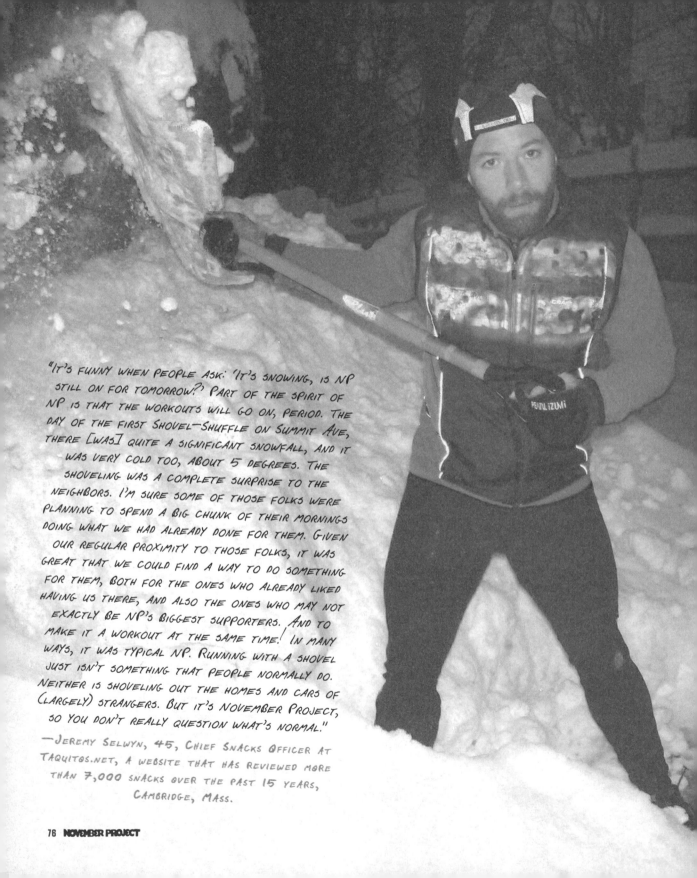

"It's funny when people ask: 'It's snowing, is NP still on for tomorrow?' Part of the spirit of NP is that the workouts will go on, period. The day of the first Shovel-Shuffle on Summit Ave, there [was] quite a significant snowfall, and it was very cold too, about 5 degrees. The shoveling was a complete surprise to the neighbors. I'm sure some of those folks were planning to spend a big chunk of their mornings doing what we had already done for them. Given our regular proximity to those folks, it was great that we could find a way to do something for them, both for the ones who already liked having us there, and also the ones who may not exactly be NP's biggest supporters. And to make it a workout at the same time! In many ways, it was typical NP. Running with a shovel just isn't something that people normally do. Neither is shoveling out the homes and cars of (largely) strangers. But it's November Project, so you don't really question what's normal."

—Jeremy Selwyn, 45, Chief Snacks Officer at Taquitos.net, a website that has reviewed more than 7,000 snacks over the past 15 years, Cambridge, Mass.

BE THE CHANGE – Do Your Homework

🕐 3rd June 2013   👤 brogan   📁 Blog   💬 3 Comments

In 2002, as Bojan and I were only a few months into our first decade here in Boston, we both had the exact same feeling as we worked to get to know Boston: The city isn't very friendly. I remember calls back home to my brother DG in Madison where I'd say just that, "Boston isn't very kind." Both Bojan and I were on scholarships for making boats move for the Northeastern University Huskies so we had no choice to go anywhere else. Looking back, this was a very good thing as we had to work harder to make new friends. Over the years this city has opened up as we continued to interact with people we didn't know, high-five unsuspecting runners during our river loops, and crack mid-level jokes at bars, bike racks, and even urinals/bathroom stalls hoping to get a laugh or even a smirk out of those serious faces.

Fast forward to 2013 and we have come to a place where November Project, the hugging, racing, and community building tribe, is ON FIRE. The good vibes that kept us warm during Boston Nor'easters, Madison winters, and San Francisco cold rains, are undeniable. The friendly faces and interactions that have taken place around our many workouts, events, and races are unparalleled. But then last Friday, for a brief moment, I lost my faith in what I/we are doing when my most valuable personal belonging was stolen as I was moving into my new apartment. And man, was I pissed . . . at the person that did it . . . the whole city of Boston . . . the world. But then I decided that instead of focusing on negatives I will make a positive change. Guide this act of evil into an act of kindness. And this is where your homework comes in to play . . .

Required Homework:
(not for an extra credit, this is for your final grade)

In the next 7 days, yes 7 days, you need to complete at least one random act of kindness. But not just any random act of kindness, it must be an **UNSUSPECTING RANDOM ACT OF KINDNESS**. Holding doors, giving up your seat for the elderly, and picking up trash on the street does not count as completed homework. You should do those things all the time! An example of an **UNSUSPECTING RANDOM ACT OF KINDNESS** could be paying the toll for the vehicle behind you, picking up a round of coffee for people you always see in the morning on the way to work, or giving your jacket to a runner that looks cold during early morning hours. But please do not tweet, post, or brag about anything you do for this homework assignment. Bragging about doing nice things defeats the purpose of that very same act. If you would like to post on our wall or send us a tweet with a simple "Homework Complete" note, that's cool, but only two people will know the exact details of what you did and that's **YOU** and the person that you surprised. Now go make your city and the world a better place!

BZZZZT...CLK...
FUCK YEAH!

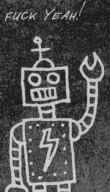

* NO HUMANS, ROBOTS, OR SLEEPWALKERS WERE HARMED IN THE CRAFTING OF THIS SECTION OF THE BOOK.

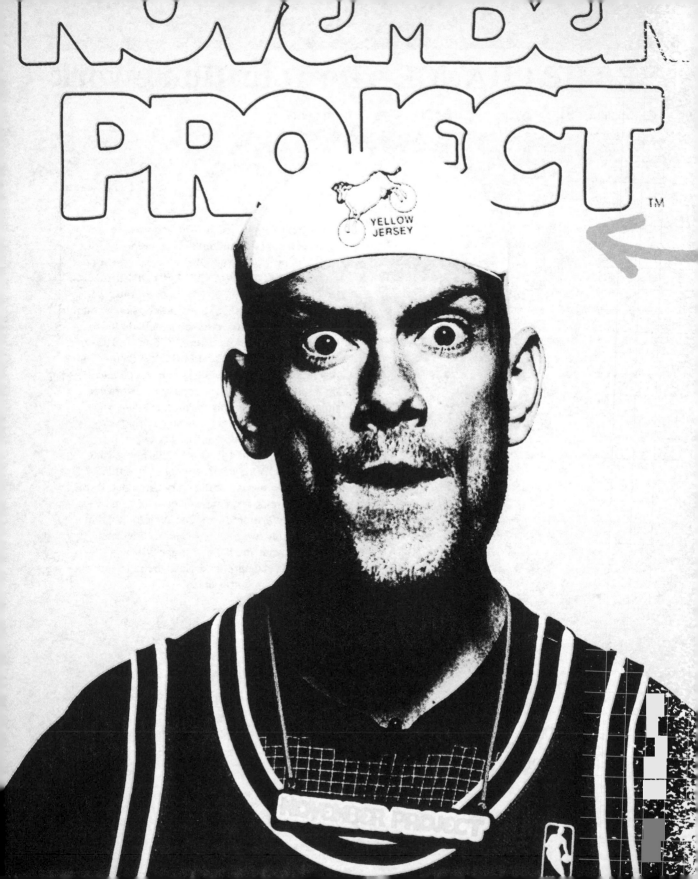

CHAPTER 4

GROWING UP GRAHAM

BY BROGAN GRAHAM

WISCONSIN NOTES:

- BLACK BEARS, BITCHES!
- A FAMILY TOGETHER, A FAMILY APART, RULES IN TATTERS
- SIZE 11 MEN'S SHOES IN THE FOURTH GRADE
- THE TALLEST—AND—WHITEST LITTLE DUDE ON THE TEAM
- MAN OF STEEL
- GRADUATION SPEAKER; WHAT?!
- ROWING TO BOSTON
- A LIFE-CHANGING MOMENT THAT LEFT BLOOD ON THE SIDEWALK AND MY MUG IN THE PAPER

"LET ME JUST STATE FOR THE RECORD, I'VE ALWAYS BEEN THE KIND OF GUY WHO FEELS PERFECTLY COMFORTABLE OWNING A MAN CRUSH. I THINK IT'S A HEALTHY THING TO ACKNOWLEDGE. I MEAN, I'M A VERY HAPPILY MARRIED FATHER OF THREE LOVELY LITTLE GIRLS, BUT COME ON! IF YOU'RE A DUDE, AND YOU KNOW BROGAN, YOU KNOW EXACTLY WHAT I'M TALKING ABOUT.

"SO, IN WALKS THIS GUY, MADE OF PURE THUNDER AND CHARISMA (ROLL THE R, FOR FULL EFFECT). HE'S TEN FEET TALL IF HE'S AN INCH, HIS LIMBS ARE COVERED IN SEVERAL SQUARE YARDS OF GNARLY TATS, HE'S GOT THE WHOLE CHISELED JAW THING GOING ON, AND AN 18-PACK THAT'S FULLY APPARENT EVEN UNDER A DOWN JACKET. SO WHEN I REACH OUT FOR A HANDSHAKE AND HE LEANS IN (AND WAY, WAY DOWN) FOR A BEAR HUG INSTEAD, WELL, IT'S PRETTY MUCH ALL OVER. I'VE GOT A FULL-ON RAGING BRONER."

—MICHAEL HOWARD, 44,
ADVERTISING CREATIVE DIRECTOR,
LEXINGTON, MASS.

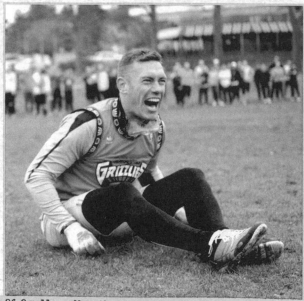

26.2 rolls on Marathon Monday 2015 and we're feeling pretty good.

Here's the deal: I've been this way my whole life. All over the map, slightly ADD, loud, the total class clown. Find the rules and bend them. Find the fun and go that way. I don't know if it was the early years of trying to impress my older brother, Dan, or if I was just the younger one with fewer rules hanging around my neck. Either way, I've always sought out the unmarked routes. That's just how my DNA helix coils (how did that sound? A+ student, right?). That little tire adventure with my dude John Vining? That was just another in a series of stunts I've been pulling since grade school. I'm not trying to tell you that my life is WILD and TURBO, but with NP and our days of creating, hosting, hyping, recruiting, and building, it truly makes tossing Goodyears and conjuring T. rex pool-party awards and whatever other nonsense went down that Friday morning, sadly, old news by the next workout.

OCTOBER 2012—

THE HEAD OF THE CHARLES REGATTA

Olympic medalists Esther Lofgren, Dan Walsh, and Will Miller return to Boston for the unofficial rowing reunion and, through word of mouth, show up at NP workouts. Their presence further cements the movement as something new—not just a run club, not a boot camp, but an all-around training community for the urban athlete.

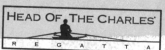

WEDNESDAY, OCTOBER 31, 2012

"Capes & Feathers," NP's Halloween theme, puts the group on the front page of the *Boston Globe*. Stone Hearth may or may not have been under the stadium cooking XXL breakfast pizzas...but come to think of it... there was no permit...so this couldn't have happened.

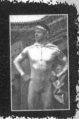

When it comes to putting the fun into fitness, we've harnessed kayaks, Priuses, even the Staten Island Ferry. And by the time this book hits shelves? We might all be serving time, who knows.

But that was the rhythm of my life as a teenage lifeguard at the Shorewood Hills Pool, as a high school idiot, as a party animal, as the captain of whatever teams, a rower for the Northeastern Huskies, on stage in Shakespeare plays in college, as a pedicab driver in Boston, as the man-with-the-mic for Boldfacers (a website featuring Boston events and dispatching a guerrilla interview squad to get the skinny on the street), as a marketing stuntman for Hubway (Boston's bike-share system), and on and on. I've worn tons of hats, but they all share the same theme: fun, intense, usually funny, and constantly moving on to the next chapter while I'm still writing the first. And this November Project ride? It's a speedy, thousand-hearted beast that doesn't have a rear-view mirror and the brakes fell off miles ago. Or something like that. Troublemaking or my outlook on life—they're one and the same. Be fun. Be a dreamer and a creator and make sure that whatever you do, you make a scene. Oh, and don't worry about shit you can't control. OR, worry only about the things you *can* control.

BLACK BEARS AND MAKING THE RULES

My story starts in Madison, Wisconsin, where I was practically born and undeniably raised. That's where I first started testing boundaries like it was a character trait and not a behavioral choice. As kids, my older brother, Dan, or DG, and I were allowed to have either two friends stay over or a night out at the movies or dinner at Pizza Hut for our birthdays, which were (and still are) 11 days apart. First, I'd see how it looked to follow the rules on November 5th because my brother always nailed the guidelines. Then I'd go to work. Turn two pals into seven, get a larger deal out of the "deal," and go bigger in a situation where it seemed to be pretty well defined. What if the options were all combined? Sleep over and Pizza Hut? This kind of scheming drove DG crazy, but the grooves in my brain just twisted that way.

Outside of the house, it was: how late to class is considered late (because that's when I'll show up)? What is the actual speed limit (not just what's on the signs)? Which trails are "closed" because there isn't enough snow and how can I get on them? How much does barbed wire actually cut your skin in a chase? How can we get the beers, the IDs, the keys to drive the cars before we're legally *allowed,* rally the good, bad, ugly, and weird, steal a 7-foot-tall gumball machine, and aim to do it all again the next weekend? How can we, the collective WE, have a better time? Even if that means that someone's parents come home early, a few of us get grounded, drinking tickets get issued, and we end up having to clean the yard of toilet paper, scrub dried eggs off a windshield, run from the police, and a car or two gets dinged in the process?

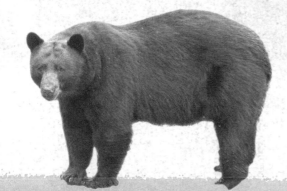

THURSDAY, NOVEMBER 1, 2012
"THE RUNNING OF THE BOWLS"
NP 1ST B-DAY PARTY
The idea: Running-of-the-bulls-in-Pamplona theme. Each participant dressed in all white, with red kerchief, runs with a plastic red bowl to a surprise location (a pub) where the bowls are filled with beer. BG and Bojan shoot each other the first of many looks that says: "Holy fuck, we pulled it off, can you believe this shit?"

LATER THAT NIGHT . . .

A lawyer friend, and solid core member of NP, Alison Hall passes off paperwork to BG & Bojan making this duo, this name, this tribe, and this soon-to-be movement, an official company. November Project LLC is born. What these two would do with it, nobody (including them) would know.

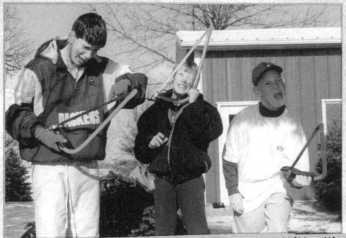
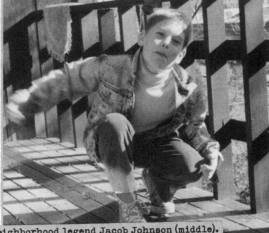

DG (left) and BG (right) cut down their Xmas tree in the mid '90s with neighborhood legend Jacob Johnson (middle). At right, BG works the camera early. #AcidWashDenim"

Of course, this way of operating wasn't without risk. In my years growing up, from K–8 through my hellion high school years to my transformational phase during my time at Northeastern University, I was thrown out of every . . . single . . . school I'd ever attended. I know, sorry, Mom. Pranks, schemes, clowning moments, fights, parties hosted and attended, you name it. I was always at the drawing board of a restless mind. What's been done? What's new? What isn't here that should be?

While working on this project: writing, rewriting, answering questions, and culling through photo archives, I realized that everything in my life up to this very keystroke goes back to the fourth grade and a report I wrote on black fucking bears. Community, creativity, late nights, fake IDs, who I see myself as, how I see others, the value of fun over most all else, run-ins with the law, leaving Madison to seek adventure in Boston, literally following my brother to the ends of the earth, and every other piece of spice worth reading on normal book pages, all starts with an overhead projector, a series of transparencies, and an oral presentation I'd been working on for weeks.

So let's jump back to 1993 and Shorewood Hills Elementary School in the West Side neighborhood of Madison, Wisconsin. This wasn't your typical camo-sweatshirt Middle American public school. A lot of my classmates were children living in University of Wisconsin international student housing. Their parents had come to learn the ways of agriculture in the Midwest. (UW has one of the best schools for this. It's located in the center of "dairyland" and the breadbasket of the country; the soil is amazing, the production large-scale, the farms robust. My father, Nelson, who works in the industry, can tell you all about it.) So, the seats in my classroom were warmed by butts from wildly far-flung places that made our minds race and our imaginations sprint. None of that, "Yeah, we have one kid from Mexico" and "We bus in the token black kids" nonsense. Asia, Africa, Austra-

NOVEMBER 2012

Puma #justshowsup campaign. The November Project Winter Kit is introduced. Show up each week and get a free piece of warm running gear, courtesy of Puma. Those still standing at the end of the month would earn a pair of gloves, hat, long-sleeve shirt, and a jacket. Colors selected by NP were light/white/gray so that "they'd take paint best."

NOVEMBER 2012

First Yearbook photos are taken, with the goal being to connect more people within the tribe. This becomes tradition and themed.

DECEMBER–JANUARY 2013

New Balance partners with NP to tell "The Story Behind the Movement" through its Runnovation video and print campaign. This 6-month "rights to your name" and authentic storytelling helps NP exposure, but makes BG and Bojan most nervous.

lia, South and Central America, you name it, they were all represented. Shit, man, our ESL program was about as full as our main classrooms were. The world was all one big, connected place, and my classrooms were proof. In the same week, I'd work on basic math, super-fun art projects, play the didgeridoo, and create Indonesian shadow puppets. Cultures, countries, nations' flags, customs, skin colors, eye shapes, accents, languages, and holidays were all fascinating to me, and it was presented to all of us at an age when we weren't yet scared not to know what we didn't know. I will die knowing that my years in elementary school shaped my vision of humans and the size of this planet.

I stood out among all this global diversity, not because I was a white American, but because I was already almost 6 feet tall and wearing men's size-11 shoes in fourth grade. (If you're wondering, I weighed 11 pounds 5 ounces when I hit the delivery room table in rural Indiana's Tippecanoe County back in 1982.)

Despite the confidence that came with looming over adults as a 10-year-old, I was fucking nervous when I stepped to the front of that classroom to deliver my presentation on black bears. Shitting bullets. The class next door was coming over, plus the parents of all the kids presenting were there, too. I'd been prepping for what seemed like

months, readying transparencies and hand-drawn illustrations, memorizing regions, the works. Black bears had been the most talked-about topic in my house for weeks. I dreamt in black bears. They were the shit, right? Who doesn't love a good info session on black bears? Anyway, I was excited to drop some serious ursine (Boom! Didn't see that word coming, did ya?) knowledge on these foreign chaps. But what I hadn't been prepared for AT ALL was "the talk" the night before. My parents sat me and DG down and told us they were getting a divorce. Just like that. This was an immediate and seismic shift in my 10-year-old psyche. It marked my introduction to the notion, and eventually the power, of disruption, and what, for me, would become a second language: rule-breaking.

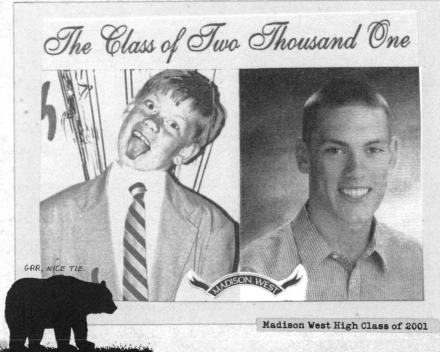

The Class of Two Thousand One

GRR, NICE TIE.

Madison West High Class of 2001

FEBRUARY 2013
Core member Lindsay Smith proposes to his girlfriend Renata at a Harvard Stadium workout. Yeah, there're gonna be babies!

MARCH 2013
BG's older brother Dan Graham (a.k.a. DG), a 6-foot-5 swim instructor, starts a November Project tribe in their hometown of Madison, Wisconsin.

FRIDAY, APRIL 12, 2013
Editors from *Runner's World* are cajoled/recruited/really cajoled at the Boston Marathon expo by BG and Bojan and show up to the hills to check out the group. Editor-in-chief David Willey is smitten.

As I stepped onto the makeshift stage, the daylight peeking through the edges of the closed curtains, the shitty news was still vibrating in my bones like the tuning fork in our piano bench at home, or more like a fucking out-of-tuning fork (I never learned much about it). Getting louder and louder. I was confused, shattered, in denial. And there my parents stood, both of them, Ann and Nelson, in the dark classroom against opposite corners of the room like boxers between rounds.

They'd met at their high school in Cleveland, fallen in love at Ohio State University, and got married soon after turning their tassels. Now that perfect story was ruined like a burn hole melting a movie frame. I remember thinking about everything in the world other than black bears as I walked to the overhead projector with my basic illustrations and keywords in my stack of transparencies. That day, that moment, for the first time, I thought clearly about authority outside of bedtimes and good manners. What are the rules, and who makes them? If my parents are getting a divorce as simple as that, a topic far more important than black bears, polar bears, the rain forest, and everything else we'd "need to learn about this year" in school, then what the fuck was all of this, or anything, really about? Was school just

something for us children to gnaw on while we grew old enough to grow beards, drive cars, tuck our shirts in, and pay bills? These were the actual thoughts running through my man-sized, fourth-grade dome. If people, normal people, can just make the rules and dump one another along the way, breaking family rules that seemed (up until the night before) to be carved into stone, how would it look if I simply gave less of a shit about school? Fuck it, let's all break the rules. No, I didn't do anything crazy. Not then. I just stepped up and delivered a weak version of my turbo-researched report about black bears, with a few tears held back.

The classroom, packed with dimly lit faces from 15 or more countries, clapped loudly as the lights came up and we switched presenters. My mom and dad were both smiling from their corners. It was a half-assed performance and I'd been applauded like I'd saved someone from a burning building. I could almost hear my teacher's pencil strokes from across the room giving me a B+, C-, A+ (or who cares, it didn't matter). To me, she was just another confused, rule-making, rule-breaking adult now.

I was seeing the world for the very first time, the bullshit burned off. It was a moment of clarity, like alco-

"HE WAS DRIVEN. HE WAS ONE OF THOSE KIDS WHO YOU'D TELL HIM YOU CAN'T OR SHOULDN'T DO SOMETHING, HE WAS GONNA DO IT. NO MATTER WHAT. IF IT WAS ATHLETIC, YOU COULD HAVE TOLD HIM HE COULDN'T RUN A MARATHON AS A 13-YEAR-OLD, HE WOULD HAVE DONE IT."
—DAN GRAHAM

MONDAY, APRIL 15, 2013
Bombs explode on Boylston Street, forever changing the city and the historic footrace known as the Boston Marathon. The sun sets on Monday with tears on a sea of faces, blood stains on the sidewalk, and mass confusion throughout the city and the running scene.

TUESDAY, APRIL 16, 2013
Dead air and sadness, anger, denial, and fear line the insides of Boston-area communities looking for answers. Ongoing fear is palpable with the perpetrators on the loose.

WEDNESDAY, APRIL 17, 2013
After some discussion, the workout at Harvard Stadium goes forward as planned. Expecting less than a hundred people, almost 500 gather to move as a community. Hugs, tears, sincere looks, and a simple workout are shared as a warm sun comes up.

holics talk about. I mean, think about it: If the reward on the other side is good enough, rules SHOULD BE bent. Even broken, right? Well, that is how I began to roll after my D-/A+ presentation on black bears came to a close and I couldn't have cared less about anything. Sounds angry, huh? Maybe even a little self-destructive? Nah, just maladjusted, distracted, and pretty bummed out. Motherfucking black bears, they were the creatures that clawed open industrial dumpsters in restaurant parking lots, and now my eyes! For better or worse, black bears.

ESCAPE HATCH

At the same time that the black bear became my power animal (I made that up just now), another factor that would define my life began showing up. I was tall enough at that point in my life that you couldn't help but wonder about my skills on a basketball court. I was a physical kid, and I started seeing that I could escape my new home life a little through sport.

In fourth grade, my mom took DG and me to our first experience with the Madison Spartans. Aside from my classroom, this was the cultural experience that expanded my world more than anything else. We were the first white family to (seemingly ever) walk into that Neighborhood Intervention Program gym. We were tall as hell, so the coaches were excited to see us. We were also white as hell, so the other boys were confused to see us. But there we were. The Graham boys. Dan and Brogan. The odd minority. The only kids from the safe West Side of town, where parents actually knew for sure where their kids were at any given moment. Where kids wore super-clean socks and underwear. The South Madison Spartans weren't comprised of just a few black kids either. This was a throng of proud, loud, witty, fierce, fast, impressively mature men who just happened to still be young in age. Most of my teammates in those years

had their first tattoos, dunked basketballs, lost their V cards, had run-ins with the law, experimented with pot and alcohol, and dodged various bullets before stepping up to West High School as ninth-grade freshmen. Life wasn't the same on the South Side, it just wasn't.

Our coach was a diesel badass named Shelton Kincade. The original drill sergeant. "Is anyone tired!?" he'd yell as loudly as any voice has ever boomed off the walls of our well-broken-in gym. "No, coach!!" If you ever showed that you were tired, even at that age, you ran. Just like the call-and-response of "Y'all good?" during the darkest of November Project mornings, you knew there was only one answer that the athletes around you and the fearless leader in front would accept. "FUCK YEAH." Together, we embraced the concept that "When you're on this court you're never tired and you're never delivering anything other than a full serving of confidence." In those 4 years, fourth through eighth grade, I became someone who could actually open his eyes and be bold, be fearless.

I walked into West High School as a freshman already knowing the legendary scary giant black dudes such as Jeff Mack and Reece Gaines like family (Jeff went on to play linebacker at the University of Wisconsin, and Reece was a star at Louisville before going to the NBA). Culture. An open mind. Fearlessness around people who didn't look like me. Wild styles. The compassion and understanding for the feeling of being an outsider. The reach of the globe and how many amazing tribes of humans are out there living life in perfect balance the way they know it. It was all born in fourth grade. I learned some of my biggest lessons at Shorewood Hills Elementary School, and with the South Madison Spartans. Fueled by my physical stature and black fucking bears. Talk about an education.

FUCK YEAH!

THURSDAY, APRIL 18, 2013

Manhunt. The bombers are on the run. MIT police officer Sean Collier is ambushed, shot, and killed.

FRIDAY, APRIL 19, 2013

Urged by Brookline police, November Project calls off its hill workout, the only time it has ever canceled. The city and surrounding towns are on lockdown. Shots are fired in Watertown. The chase is nearing an end.

SATURDAY, MAY 4, 2013

November Project San Francisco launches with Laura McCloskey leading the charge, solo, as the new kid in town, the first female, changing the face of the movement.

MY FAMILY OF STORYTELLERS AND ARTISTS

From an early age, I remember the power of hearing stories, telling tales, the value of word-of-mouth. At Graham family gatherings, someone was always making a scene, putting on a show, pulling everyone into one room. My dad came from a large family and grew up sharing space and cranking the volume knob to be heard. The Grahams were a church-going, musically talented, polite, educated, penny-pinching clan driven by my grandfather, George Graham.

At 6 foot 3, he'd been a three-sport college athlete at both Clemson University in South Carolina and West Point, and was the kind of man who lived his life the way he hoped others would. He was known for opening or closing a conversation with the words, "You know what you need to do." And because of his usual posture or military way of life, you knew to listen.

When we all got together it was giant sing-alongs, gatherings around the pianos, guitars, tambourines, and whatever other instruments were around. There weren't many shrinking violets or wallflowers among us cousins, uncles, and aunts. From an early age, I saw closeness in the form of beautiful noise. Being loud to be heard over the other family members seemed to be a thing. I listened to the aunts and uncles on the Graham side pick up an instrument and play it without sheet music, while others sang along in harmony. Performers, artists, and friendly, loving family. That was the Grahams.

My mom's side couldn't be more different. The Doodys were a giant, Irish-Catholic family from the other side of Cleveland. The alpha male of the Doody clan, not unlike the Graham family, was my grandfather, Captain Bill Doody. The similarities ended there, however, as the men were opposite in all personality traits. They were both tall, good-looking men who were in charge of the room and called the shots. But the Captain was the life of the party and *was* the party his whole life. Bill, Captain Doody, The Dood, he was a living legend. He lived as a man of the marina, always in boat shoes and weathered sailing shirts. He was unfazed by weather and appropriate bedtimes, didn't change his language in

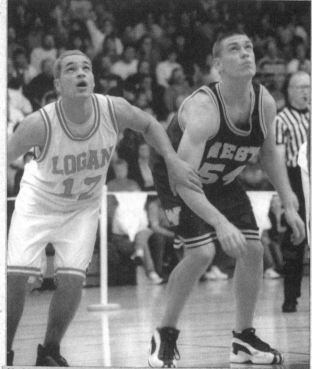

Madison West at Lacrosse Logan for a trip to the state tournament

front of children, and found inappropriate occasions to start dancing in public. He was loud and had the ability to charm strangers before they'd even shaken hands.

The Dood would have loved November Project because of the hugs, the loud Fuck Yeah greetings, the positivity, and the good-looking women who come through on the regular. He was a storyteller like none of us could ever be. Large hand gestures would take over your full field of vision as he led you through his tale, not only with his words and his voice, but his eyes, his vibe, and his entire body. He was performance art and slam poetry before those were even things. From the Captain I learned how to be loud, to tell (and later WRITE IN A BOOK) long stories about nothing, how a giant gesture can capture an otherwise partial listener, and that good friends could be gathered and friendships tightened over a cooler full of beers.

So the scene was set at the Doody family reunions, or Camp Doody, as we called it. Shirts? Of course we had Camp Doody shirts printed, which in the 1980s wasn't nearly as easy as it is now. But one of our aunts or uncles thought it was an important enough gathering for souvenir shirts. I mean, when the event has a shirt with a logo and people are wearing them, it almost feels as if you're a part of something that is actually something. I was all over it.

I've always had a connection to customized shirts and printing images. My high school and college friends would always riff on what phrases would make a funny shirt. Arts and crafts are something I can pretty much always get lost in, especially when the creation is going to be funny. Some of my favorite shirts, well before the now regular November Project image, were, "FRIEND-SHIP" all in the same, overlapping letters. Also in the same font were, "PORN ON THE COB," "SPANISH HOME-WORK," "MODERN TIMES," "WAREHOME STRONG," "GENERAL CHICKENS," and "POPULAR GUYS" (this was to poke fun at my high school girlfriend's matching hoodies that she and the rest of the pack of popular gals all bought as a gang). We got a laugh, we kept making them, and the creative vibes kept rolling.

Years later I'd lay the letters over a three-pack of

Hanes V-neck undershirts from CVS and paint November Project on them as they were laid over some bushes outside my apartment in Central Square. Bojan didn't even flinch when I pulled them out at the next stadium gathering. He knew me well enough by 2012 that this wasn't a surprise in the dark, 6 in the morning hour at the bottom of section 37.

Back at Camp Doody, we'd stay up late into the night with our cousins and listen in as the adults powered through giant stories with even larger, booming rounds of laughter. In these times, I was hearing my very first sounds and sights of what it took to gather a fun group, what it looked like to hold the attention of a crowd, and how it felt to hear an entire room sharing a solid evening of explosive laughing. These gatherings also always involved organized games of football, running races, long open-water swims, and of course, high-speed boat rides on my grandfather's motorboat named "Doody Free." These Camp Doody events always turned into a full-scale triathlon or a long swim across Devil's Lake. Physical activity seemed like, without it ever being too advertised, the work and play that you did to earn your party and play. We always partied hard when the race came to a

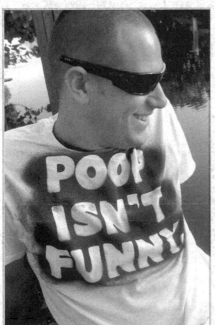
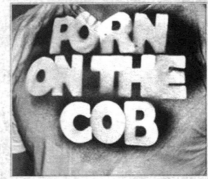
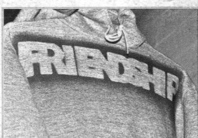
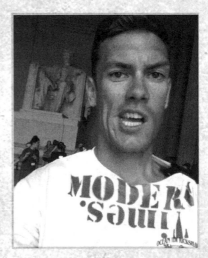
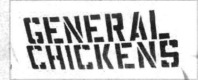

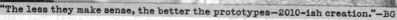
"The less they make sense, the better the prototypes—2010-ish creation."—BG

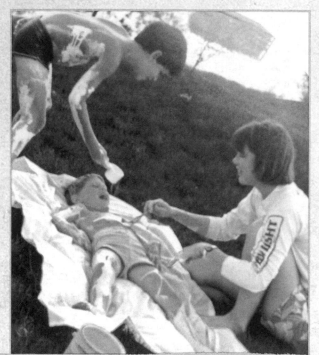

Ann Doody shows sons Dan and BG how to think large scale with their artwork. Primary colors only, these canvases became giant wall art in the boys' bedrooms. Weird? Cool? She didn't ask you.

close. Family and fun and fitness were twisted together into one strong rope—to pull a car from a ditch or knot loops around a tree branch over lake water.

CAMP DOODY

In our house on Tally Ho Lane (perfect name, right?) in Madison, my brother and I grew up looking at things differently. This tilt to life was driven by my creative mother, who some people thought was insane and others thought was a genius. We would gather around the table at our favorite pizza joint, two giant boys over 6 feet tall in sixth grade, ready to feed. Mom would get the classic salad bar meal and we would dive into a few large pies without missing a beat. MAN, sometimes when I think back to how she kept us fed on her design firm paycheck . . . fuck, man, what a job.

Anyway, when the meal was on its way or we were digesting it before heading home, the basic crayons were dropped onto the table. You see, DG and I pretty

much never looked like kiddies or even children, the kind that would need crayons to stay entertained. The interesting part of this dynamic is that our mom, an artist her entire life, would ask for them. But this isn't going where you think; no simple coloring sessions here. Oh no, the standard candle that was set in the center of each table, guarded tightly by the salt and pepper shakers, became the gas pedal for the artwork that she would crank out.

By flipping the generic placemats over to see a full 11x17 blank white canvas, the wax crayons could become paintbrushes when held under the small flame for a few seconds. My mom, a master of water color and design, took these opportunities to tell both DG and I how AMAZING and BEAUTIFUL our artwork was, never criticizing a thing along the way. EVERYTHING WAS AWESOME in the Ann Doody School of Art . . . and that enthusiasm extended beyond the crayons and into the little school work we actually did get done over the years.

But this positive vibe, this complimentary attitude, this overwhelming boost in confidence that could be seen in Artwork By Pizza (1995) would best show itself in athletics. Mom taught us all how to ski, and when I say WE, I mean all of our cousins on her side, and half the neighborhood. She led kids into their lifetime love of skiing (something that she does to this day as a pro at Aspen Ski School) by simply setting them up to try. Don't

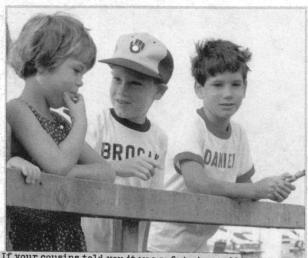

If your cousins told you it was safe to jump off the bridge . . .

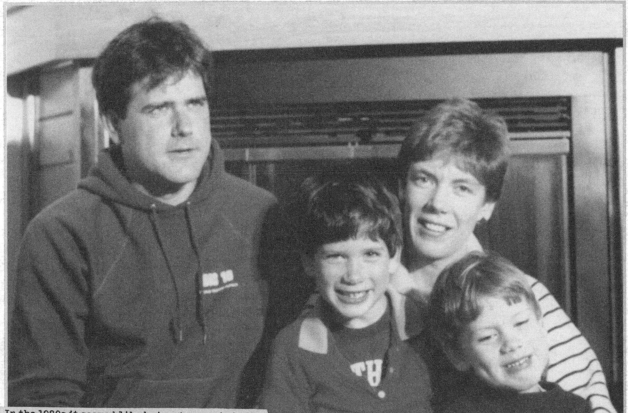

In the 1980s it seemed like haircuts came in bulk.

complain or doubt yourself, she'd say. Just try. You have to try or you won't ever know how awesome you are. Not: You have to try in order to know how good you are OR how bad you are. She leads people into art, skiing, and anything else by encouraging them to TRY so that they'd KNOW how awesome they are. I know, I know, it sounds like a fucking emo greeting card that would sell at Urban Outfitters or something . . . but it is true. She was ahead of her time.

Ann Doody was NP before there was an NP. At our workouts, you don't just cheer the badasses, the Scott Gilroys, the Shira Klanes, the Ian Nurses, you yell and scream for anyone who has the balls to toss off the covers and just show up. You're 300 pounds? You just quit smoking? You haven't broken an honest sweat in decades? And you're bouncing with us, attempting just 4 stadium sections? Well, you are a fucking badass and we fuckin' love you.

A STIFF SPINE

At age 12 or 13, during a required camp physical my brother and I both took, it was detected that I had scoliosis. DG went in first and they were all up in his ears, nose, throat, and, most likely, balls. When it was my turn, I figured I'd fly through all of the testing just like DG had. But at the end of the exam, when they asked me to bend over so they could look at my spine, they discovered that it was curved from side to side. Scoli-Oh-Shit! With more vertical inches in my future, based on growth projections, this was going to become an issue. Over the next two years it got progressively worse, as yoga, full-body back braces, and chiropractic work didn't seem to help. The only option I had left was some seriously invasive, out-of-state back surgery.

After several second and third opinions, we landed on Dr. Shaughnessy, a surgeon at the Mayo Clinic in

NOW I SEE WHERE ALL THOSE NOTHING STORIES COME FROM! BG - THE MASTER OF ATTRACTING CROWDS TO TELL STORIES ABOUT ABSOLUTELY NOTHING !!!

Rochester, Minnesota. The two of us wheeled and dealed about dates for this major reconstruction of my spine like we were bidding at an auction. My end game? To get back on the basketball court as soon as possible. His end game? To collect the correct number of self-donated blood transfusions before we rushed into this marathon, 8 to 12 hour surgery. I was dialed in, eager to look past the scary piece of what I was facing and right into the "we're going to be fine and past this" piece. We set the operation for February of eighth grade, which would be followed by several months out of school and off the court.

Want to change your perspective on stress levels, how "busy" you are these days, or what's truly important in life? Visit the fucking pediatric unit at the Mayo Clinic, because those noncomplaining champions in there are sitting around bravely enduring some of the most debilitating illnesses and injuries your mind could ever imagine. They're 6 years old waiting for a lung. They're 9 years old with the tumors removed and the third round of chemotherapy whaling on their small frames. Speaking of frames, what about the 5-year-old in one of those steel head/neck braces following a massive car accident that he was buckled in for? Again, if you need to feel great about your unpaid bills, your dissatisfying love

"FIVE YEARS AGO, I WAS CONFINED TO A WHEELCHAIR, AND MY NEUROLOGIST NEVER THOUGHT I WOULD WALK WITHOUT AN ASSISTIVE DEVICE OF SOME SORT. I WORKED MY ASS OFF TO PROVE MY MEDICAL TEAM WRONG. SINCE THEN, MY FRIENDS HAVE TREATED ME WITH KID'S GLOVES BECAUSE THEY DON'T WANT ME TO GO THROUGH THAT EXPERIENCE AGAIN. TO BE HONEST, THE ONLY PEOPLE WHO HAVEN'T TREATED ME LIKE I WAS 'SICK' HAVE BEEN THE DC AND BOSTON NP TRIBES, AND I CANNOT APPROPRIATELY CONVEY THE DEPTH OF MY APPRECIATION FOR THAT."
—MEG GUILFORD, MAY 16, FROM FB, 46, TUFTS PHD CANDIDATE

BULLSHIT !!! HE HATES IT!

life, or the petty shit you think is bringing you down, head on down to Rochester, Minnesota.

My 9-hour surgery went well. The Harrington rods, like two extra-long pieces of stainless steel shaped like drinking straws, were latched at the top, middle, and bottom of my thoracic spine, making 11 individual vertebrae into one giant, interconnected piece of metal and bone. A bone graft was taken from my left hip and added to the metal tower to pack tight what would eventually heal into a Robospine that I have had with me ever since, even as I type this story for you now. I was a full 1.5 inches taller after the surgery, I kid you not. From just below my neck to the top of my lower back, there's one enormous piece of hardware. Since your next question will totally be, "Do you set off metal detectors at airports?" I'll tell you this: People ask me that all the time, and I don't get annoyed. It just reminds me not to ask people the thing that is the most obvious THING in the conversation. The waitress with pink hair has been asked 10,000 times today how she gets it that pink. But since you're still wondering: When I go through the TSA, I smile, drop a yes sir/no sir, and hope they don't make me check my skateboard. The metal in my spine doesn't set anything off in airports, not at all. And I fly all the time.

The recovery was insane and all over the map. It took almost a year. While relearning to walk, I attended one of my brother's basketball games. I sat in a wheelchair in a special section with my mom and the mentally disabled kids, most of whom had full-time aides. Want another reality check on how awesome your life is? Go sit at a basketball game in a wheelchair with the mentally handicapped kids and view the world from their perspective. The seats are great, sure (almost courtside), but the connection to community couldn't be more remote. What I took from that experience is that a simple greeting to a person in a chair, or on crutches, or who is unable to control their own body, even with no response, can forge the tiniest connection to that person and help bridge the social chasm between them and the "normal side" of the room.

You'll find that bridge at NP, too. One of our earlier members, Ashley Brow, is visually impaired. She showed

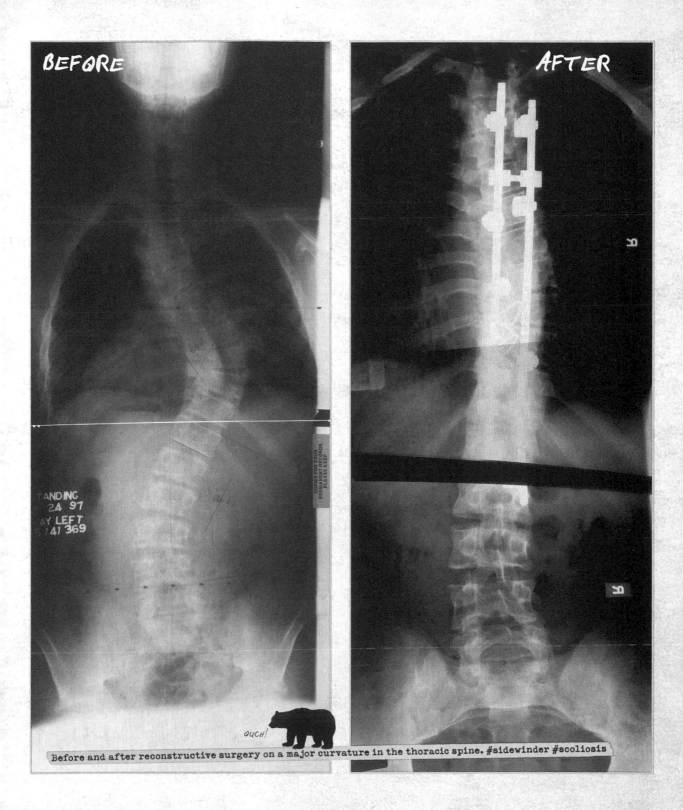

BEFORE

AFTER

STANDING
24 97
AY LEFT
141 369

COPIES FOR YOUR
PERMANENT RECORDS
PLEASE KEEP

OUCH!

Before and after reconstructive surgery on a major curvature in the thoracic spine. #sidewinder #scoliosis

up to Summit Ave to walk the hills holding her friend's arm in one hand and her cane in the other. She eventually found a way to actually run the hills with almost no assistance. In Kansas City, fierce, adaptive athlete Tatsiana Khvitsko helps lead that tribe on two Cheetah blades. Our members have faced medical procedures that make mine seem like child's play—brain surgery and open-heart surgery—and then returned to their respective NP workouts. Female members have trained into their ninth month of pregnancy, and even have had their water break on Summit Ave. Everybody and every type of body is welcome in our house.

MY PODIUM DANCE

In the history of West High School, I think I'm the only student to be named commencement speaker, prom king, and leader of Bike Day—a two-wheeled rally I started because my car had shit the bed and I needed to make carrying around a helmet at school seem cool—while quietly flunking out of school at the same time. Through a popular vote, I was elected one of two commencement speakers. I was pumped but also terrified that it was all going to blow up in my face. I remember working with the teachers in all of my classes to figure out if I could actually pass. Each week brought a sigh of relief when I found out that German would be a pass . . . that Dance 2 would be a pass . . . and somehow, through some wheeling and dealing and pleading and negotiating, plus an extra dance class that desperately needed males, I locked down my name on a bona fide high school diploma.

"BG was bigger than life . . . and crazy in that big brother/I want to grow up like that one day kind of way. He pushed limits, poked at authority, and was too damn cool."

—Joey "Big20" Kile, 26, product developer at New Balance

On graduation day, I had no idea how heightened my senses had become, how much of a sponge I'd grown into, or how life's lessons had already become embedded in me. I'd done a sound check with Rodney, the other student speaker, and knew he had his words on lockdown. Rodney, now known around the globe as the spoken-word poet and hip-hop artist F. Stokes, spoke in his usual "top of the mountain" style voice. He didn't hold back, either, as he spoke of being black and being proud. Rodney, or Rodzilla as I called him then, was one of my teammates on the Spartans. He had sleeve tattoos that were as legit back then as they are now. Rodney killed it in rehearsals, and I was only okay. I worked a good deal over my words, my plans, my pauses, the night before and that morning.

And while I don't know if I killed it that day, I definitely had an amazing time delivering my speech. A beautiful, always-smiling gal named Angelique introduced me. She said, "You may know Brogan Graham as the captain of the basketball team, you may know him from Bike Day, and you may not know him at all. His friends call him BG, so ladies and gentlemen, here's BG." My life had changed only a million times since I stood up to talk about black bears 8 years before. Rules had definitely been bent and broken along the way. The grades were alright, good, and sometimes very bad. Like my brother, I'd left a mark on many of my classmates as I dodged school work, and got better and better each year at standing tall.

My speech was fun and didn't follow any rules, but it did have a theme. I homed in on a board game that my

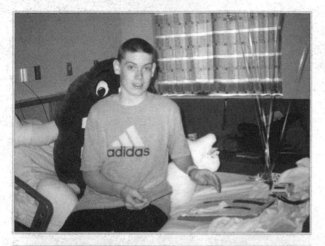

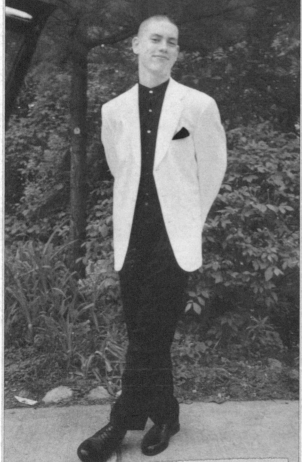

Leaving Mayo Clinic (top) to get back to 7th grade schoolwork at home. Looking '90s fresh one year later (bottom) as commencement speaker for 8th grade graduation (was that even a real thing?)

brother and I used to play when we were young called Off and Running. The game was as simple as it gets. (As I sit here typing this, it occurs to me that it almost exactly outlines the values of November Project as a movement and as a weekly activity.) I mentioned how we, as students at West High School, were all moving one another around the board, a shared board, around the track and over the years. Though we weren't all teammates, or bandmates, or in the same theatrical productions, we all looked to one another for greatness and motivation as we, the collective WE, moved around the board, the shared track of life.

"Off and Running," I told the thousands who had assembled in the Kohl Center that day, "was about moving one another forward."

In the actual board game, there was a giant spinning wheel (only one) that was passed around from player to player. The arrow on the wheel would direct each person who spun it to move any of the four characters on the board toward their goals, starting in the center. No one was in this race alone; in fact the entire group was pushing each other along toward their finish line. After your spin told you who to move forward, you reached to the board, moved that character ahead, and passed the wheel to the next player.

I used the game that DG and I had played years earlier in our tiny home in Sun Prairie, Wisconsin, to explain how the students at West had been moving one another along the way, pushing one another with support and high expectations. How we, the collective WE, were moving us, as a group, forward. Off and Running wasn't even a game you could win, the same way you can't win at high school, life, or anything else that really matters. What you can do is push those around you and grow rich in experience by being a part of something great, some kind of movement that achieves a collective gain. Come to any November Project workout in any of our cities and you'll see what I'm talking about.

But the highest moment of my high school graduation wasn't about me, my performance, or the unlikely fact that I was standing there at all. That didn't come until the headliner. J. D. Walsh, an actor who'd attended

Yale School of Drama and was a proud West High alum, stepped up to the mic and brought the house down. The crowd didn't just listen to his words, they were on a ride with him as a tour guide. You just held your breath. He was a matador guiding the giant wave of laughs and pauses and deep, thoughtful moments all at once. He was the Captain Bill Doody and all of the best storytellers I've known wrapped into one. And he seemed to do it with ease and rhythm. J. D. changed the way I saw public speaking and comedy, and I wanted to be that.

"If you see someone interesting, go speak to them, you won't regret it. And don't just go for looks either because . . . beauty fades, annoying is forever!" I was spellbound. I can still hear his voice, and the words and phrases he used to close out his nonstop rant of reality and jokes and truths about being yourself and being fearless.

"Be a hugger, not a shaker," he said (and I'm paraphrasing here; actually quoting myself paraphrasing J.D., because I've rolled his ideas and phrases into so many of my newbie spiels at NP). "Huggers live better lives. They risk more. They live more and they don't live with regret! Regret! That's a big one, you need to fight it. You need to fight it every day! Shakers follow the rules. They play it safe. They risk nothing and they gain nothing. Shakers risk the chance to live more in each moment. And be a dancer, not someone who watches and judges. The people watching are scared. They're scared they'll look stupid, so they sit and watch. Dance, risk, live, and you'll never live with regret. Regret! REMEMBER THIS ONE AND FIGHT IT EVERY SINGLE DAY! And I'm not just talking about some metaphorical party way off in your future where you'll have to decide! I'm asking you to decide right now, because life is happening right now, and I'm GOING TO DANCE! And you can sit there and watch me and risk nothing, or you can join me."

His voice had now climbed to an emotional yell. He took two steps back from the podium, the crowd in the palm of his hands.

"So what's it going to be!?" he shouted. "Will you dance!?"

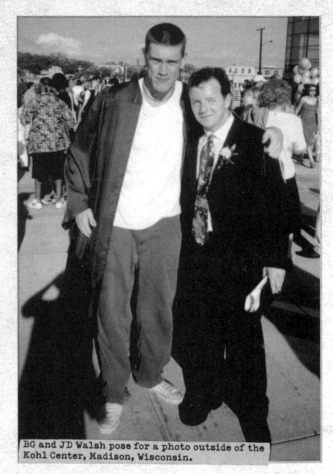

BG and JD Walsh pose for a photo outside of the Kohl Center, Madison, Wisconsin.

GOODBYE MAD TOWN, HELLO BEANTOWN

Time sped up in the months that followed. A group of my best friends all left for Arizona on the same flight to begin their freshman year of college. We were all shot into the world of choices and responsibility. We were Off and Running.

But life is a weird thing, and we never know who we'll let drastically impress us, influence us, or guide us. In my senior year in high school I'd picked up rowing with a very dorky, intense, fun, cult-like athletic group of driven people at the Mendota Rowing Club. Being 6-plus feet tall, they'd been trying to recruit me for years. At the time, I was looking for a fall sport and was curious what they saw in me exactly. That curiosity changed my life. My options for colleges multiplied almost immediately.

And as fate would have it, another life-changing path

opened up. That same year I auditioned for a few acting groups and plays at school. By this time, I'd ditched a lot of my bad-kid antics and was getting my shit together. But I definitely still liked to joke and be a wiseass in public and could project my voice like a souped-up megaphone. Just like rowing, I was looking for something new, something outside of my wheelhouse. The theater crowd at West was super creative, open, funny, very passionate, very tight. I made friends with musicians, dancers, writers, and directors who I'd passed as nameless faces in the halls for years. As the captain of the basketball team, I was suddenly the outcast. But the group accepted me right away, and I've never forgotten how that feeling of inclusiveness can allow you to reach your full expression. And the stage wasn't just a one-off experiment. Later, at Northeastern, I was the only dude on my boat, hell, the whole boathouse, who was majoring in theater. I love entertaining, cracking jokes, throwing out weirdness. With November Project, I definitely bring a big dose of performance art to the workouts. Why the fuck not? Who said hardcore fitness has to be hardcore boring?

NU DAZE

The biggest shift in who I was as a young dude, an athlete, a competitor, fuck it MY ENTIRE IDENTITY occurred in 2003, when I was a sophomore on John Pojednic's mighty Northeastern University Men's Rowing team. As you know if you've hung in with me so far, I was a bit of a bad kid, a creative troublemaker, and a person who moms told their kids to stay away from (I see you, Lynn Johnson) during certain, more explosive summers.

John saw potential in the 6:26 time I posted for the 2000m test

that I took at the Mendota Rowing Club during my senior year of high school, before I really knew anything about the sport. He saw potential in my athletic build and loved the fact that I could be swept out from the Wisconsin Badgers' hometown. John, one of the most intense dudes I've ever met, saw a rower in me and wanted to bring me out to Boston. With a generous enough scholarship to make the decision, my acceptance, and a 17-hour van ride with DG and my mom, I arrived in Boston for the first time. Huntington Avenue and Forsyth. I was moving into White Hall as a dude who didn't know anything about college and even less about rowing. And I was freaked out.

My teammates, who I met within the first few days on campus, all had years of rowing experience under their belts. I had one. They all seemed to have raced one another over the years, and they knew former high school

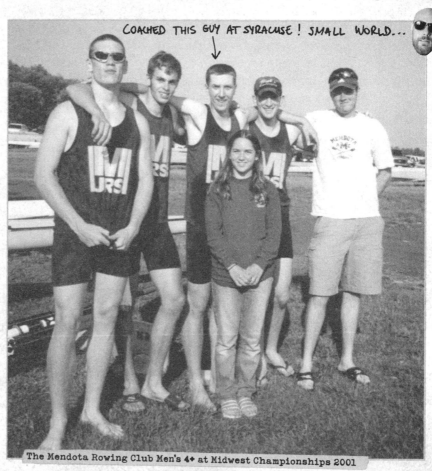

COACHED THIS GUY AT SYRACUSE! SMALL WORLD...

The Mendota Rowing Club Men's 4+ at Midwest Championships 2001

teammates who were now sprinkled around the Eastern Sprints league. As a freshman, I was the biggest guy on the team but also the least experienced. A dumb fuckin' mule. The feeling of being tested every day was in my head all the time.

Freshman Coach Seth Brennan pushed the team until we cracked. More work. Harder work. Don't talk back. See you tomorrow. Those seemed to be the main themes throughout the fall. My second day of practice under coaches Pojednic and Brennan was on September 11, 2001. We listened to the radio in the van as we returned from our morning row. Nobody spoke during our shotgun-speed dash back to campus, and we sat glued to our miniature dorm TVs through the lunchtime hours, watching the remains of the towers and waiting for updates.

Being as close as we were to NYC, I was now watching big news on TV that affected people in my building. The fall of the Berlin Wall, the Oklahoma City bombing, the death of Princess Diana were all real, but off in Wisconsin, in a kid's mind, they pretty much occurred within the frame of the TV, the pages of the newspaper, and so on. They didn't seem close enough for me to feel the ripple. But on 9/11 I was listening to people up and

down the halls talking about dead phone lines and how they still hadn't heard anything from their family who works or lives right there.

The most intense part of that surreal day was when we went, at the planned time, to quietly load into the van and drive upstream to Henderson Boathouse to row again (what?). The weather was great and the van was on time and there was nothing said about practice being canceled. So we went out to row miles and get ready to race. We were there to train, and that is what we did. None of the newbies, the freshmen, were going to speak up and ask if it was insane to head out and practice against the background of serious fucking world-changing national trauma . . . we just went out. That was my first giant dose of "FUCK YEAH WE'RE GOING TO GO TRAIN." This was the ultimate, and extreme, example of the #justshowup philosophy that would later become a cornerstone of November Project. (At NP we created an "Injury Deck" for busted-up athletes and bruised runners—even broken bones and stress fractures are no excuse not to show up. Get crunching with your booted feet in the air, motherflicker! I have led workouts while wearing a leg cast. The accountability of rowing is drilled deep into my DNA. The rest of the team, and the workout itself, depends on your ass being there.)

Roughly 6 weeks later, we raced in an 8+ at the Head of the Charles Regatta (or HOCR) in October. *(Editor's note: The "8+" is the name for the 8-person-powered rowing shell. Each athlete rows a single oar that is placed on one side of the boat. The "+" part means that there is a coxswain, or a jockey, who steers the boat.) (Author's note: What is up Rob Dalton!)* The HOCR is

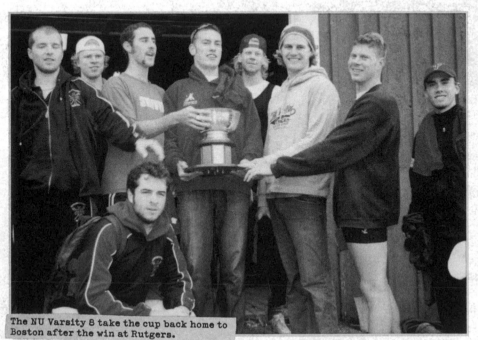

The NU Varsity 8 take the cup back home to Boston after the win at Rutgers.

ONE TIME DALTON ALMOST GOT KILLED BY A BAG OF NUTS. TRUE STORY!

Brogan's Abs @brogans_abs · 18 Jul 2014
Did you know that my Latin name is Rectus Abdominus? Anagram of that is Unbiased scrotum. You're welcome!

Brogan's Abs @brogans_abs · 14 Jul 2014
My gut tells me, that I'll be pushing out some serious burrito poops today. Excited for the workout!

Brogan's Abs @brogans_abs · 13 Jul 2014
Today I didn't do shit and I still look amazing! #SucksToBeYou

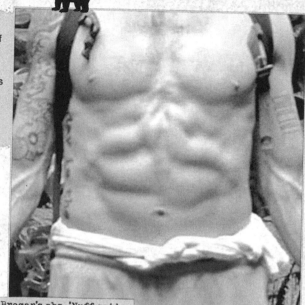

Brogan's abs. 'Nuff said.

one of the more twisted courses, and it brings most of the rowing world to Boston each year for what looks more like a boat parade than a race. We finished second that day behind some studs from Harvard, which is located just a mile down the river on the same side, our side, of the Charles. Later that fall, at the last race of the year, we beat the same lineup of guys (and everyone else) at the Foot of the Charles, a much smaller race for college crews mostly. I felt like I was going to survive this rowing thing, this college thing, this big East Coast city thing.

Just barely, as it would turn out.

It all started with Seth, a diehard Princeton rower, who had a hate for Harvard that ran deep. Seth was a lumberjack-looking fellow who we all feared. Though he was in his mid-to-late 20s when he coached with John at Northeastern, we all thought he was 40 or 50 or 200 years old. Going in for the winter (the Charles freezes over, putting BU, NU, Harvard, and MIT on the rowing machine and indoor tanks for the winter to work like animals), we trained to beat Harvard. They trained to beat everyone. By winter break it began to feel like I could actually make a go of this college thing, this D1 athletics thing, and that with enough day-to-day hard work, I could actually do this. With help from my coaches, my family, friends, trainers, professors, tutors, and what felt like all of the positive vibes in the world, I was turning my life around.

During my hoops-playing days, I never bought into the whole "let's compete and then we'll be friends after" concept. No way. I was all about the real-life hatred we had for "ABC" or East High or whoever it was that we met on the court. There were fights, on the court, off the court. There were suspensions. Some sports do the sportsman-

ship thing really well. Rugby, for example. Those dudes nearly kill each other every single play and then hug it out and make their way to drink a trillion beers within a few minutes of their matches being over. Rowing is closer to rugby than it is to hoops in that regard, but I wasn't a real rower. I loved racing and fell in love with it on the rowing machines inside Henderson Boathouse and out on the many twisting miles of the Charles River. But personally I was more like Happy Gilmore (the fictional hockey player turned golfer) in the way that I connected my identity to rowing.

Rowers are rowers. They'll wear the shirts and pants that say ROWING, just ROWING, the name of the fucking sport. ROWING, down one leg of their sweat pants. ROWING. Rowers are traditionally preppy, and the best schools in the country for men's rowing will no doubt continue to push this terrible-but-all-too-real stereotype. There are the pillars of the sport, both historically and currently: Brown, Princeton, Yale, Dartmouth, Cornell, and what's that one in the West? . . . Oh, right, Stanford. And then there's the one we all hated as a group. Harvard. Harvard Rowing is like the New York Yankees with less ethnicity and more winning. Harvard Rowing is so easy to hate because the hate continues to stoke itself as a hot fire that loves to burn. The team is giant, their boathouse 11,000 years old. They have another boat-house for their women's team just so you know how much money they have, and, this is the worst part, they're usually really fucking strong and fast. Harvard Rowing.

EXTREME TURNING POINT

Saturday, March 8, 2003. Some of the friendly Canadi-ans on our NU Husky team were invited by their high school teammates—now Harvard guys—to share a night out at the Radcliffe fundraiser in Cambridge.

The fundraiser was the kind that Harvard rowers on the men's and women's teams both looked forward to. The men JUMPED at the opportunity to wear their tuxes, which all seemed to fit suspiciously well, and the women were able to wear heels around the only group of men on campus who would be into women who stood 6 feet or taller.

We rolled into the event with mixed emotions. The Canadians on our team, like all Canadians, were the nic-est people in the world, and felt that all rowers were family. The rest of us, as devoted sons of the Seth Bren-nan Fuck Harvard Camp, weren't quite as hyped about fraternizing with the enemy. But we went anyway. I owned a pair of nice black shoes, which I wore along with my Northeastern felt dress jacket. I had no idea that this night, 20 years after I had reported on black bears, lost faith in the rules, piled on the troubled years, and FINALLY got things back together, would become the most pivotal moment of my life.

The vibe wasn't good. Trip, Yossi, even Dan (who was a friendly Canadian) couldn't naturally mix in with the Harvard men or women, even though both groups (espe-cially the men's team) were overly nice to us. The event was actually a date auction for which we pushed our thinnest coxswain up onto the bidding block. He actually went for a few bucks and won a date to the bowling alley with future Olympic gold medalist Caryn Davies.

Unfortunately, that was the only positive or fun thing that happened the entire night. We read the vibes well and knew that after only a few conversations with the Harvard dudes that if we stuck around too long, Trip or

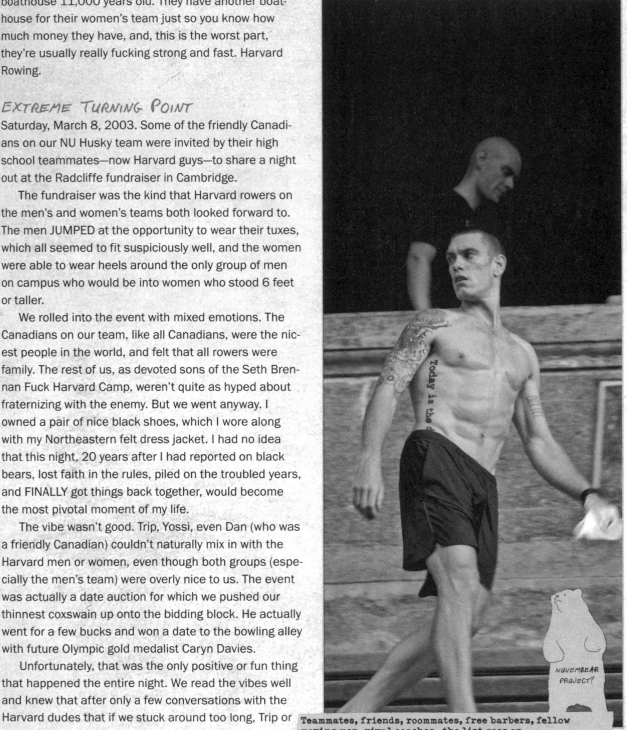

NOVEMBEAR PROJECT?

Teammates, friends, roommates, free barbers, fellow moving men, rival coaches—the list goes on.

one of the other dudes on our team was going to get into a fight. So we decided to leave, and that was when it all came melting down. Trip, my wildest college friend, teammate, and the most fearless/stupid guy I've ever met, turned around halfway down the giant staircase leading out of the boathouse.

"I'm going to get Malcolm's sunglasses and wear them to our dual," he said, "because fuck that guy."

Now, there was a bit of inside rower-speak there, so I'll quickly translate: Malcolm Howard, one of the best guys on Harvard's men's team, would go on to become one of the best in the world. That night he was wearing Elvis-style shades as an ironic twist to his tuxedo or suit or whatever it was he had on.

The "dual" races that happen each year have been etched into metal trophies for decades. These races pit two universities against one another on decided week-ends each spring. The course covers a distance of 2000m. Dual races are a side-by-side race between each school's freshmen, then JV, then varsity, and so on. What made dual racing cool was that you knew your opponents and when you would be racing them, head-to-head, months or even years in advance.

If we went to Providence to race Brown on their home water one year, they would come to Boston the next. The cup between two teams in a certain dual would be kept inside the boathouse trophy case of the team with the faster Varsity 8+, and the team name and year would be added to its placard. At the end of a dual, the teams pull their boats together so that each of the nine seats line up, and the losers take off their matching racing shirts and give them, along with a traditional handshake, to the champions before pushing away and free of the intertwined rows of emotions. In my experience in sports of all kinds, racing, playing, training, and whatever else, there is no better feeling than taking your opponent's shirt, shaking his hand, looking into his eyes—fuck it, his SOUL—and saying good race. On the other hand, losing

your shirt and rowing back to the boathouse topless . . . there is no worse feeling. The sport has been doing it forever and the tradition is widely known and heavily respected.

Again: "I'm going to get Malcolm's sunglasses and wear them to our dual . . . because fuck that guy."

I kept walking, shook my head, and thought nothing of it. In fact, I clearly remember thinking, "Wow, we're actually leaving this event without anything happening. I thought for sure someone would do something stupid and we'd be asked to leave."

I pushed through the giant wooden doors and stepped down the small, simple staircase into the night. The boathouse is right on the Cambridge side of the JFK bridge, where JFK Street would lead us to the red line, green line, E train, and back home to NU.

Thirty feet away from the boathouse I heard a noise and some laughing. Then Trip blazed by me wearing Malcolm's gold frames, laughing and springing with his usual bright red face. Then the door was opening again. Malcolm was giving chase at full speed. He was on a beeline course, in hot pursuit of Trip. When I heard a "Get back here, Trip!" I turned quickly to see what looked like an attack, and within one-tenth of a second my whole world came to a halt.

"BG is for many of the men in NP their first 'bro-crush.' That dude must have swallowed a shit-ton of magnets growing up because he has an incredible ability to attract people!"
—Ryan Komaiko, 31, marketing professional, Boston

> "Did I take Malcolm down that night? Yes. Was it bad?
> Fuck yes. Did I intend for him to land face first, get
> knocked out, and spend a night in the hospital? No way."
> —BG, one-time cocky rowing jock, full of piss and vinegar

You have a flight-or-fight response. You do. You may not know it, but you do. Do you hold your ground? Do you flinch and step back? I didn't step back. I stood hard. In fact, though I've replayed this moment in my head at least 10,000 times, I still can't say for sure which body parts hit what. I can tell you that as I braced myself and brought my forearms up over my face, Malcolm (another 6-foot-6, 220-pound guy) was at a full sprint when he and I connected. Hips, head, shoulder, and all. It was like the crack of an open-ice body check that I'd later see in Andrew Ference highlights. The only difference in the two brick walls that smashed together in that brief moment of physics was that one was propelling himself at significant velocity in one direction; while the other was scared stiff, holding his ground, and without intention, checked the oncoming rowing stud into the dark night where nobody could see.

Malcolm was knocked out cold, and he hit the ground face first. His hands didn't come up to protect his face, and a pool of blood began seeping out around the shadow of his face on the sidewalk. Trip, Dan, and I . . . none of us knew what to do or what to say. A few Harvard guys walked out the door, then ran to the scene. The police were called (they come quick on that campus). My teammates told me to scram. I was afraid. I didn't know what to do, what was right, what had just happened, and I took off.

As I walked to the red line station at Harvard Square I was tracing the outlines of my shoulders, elbows, and even my face and forehead. Where did the connection, the contact, the blow come from? It was like a magician's sleight of hand. If I'd been given a million punches in a row, I'd have never been able to take this guy out with a single blow. Scuffles and dust-ups had vanished from my life, and yet I had put down an elite athlete and future Olympian. My friends boarded the same train that I was on at Park Street and we rode the green line outbound E line as a team. Nobody spoke.

Over the next few weeks I was suspended from the team, brought in front of the Middlesex County Court, and had to face a felony charge for aggravated assault. (I was told that this was the most reaching charge the Harvard PD and Harvard Detective Unit could hope to get me with. Charge him with this and he'll plead to a lesser charge was the idea.) Just a side note: Most first dates and job interviews start with my having to explain the "Rower Pleads Not Guilty" headline that comes up in Google searches of my full name. Go ahead, take a minute if you want to dial it up yourself. Although the *Harvard Crimson* piece isn't fair and fails to include many/any of the actual facts, it is a good piece of dramatic writing.

Okay, back to the story. Where were we? Right, totally fucked and sorting out what might come next. After the *Harvard Crimson* published the article, I went before the student board of the Office of Student Conflict Resolution. Northeastern had to take action now that the story was picking up steam. With Malcolm watching, I told my story. It ended with an incredibly long apology. That was the last time I ever saw him outside of racing.

Not only was his recovery fast but he didn't ever press charges. He was rowing with his elite 8+ that would go on to win everything that year. Malcolm, in 4 years of racing for the Crimson, won every single dual, Eastern Sprints, Harvard/Yale, and IRA. The dude never, ever lost. He went on to the World Championships, and followed that up with an Olympic gold medal at the Beijing Games in 2008. As our boats passed over the years on the Charles River or during the many races we both lined up for, I always wanted to tell him how the accident changed my life, how it dealt a blow to my psyche, and it developed my love for community.

After taking a 1-year "proof of person" plea, which showed the court system that I wasn't an axe murderer, that I had no interest in getting into any more trouble with the law, and that this had been simultaneously an accident and a turning point, I was able to prove that I was worthy of not having a felony on my record.

Did I take Malcolm down that night? Yes. Was it bad? Fuck yes. Did I intend for him to land face first, get knocked out, and spend a night in the hospital? No way. Was it a fight? NO way. Did I wish there was a camera that caught all of this on video? Absolutely. I was stripped of my scholarship and thrown out of school, at least for a while. I lost a lot of friends. And on top of becoming an outcast in the scene that I'd fallen in love with in Boston, I was handed 100 hours of community service from Northeastern and 100 hours of community service from Mid-

dlesex County Court. My attorney told me to get a job, nail my hours of community service, meet him for the regular hearings that would come up every few months, and that if I truly was sorry and that I truly wasn't this bad guy that was written about in the paper, that I'd come out on the other side as a better guy.

Doing my Time

Some of my jobs took me to the basketball courts at City on a Hill Charter Public School, which at the time was located inside the Huntington Avenue YMCA. Proud, loud, and super-funny high-school-age black girls playing ball and talking trash. It was a scene I knew well. The 100 hours flew by, and I became connected to the team and the culture and the athletes. The YMCA is also one of those iconic places in the Back Bay that you may

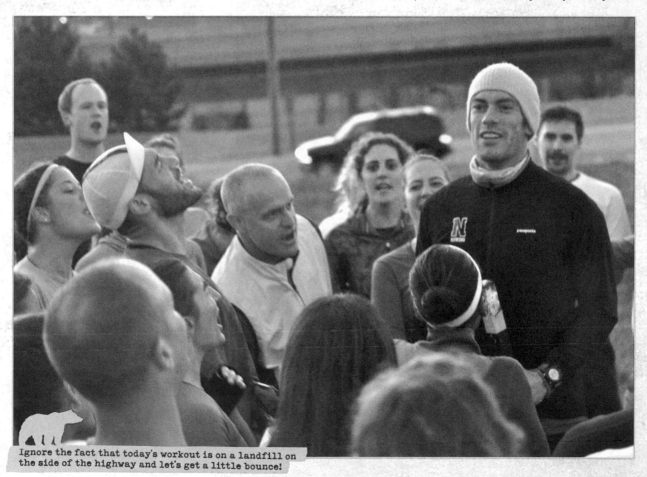

Ignore the fact that today's workout is on a landfill on the side of the highway and let's get a little bounce!

never actually go into. I was all over that building. Hosting events, shoveling the sidewalks, teaching swim lessons in a 100-year-old pool that required everyone, I mean every ONE of us, to wear swim caps because the drainage system was beyond repair.

Now I want you to understand something. This time was hard and long for me, and it didn't seem to have an end. My future at NU was uncertain, but for the time being the university required me to stay connected to the community through service. The b-ball and swimming were great, but most of my time was spent next to the jail by Interstate 93, where I sorted cans at a Boston Food Pantry. Remember the last time that you cleaned out your shelves for a canned food drive? You gave creamed corn and a bunch of other shit you wouldn't ever eat. From that drop box/bin to the mouths of the people who need it in Boston is where volunteers come in to sort, package, load, and unload the right combination of good, bad, and expired food.

That was one of two spots where I volunteered in the Roxbury/South End/Southie neighborhood. The other, the well-established Pine Street Inn, was a place where I had the privilege to walk with those who needed a hand, those who were a little off their track, and those who'd lost faith in the collective "we." The Pine Street Inn is a homeless shelter on the line between the South End

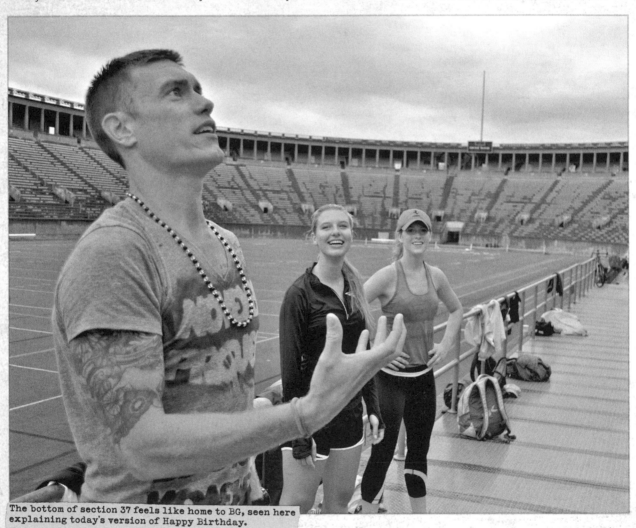

The bottom of section 37 feels like home to BG, seen here explaining today's version of Happy Birthday.

and South Boston. (This might sound like the same thing to those not from the area, but it's comedy to those who know the two places because of how different they are.) This shelter has been aiding the homeless community since 1969 and is a grounded, historic, and proud institution.

But with my hours logged, my new destinations and routes through the city mapped, and my connections made, I was able to fight for my scholarship and my clean record. I never missed a day in court, a call with Mr. Marty Kane, or a session in the pool, in the gym, on the trucks, or at the Inn. My life had become rich as I matured through the ordeal. I let go of any anger and any disconnection to family that had resulted from my parents' divorce. I never lost the feeling of debt I owed to Malcolm or his teammates, even though I'd tried a few times (against my attorney's wishes) to reach out. I'd become able to see the full city. I took jobs during my time away from school that had me moving furniture for the Gentle Giant Moving Company. I'd seen how Boston looks for high school kids, for teachers, for swimmers, for the rich with plans to move their grand piano, and for the homeless hoping to find a place to lay their head at night. I'd become better through my mistake and I'd grown from the rebellious kid who always needed to stir shit up to a man who made good on his absolute last chance to pull his ass out of the fire.

Even though at the time this was just my day-to-day, some of these revelations would later drive the creation of the Destination Deck workout on Mondays at NP. We all lived in this city, but many of us hardly knew it at all; we just knew our little plot, our grocery store and pharmacy, our work and home subway stops. Why not inject the workout with a cool geographic twist? Start your week in a new place, with a new vibe? There's no rule that says you can only work out in the same one or two places. Get fit and get to know your city at the same time, your entire community—what could be better?

Bojan and I have gone back and forth on this. Is this the reason that he and I built NP? No way. Is it the reason behind all of the community drive? Nope. Then what

"Got a bad rap? I don't care. Are you at November Project to be kind, work your ass off, and start your day right? Then that's all that matters."

—BG

the heck does any of this have to do with anything? It is simply the moment that defined who I am and who I transitioned into. Two years and 31 days after that night at the Weld Boathouse and the Radcliffe Date Auction I was reset, reframed, and given a life that I could take in the right direction. It was also my first time being judged by the news, be it real, fake, or somewhere in between. It was the first time I had to go explore and connect with people in Boston who were outside of the normal college kid stuff on Huntington Ave. It's the reason that I give people multiple chances to prove who they are. Got a bad rap? I don't care. Are you at November Project to be kind, work your ass off, and start your day right? Then that's all that matters.

And Malcolm, if you or anyone from your Harvard Community are reading this, including Zuckerberg, the Twins, your undefeated teammate, Butt, Linda, Burger, Blocker, even the family of recently deceased Harry Parker, please know that I am sorry. If I'd had a full second to make a choice, I'd have stepped back and let you pass.

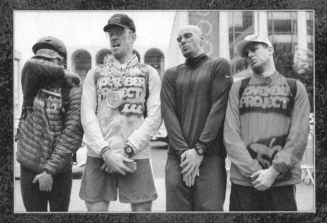

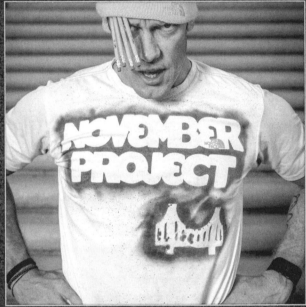

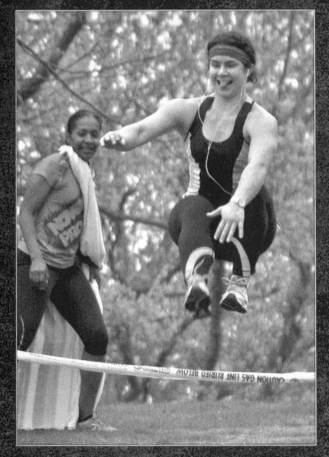

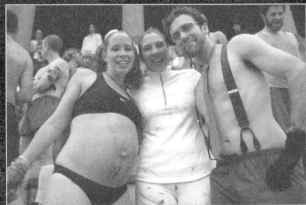

What's so weird about NOVEMBER PROJECT

"NP redefined Weird. Hugging strangers is totally normal at this point."
—Joey "Big 20" Kile, 26, product developer at New Balance, Boston

"The weirdest thing about NP is convincing yourself that spray paint is fashionable."
—Marinna Marotta, 25, counselor, Antioch, Ill.

"The whole thing's fuckin weird. Some of the clothing get-ups they come up with are pretty interesting. For an outsider to watch it, it's completely weird."
—Dean Karnazes, 53, renowned ultra runner and bestselling author, San Francisco

"The serious faces when taking pictures at the end of a workout. We're Minnesota Nice over here, it's hard for us not to smile!"
—Heidi Ylvisaker, 26, graphic designer, Minneapolis, Minn.

"The fact that otherwise 'normal' people will lose all inhibitions, put on costumes, and make complete fools of themselves without a moment's hesitation."
—Mary Anna Yram, 50, research compliance coordinator, Medford, Mass.

"This sh*t is totally normal."
—Bobbie Werbe, 34, "fulltime yahoo," co-leader, Indianapolis, IN

"Chanting weird noises and taking, tagging, and posting SO many running photos to Facebook."
—Alice Nelson, 28, geologist, Brookline, Mass.

"I don't find anything weird. Everything is awesome!"
—Deniz Karakoyunlu, 34, senior software engineer, Boston

"No morning at November Project is normal, and if it is, we're doing something wrong. We don't want to be normal because normal is boring. Normal is what you do for the rest of the day while at work, or school, or at home. We want to be the most abnormal thing you do on a Wednesday or Friday morning."
—Patrick O'Neill, 24, medical student, co-leader, Baltimore

"#Paulleak"
—Emily Faherty, 29, web editor, Hoboken, N.J.

"#Paulleak"
—Katherine Shea, 35, stage manager, Brooklyn, N.Y.

" The fact that BG and Bojan can get us to do whatever they say. Go running around Castle Island in the dark in freezing weather? Dress up like a dinosaur? Be inappropriate? Fuck yeah."
—Daisy Chow, 38, baker, Allston, Mass.

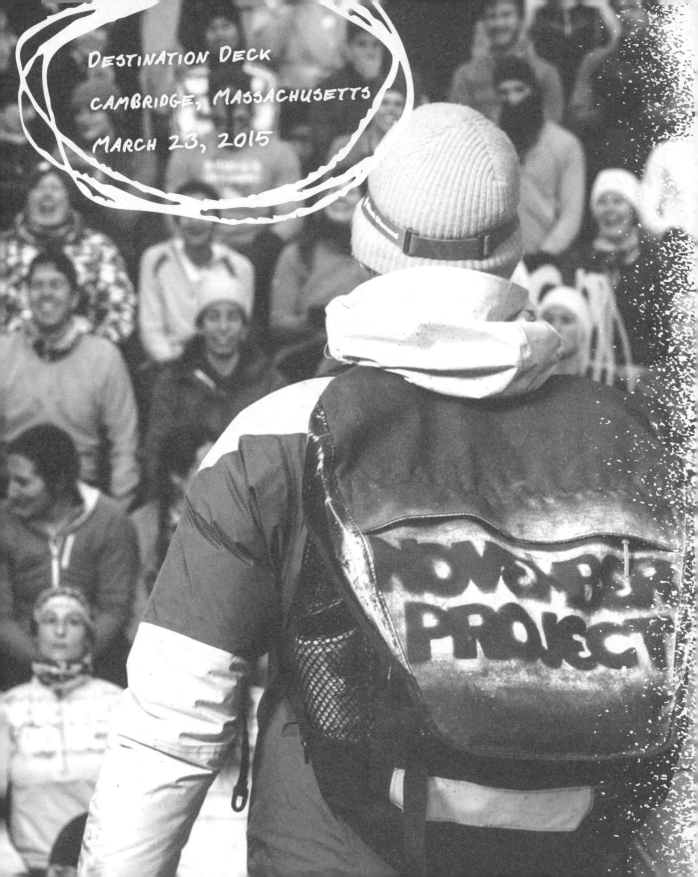

DESTINATION DECK

CAMBRIDGE, MASSACHUSETTS

MARCH 23, 2015

CHAPTER 5

"THIS IS WHERE EVERYTHING CHANGED FOR ME"

WISCONSIN NOTES

- #RUNDECKRUN

- HOW TO FALL IN LOVE WITH YOUR CITY

- WE RAN TO WHERE THE SMARTEST PEOPLE IN THE WORLD MEET AND DROPPED SOME INTENSE FITNESS KNOWLEDGE

- THE TRIBE IS TAKEN ON A JOY RIDE

- THAT FRANK GEHRY HAS ONE FEVERED IMAGINATION

- HOISTEES AND BURPEES AND PUSHUPS, OH MUTHAFUCKIN' MY!

- ONE TRIBE MEMBER STOPS MOVING AND GETS IN MOTION

Jesse Ledin swiped off the alarm on his phone on the second snooze, pushed away the covers, and padded across the dark room, doing his best not to wake his girlfriend, Katie. It was 4:48 a.m. She liked to sleep until the last minute, her clothes carefully laid out the night before. Ledin walked to the kitchen and poured himself a bowl of Honey Nut Cheerios. For a moment, the 37-year-old stood in the living room on the eighth floor of his condominium in Boston's Seaport district, taking in the lights of World Trade Center Boston, the rows of flags fluttering hard. He checked the weather app on his phone: 16°F. Then he pulled on his gear—dark blue leggings, a long-sleeve compression top, his orange 2014 Boston Marathon jacket, his November Project neck wrap, and a blue knit cap.

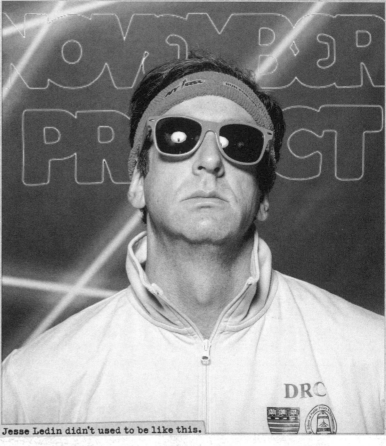

Jesse Ledin didn't used to be like this.

Even though he'd been attending November Project workouts for almost 2 years, Ledin still felt nervous before NP, especially Destination Deck. What would the workout be? A circuit? Seven minutes of burpees? He loathed and loved (loaved?) burpees. Or a surprise, like the time they ended up kayaking on the river, or the unfolding of zany fitness commands that were hidden in Easter eggs? Who would be there? How would he perform? He placed his empty cereal bowl in the sink and took a long drink of water.

Added in July 2012, Monday's Destination Deck (DD) was the last workout to join the NP menu. The idea: run to a random spot in the city for an intense round of calisthenics and then back home again, adding distance if you lived less than 6 miles away. The location was posted on social media and a day or two later, bodies converged, flash-mob-style, on college campuses, maligned neighborhoods, city beaches, municipal plazas, alleyways, even on top of an old landfill by the highway. The workout, always a surprise, might last anywhere from 7 to 21 minutes. Initially, Graham and Mandaric greeted tribe members with decks of cards to flip, suits and numbers dictating pushup, sit-up, and reps. As the membership swelled, the decks were more or less replaced with high-octane exercises that utilized public spaces as gym equipment: walls, ledges, benches, statues, steps, tennis courts, playgrounds.

SUNDAY, MAY 5, 2013

Runner's World contributor Caleb Daniloff, now known on the team as "Ethan Bookman," is given the assignment of telling the story of November Project in 1,000 words or less. The dude falls into our trap, and he develops a larger story as he JUST CAN'T NOT SHOW UP and JUST CAN'T STOP WRITING.

WEDNESDAY, JULY 10, 2013

Andrew Ference leaves Boston as his pro hockey life takes him to his hometown of Edmonton, AB. At his last workout, the whole Boston tribe sings the Canadian National Anthem: www.youtube.com/watch?v=YrsCZBUxyI0. In Edmonton, Andrew's sister Jen, and Nadim Chin, a die-hard Oilers fan, take NP international by becoming the fourth tribe to come on board.

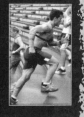

Today's DD was at MIT, about 4 miles away in Cambridge. Ledin took the elevator to the lobby. He and Katie liked to run at different paces and often set out separately. Ledin looked at himself in the reflection of the doors. He stood just over 6 feet and weighed a solid 230 pounds. His legs and backside were thick, like they belonged to a different, heavier torso. The skin around his cheeks was loose. A body in transformation. There was also a looseness in his dark brown eyes that hadn't always been there, where the grip of a troubled past had once clung. He stepped out of the atrium and onto the darkened lane, the wind bullying a torn coffee cup down the sidewalk. He jogged around a couple stubborn mounds of snow that were studded with fossilized cigarette butts (it had been a brutal winter in Boston; still was), zipped his jacket up to the collar, clicked on his GPS, and set off.

About a half mile up the boulevard, Ledin came upon a long line of news vans, satellite dishes sprouting up from rooftops like mushrooms. Through the windows, he saw occupants inside reading, blowing on coffee mugs, catching sleep. All of them waiting for testimony to resume at the nearby John Joseph Moakley Federal Courthouse, where the trial of admitted Boston Marathon bomber Dzhokhar Tsarnaev was taking place. It was week three. Like many in Boston, Ledin had a connection to the finish line attacks. On that fateful afternoon, he had left his spot in front of Marathon Sports, the site of the first bomb, which had killed 29-year-old waitress Krystle Campbell and maimed hundreds, 15 minutes before the explosions. "A lot of people I'd been standing with there for several hours, talking to, I later saw on TV injured," he said in a soft-spoken voice. "That easily could have been me."

Warmed up, Ledin picked up his pace as he strode across the bridge spanning the Fort Point Channel and headed toward Downtown Crossing, the open wind using his face for a speed bag. Across Atlantic Avenue, steam poured from a pair of manhole covers like sleeves. A few trees were strung with white lights. The occasional hooded figure, a construction worker perhaps, strode across the road. Otherwise, the city was quiet, dark and still, like a movie set. Ledin, the China Programs coordinator at Harvard's Kennedy School of Government, relished this peaceful time, that feeling of promise, when Boston had not yet revealed itself, that it was somehow his to shape now that the rest of the world had loosened its grip. He took such moments as a reminder that he was free, too, his life finally his to determine.

Ledin cut through Boston Common, into a deserted Public Garden, across the twisting Fiedler footbridge, and onto the Esplanade along the Charles River. He was striding at a tidy 9-minute-mile pace. Two-plus years earlier, when he was carrying some 312 pounds on his frame, his miles were measured strictly by car odometer. Aside from some snowboarding back in Wisconsin, he'd never been one to consciously break a sweat. It wasn't in the family DNA. But determined to get his weight under 300 pounds, he'd begun dipping his toe in the local fitness scene. It was then that Ledin came across November Project on social media. He followed them for a few months before he got up the nerve to show up.

"Stepping into Harvard Stadium that first day with Katie, I thought we were in the wrong place. I had very low self-esteem and was really intimidated seeing all these crazy, insane fit people. Everyone had their shirts off. My anxiety was running high. I was ready to walk right out. But I stuck around for the newbie meeting. I was completely scared of Brogan. But as soon as he started speaking and mentioned that he was from Wisconsin, my home state, I felt a wave of easiness. His passion came out instantly. I got through a few sections and was dying. I was probably 60 pounds heavier than I am now. But I did it. Now, I'm about to run my fifth marathon."

SATURDAY, AUGUST 17, 2013

Driven by media wins, interest in expanding November Project to more cities is obvious. To preserve core values and maintain quality control, BG and Bojan develop intense guidelines that every leader should possess and use to create a rigorous pledge process. Pledge Zero is a young triathlete, Danny Metcalf, from Washington, DC.

NOVEMBER 2013

November Project DC (Danny Metcalf and Steve Christensen), Denver (Dan Berteletti), and San Diego (Jessie Craik, Ashleigh Bordwell, and Lauren Padula) all come into the family. #Powerful7

FRIDAY, NOVEMBER 8, 2013

The Boston tribe has the full unfolded cover, front, inside, back cover, and 10 pages inside the December issue of Runner's World magazine. BG's "presentation" at the Runner's World gathering during the New York City Marathon, which includes roughly 20 F-bombs, lights up the room and untucks a lot of shirts.

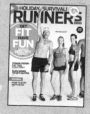

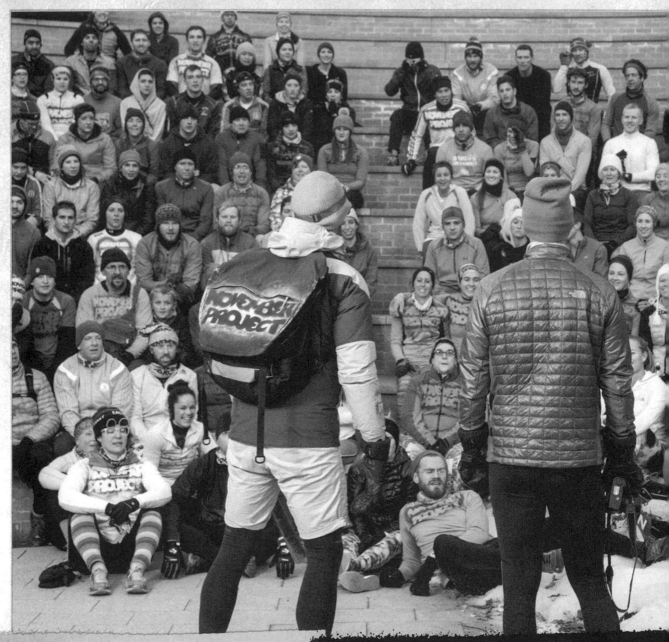

SATURDAY, DECEMBER 14, 2013

The First Annual November Project Summit (#NPSUMMIT) is held in Edmonton, AB (Canada), bringing ten coleaders together for a powwow and assorted antics. BG and Bojan pay for the event along with generous discounts from Westin Hotels (huge love for runners via the RunWestin concierge program, which is seriously legit).

#NPSUMMIT

WEDNESDAY, JANUARY 29, 2014

November Project family expands into Baltimore, MD (Nick Rodricks), Philadelphia, PA (Suzanne Allaire), and Indianapolis, IN (Bobbie Werbe). #Power10*

*No, we weren't "power" tripping with similar hashtags. Power10 is a rowing move where the crew tries to overtake or pull away from another boat.

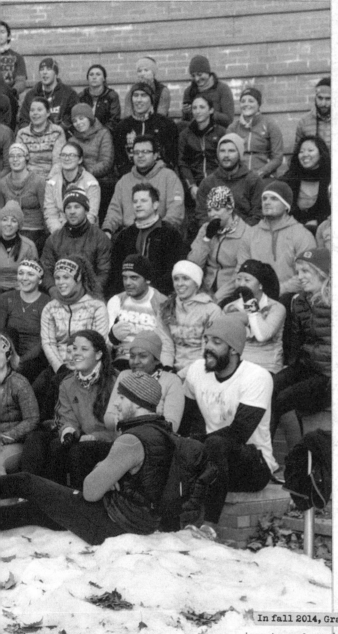

Headlights from Storrow Drive washed over Ledin's face as he sawed his arms against the darkness. The Harvard Bridge, which connects Boston and Cambridge, began materializing through the mist as he strode closer. "Someday, I'd like to do a full Ironman triathlon," he continued. "Being around all these other people who are super athletes, doing marathons, really motivates you. I had never really challenged myself before November Project."

As if on cue, out of the darkness, another figure in the same orange Boston Marathon jacket appeared, moving at a rapid clip. It was Seth Waltz, a tall 26-year-old 3:03 marathoner, who was training to qualify for the elite field at Boston (sub-2:21). A core tribe member, he gave Ledin a high-five as he passed. "I'll be there, buddy, just getting in extra speed work," he yelled over his shoulder.

"See ya there," Ledin called and smiled, as he wheeled onto the bridge's access ramp.

As much as November Project had transformed Ledin's body (his marathon PR is 3:53.02), it had, more importantly, jump-started a battered spirit.

"I've always been extremely shy. People thought I was a mute growing up. Teachers would call on me at school and I wouldn't answer. I always cared what people thought about me. If I kept quiet, people couldn't judge me based on something I say."

Ledin grew up in Mellen, Wisconsin, a small town in the northern reaches of the state. With a population of 800, everyone in town knew each other, especially the Ledins.

"We were a large family. My brother and sister are morbidly obese. My parents were pretty large. We were the family that everyone teased to make themselves feel better. We were all bullied relentlessly growing up. We were not liked at all."

It got so bad, Ledin revealed, that they were eventually driven out of town.

In fall 2014, Graham and Mandaric handed over the reins of the Boston tribe.

WEDNESDAY, MARCH 5, 2014

After leaving his hometown of Madison, DG decides to start November Project Milwaukee. In this class, he's joined by Los Angeles, CA (Orrin Whalen), New York, NY (John Honerkamp and Paul Leak), and Minneapolis, MN (Ben Bauch). #Turbo15 #PaulLeak

APRIL 2014

November Project members solidify the tradition of volunteering at the water station at mile 18 of the Boston Marathon. Across the road, a separate, raucous NP cheer station celebrates everything that moves. #cheereverything. NP volunteer and cheer stations at marathons and half-marathons in NP cities become the norm.

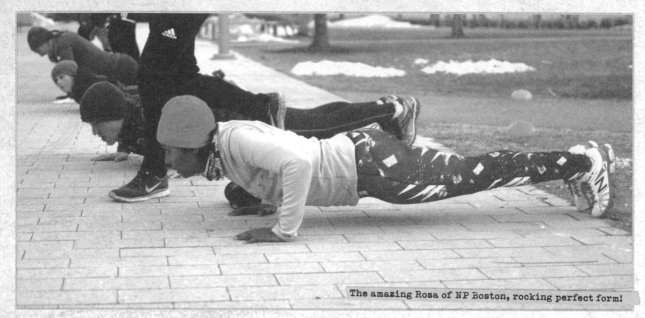
The amazing Rosa of NP Boston, rocking perfect form!

"No one would rent to us, so we had to move a half hour north when I was in middle school. They actually had a celebration at a local bar when we left."

The family moved to Ashland, a port city on Lake Superior with a population of almost 10,000. But things didn't get easier.

"When I was 14," Ledin said, "I was working at the local library and I got sexually assaulted by an older man. That brought me down even further. I gave a statement to the police, but I lied about what happened, just that a guy had made advances. I didn't tell anyone the whole truth. I just put it out of my mind and tried to move on."

Corroding under a buried secret and fevered with shame, high school was a barren existence for Ledin. He spent most of his time alone, in front of the TV or hunched over a sketch pad. His family didn't have much money, but he was desperate to go to college, to escape. He managed to get into the University of

Wisconsin-Superior, a school known for graduating future action star and California governor Arnold Schwarzenegger.

"I wasn't prepared at all. I failed out after one year. I tried again at another college and failed out again. I became deeply depressed. I tried to commit suicide. Where I grew up, there were a lot of suicides, and I just looked at it as a solution other people had tried. I was just about to kill myself when the cops arrived and talked me down."

Ledin moved in with his sister in Eau Claire, a town located in Central Wisconsin. There, he met Katie. She helped him get back into school and graduate, becoming the first in his family to finish a 4-year school. Then they moved to Milwaukee. Despite the hard-won college diploma and a supportive girlfriend, Ledin wanted to stay on the move, never letting anyone get to know him. "It was just easier to be a stranger," he said. But severe depression kept him company everywhere he went, with particularly dark bouts after his father's death in 2006,

APRIL—MAY 2014

Newest additions Chicago, IL (Brent Cunningham) and New Orleans, LA (Cameron Gilly, Kate Gilly, Preston Reader, and Will Booher) blow the tribe up to 17 locations. Tribe is rated #NP17 for mature audiences, though children are allowed with adult supervision.

NP-17 | NO ONE 17 AND UNDER ADMITTED

MAY 24, 2014

BG marries his yoga instructor, long-time member of November Project, Goldie Kaufenberg, making her Goldie Graham...which sounds a lot like Golden Grahams, the popular children's cereal that is neither healthy or free (#Irony). Former creative director from Arnold Worldwide, who oversaw the New Balance Runnovation video, and now loyal friend, Mike Howard performs the service in Southern California.

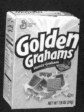

and again in 2011, 2 years after moving to Boston to attend a graduate program in architecture. No matter where he turned, his heart kept pumping out waves of shame, weakness, and failure, and he spent enormous energy keeping it below the surface.

Until those first painful steps at Harvard Stadium.

While he still tended to stand off to the side of the group and waited for others to approach him, over the next few months he was meeting new faces, learning the names of folks who didn't seem to care what he looked like or how shriveled he felt inside.

"NP was where everything changed for me. I was in this community where they didn't need to know anything about me. They'd give me hugs. They wanted to get to know me. I'd never experienced that before. I'd never experienced community before. I don't want to be a stranger."

Soon invitations came for social events. He joined off-shoot run groups, began signing up for races with other NPers. "I've finally found a place where I feel accepted, and know that I could go to a few different cities and there's an NP there and I'd be accepted there, too. My perspective on life has changed 180 degrees. My depression has completely gone away."

As Ledin crossed Memorial Drive and strode up Mass Ave, he saw neon figures emerging from the darkness, like a colorful zombie apocalypse. Clouds of breath arrived a moment before wind-chapped faces, gloved hands wiping at watery eyes and dripping nostrils. A group had gathered on the stairs in front of the MIT dome, with more runners joining every few moments, steam rising off their shoulders and hats. Watches and phones were paused and embraces delivered with the gusto of airport reunions. A few people pulled Ledin into their arms. Katie wended her way through the bodies and hugged her boyfriend.

"I don't need to hide from my truth anymore," Ledin said. "I'm not embarrassed. If people are going to judge me because of my past, then I don't need them in my life. Everyone's got a history. I've buried my real self my whole life. But I've found a comfort level now where I can share with people I trust. And I do trust people at NP. That's one of the coolest things about this whole thing: They're really true and genuine people."

"All right, people, bring it in," a thin voice rose into the air. "Top steps, everyone."

The voice belonged to 31-year-old Evan Dana, a web developer and one of the Boston tribe's new leaders. Standing 5 foot 6, the wiry Dana was almost a foot shorter than his predecessor. But he was a 2:54 marathoner who could knock out 150 burpees in 7 minutes, and had been a core member from the get-go. "Let's—" he screamed, leaping into the air, "—getalittlebounce!"

Five months earlier, Ledin and Katie, along with the rest of the Boston tribe, were jolted when Mandaric and Graham announced they were turning over the controls of the Mother Ship. The pair were quitting their jobs—Graham at New Balance, Mandaric as a freelance graphic designer, to hit the road and focus their energies on spreading November Project, which by that time had grown to 16 tribes around North America. The movement had taken the shape of a spear tip in the grassroots social-fitness trend. Knock-off groups had sprouted, some borrowing heavily, and unabashedly, from the NP playbook, especially when it came to photography and social media. And for the past year, Graham and Mandaric had been courted by high-profile athletic brands seeking a partnership. If November Project was to continue to evolve, they reasoned, then they needed to redefine and expand their roles. There were worries and grumblings, of course: Would NP sell out? Would the fitness level get watered down? Would membership shrink without The BG & Bojan Show?

"Okay, this isn't the site of today's workout," said Dana. "Follow Deniz and get ready to run. Now!"

SUMMER 2014

Talks with Major Brands take place throughout the summer. Both Bojan and BG are ready to let someone help them with November Project. Co-branding, acquisition, and other big-kid phrases are not options. What they need is the freedom to manage this movement at a time when TIME isn't something that either dude has much of.

SUMMER 2014

A "tester" partnership between November Project LLC and The North Face, spearheaded by TNF marketing director Katie Ramage, begins. In exchange for comped entries and travel to TNF ECS races, along with resources for the next Summit, BG and Bojan open their brains about free, grassroots fitness. BG, Bojan, and assorted tribe members begin racing all eight North Face Endurance Challenge Series races. NP racers sweep the podiums and most of the top-20 spots.

THE NORTH FACE

Deniz Karakoyunlu, a member of the B.A.A. running team and an Ironman (3 years earlier, he was a back-of-the-pack 5-Ker), blasted down the steps to the sidewalk, legs kicking wildly, arms swinging every which way. ("He runs like Pre," Mandaric once said of Deniz, a Turkish-born runner. "Total joyful abandon."). Karakoyunlu, along with former Harvard strength and conditioning coach Emily Saul, had also been tapped to helm the Boston tribe. Karakoyunlu rounded a corner, the lead dogs on his heels, down a delivery driveway, past a length of wooden construction-site walls, and around another corner. The rest of the tribe trailed behind him like a hopped-up centipede, turning the heads of surprised hard-hatted workers and early-morning professional staffers. Rising into view came MIT's surreal Stata Center, designed by renowned architect Frank Gehry, with its fairytale vibe, all bent angles and stainless-steel box windows that jutted off the building's silvery skin.

Hugging one side of the building was a brick landing that overlooked a stone-rowed, outdoor amphitheater. At the bottom, between several piles of snow, stood two large silhouettes, like Greek actors on a stage. Graham and Mandaric. The original gangsters were back. The Serbian was dressed in black tights and a green Larry Bird jersey. In one hand he held a music player, in the other a camera. Graham was sporting his trademark orange-knit farm hat that was cinched with a headlamp, khaki hiking shorts over black running tights, and a yellow puff jacket. On his back, a giant pack spray-painted with the NP logo. It was Throwback Thursday on a Monday. You could almost feel the chill drain from the air as a collective warmth washed over a hundred-plus wide-smiling faces. Ledin and Katie made their way down to the front.

"Okay, Okay, O-motherfuckin'-K! Hello, my name is Brogan Graham and this is my good Serbian friend and personal astrologer Bojan Mandaric. Am I pronouncing that correctly, sir? Manda-rick? Manda-rich? We've been friends 10 years and I still don't fuckin' know your name."

Mandaric smiled, stroking his ginger beard. "Just stick to the single syllables, my dude."

"Okay, we asked Deniz, Emily, and Evan a big favor this morning—to take their badass tribe out for a spin. We promised we wouldn't scratch their ride, so let's bang out some squats to keep warm while people take their seats. Down. Up. Down. Up...Okay, for this morning's workout—this is just too fuckin' cool, I miss this

shit—there's gonna be four stations. We're going to split you into groups and put 20 minutes on the clock."

"A couple of quick demonstrations for the new kids," Mandaric said. "First, a hoistee."

Graham and Mandaric faced each other, grasped opposite hands, leaned back, and squatted in unison, 500 pounds of yin and yang. Then they burst up off their feet together, yelling "hoistee!" at the top. One of a handful of NP-created exercises.

"Very important, ass all the way down to the ground," Mandaric said. "You'll do 10 of these at the hoistee station across the quad behind me."

"Then run diagonally across the lawn," Graham said. "Over here to my right, you will do something we like to call a pushup. Five of those, perfect form. If you want to do them from your knees, or 'boy pushups,' then do them like this. If you're feeling cocky, put your feet up on the bench. That's for our Extended Warrior people. From the pushup zone, we're going up these rows of seats, two-footed hops, all the way up the center. If you want to scale down, march it up, but stay to the left. If you want to scale it down more, use the exit row. If you want to scale it down even further, just take a seat. We'll be done in 20 minutes."

"After the steps," Mandaric jumped in, "by that warped mirror, there's a nice little pi graffiti. Touch that and do five—yep, you guessed it—BURPEES! Chest all the way to the ground. From there, you're gonna run down the stairs, round the corner, and sprint your ass off back to the hoistee station. Repeat for 20 minutes. Race every single person alive. Cool?"

"Cool," Graham said.

Graham divided the group, sending the clusters to their respective stations. Mandaric threw on the music and began shouting, "Three! Two! One! Go!"

And with that, four explosions of neon bodies burst into the frosty air like buckshot. At the stairs, runners hurled themselves up two-footed, arms swinging, ponytails spraying overhead. Fifteen rows in all. Graham took a position at the top, egging everyone on. His voice canyon-deep as if forged in the earth's molten core, words hurtling out in bold, capital letters:

"ALL THE WAY, ALL THE WAY! HIT THE DECK AND GO! FULL SPEED OFF THE STADIUM. ADAM SOGOLOFF, TURN IT UP, BUDDY! NO ROOM TO BE POLITE! LET'S GOOOOOOOOOO!"

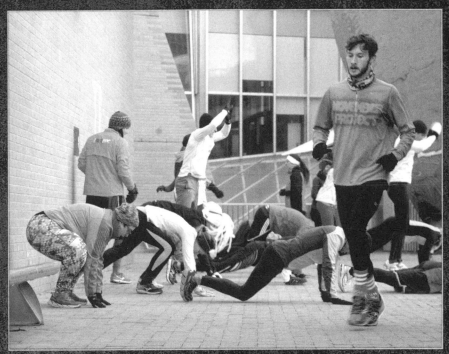

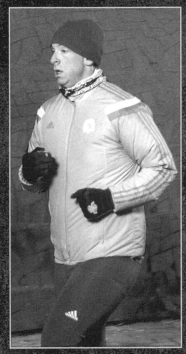

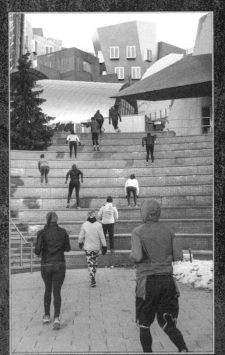

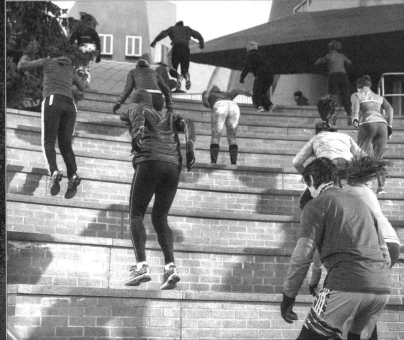

7 minutes in ...

Beyond his shoulder, the mirrored lower panels on the Gehry building shimmered with color and motion, reflecting fun-house images of jump-backs, pushups, and leaps. Ledin knocked off his burpees and took off down the stairs, around the corner, and turned on a full-on sprint to the hoistee station, where Mandaric was jumping and shouting, channeling his old coaching days on the Onondaga Lake at Syracuse University.

"IF YOU'RE WAITING MORE THAN TEN SECONDS FOR A PARTNER, START DOING AIR SQUATS! DO NOT STAND AROUND! REST WHEN YOU'RE DEAD! YEAH, BUDDY, NICE WORK! LET'S SEE THOSE HOISTEES! ASS ALL THE WAY DOWN! EIGHT MINUTES! EIGHT MINUTES DOWN! THAT'S IT DENIZ, YOU'RE WINNING, BUDDY, YOU'RE WINNING!"

Ledin hopped up the steps, clouds of steam curling from his face, as staffers came to the windows to explore the commotion down below. Graham clapped Ledin on the back as he hopped down to the top landing, tilting him toward the burpee station for another round. Ledin loved that impossible voice. Against that soundtrack, he felt like he'd never slow down.

"COME ON, GUYS! WHEN YOU SEE ME, GO TO WORK! TAYLOR, YEAH! HOW ARE YOU, DUDE? GO, GO, GO! JAMES BROAD, LET'S GO: BIG DOUBLE ARM SWING AND GO! THAT AWAY, MORGAN BROWN! WHAT YOU GOT, JESS? ARMS ALL THE WAY THROUGH! BOOM—AND THEN YOU'RE GONE! JOEY KILE! YEAH, BOSS! YOU'RE KILLING IT!"

Flying up the steps was a lithe blond woman, springing like a feather, her hair whipping upward. For the past

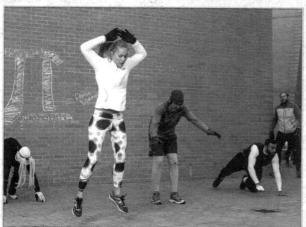

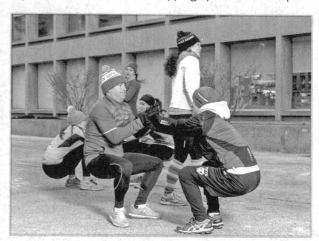

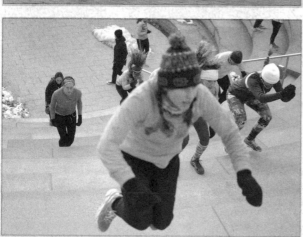

9 minutes to go . . .

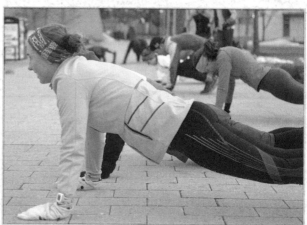

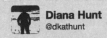
Diana Hunt
@dkathunt

⚙ 👤 Follow

When your arm gets tired high-fiving the entire tribe. #novemberprojectproblems #milelonghighfive #AllMayMon @nov_projectprob

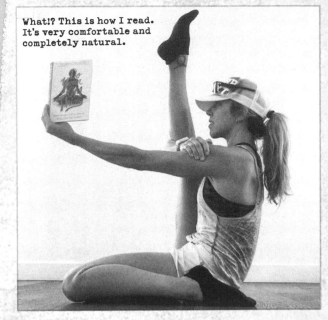

What!? This is how I read. It's very comfortable and completely natural.

4 years, she'd been one of Boston's top yoga instructors, known for a popular blacklight, hip-hop practice. Beneath her puff jacket and long-sleeve top, on her inner right bicep read a tattoo: "A good name is cool, but pairs of them are better." Graham had the same line inked on his chest.

"THERE YOU GO, GOLDIE GRAHAM! NO JOGGING AT THE TOP, GOLDIE GRAHAM! WE'RE NOT CELEBRATING WITH A NICE JOG! CELEBRATE WITH A DASH, GOLDIE GRAHAM!"

Goldie tossed her husband the bird and said, "Love you." He grinned ear to ear. Across the quad, Mandaric had dropped to his knee, proposal style, and was snapping pictures while Saul, wearing a bike cap over her long curly hair and sky-blue flip-up glasses, was pairing up partners and pulling anyone who looked lost into her hoistee hands. She had a powerful rower's build, and her guns were the envy of both the guys and the ladies of NP. "Ass all the way down!" she yelled. "Cheeks to pavement!" Mandaric sprung up and wove himself into a group sprinting back.

"YEAH SHIRA, THAT'S WHAT I'M TALKING ABOUT! LET'S GO, DANNY, YEAAAAAAHH! PARTY'S HALF OVER! TEN MINUTES DOWN! IF YOU'RE NOT BREATHING HARD ENOUGH, I'M NOT GONNA TELL YOU WHAT! LET'S GO, LADIES, RACE IT THE FUCK OUT! TEN MINUTES DOWN!"

At the pushup station, Dana was demonstrating form, planked as straight as a board, arms against his chest, yoga style. To the side, a tribe photographer was shooting. At the top steps, another shutterbug had her lens trained on the steps. From the beginning, aside from Mandaric, a handful of other NPers showed up to the workouts with cameras to spread the imagery through unofficial NP photo sites. Top-notch photography has always played into NP

strategy. Post killer pics, tag the hell out of them, watch newsfeeds swell, change profile and cover shots, and let the comment boxes fill: "What the hell is this November Project you keep posting about?" Beautiful, viral simplicity.

"NINETY SECONDS!" MANDARIC SHOUTED. "LAST MINUTE—THIRTY! YOU GOT THIS! LAAAAAAAAAAST MINUTE!"

Suddenly, the two booming voices were harmonizing from different parts of the quad.

"IT'S THE *WORK!* **ALL ABOUT THE WORK!** *BANG IT OUT!* **WE ONLY GOT THIRTY SECONDS!** *BEAUTIFUL! BARELY ENOUGH TIME!* **FIVE BURPEES!** *HIT THE DECK!* **AAAAAND TIIIIIIIIIME!!!"**

"Okay, guys," Graham said, turning to the burpee station. "Go to someone in your area, touch elbows, look 'em in the eyeballs, and say, 'Good morning.' Then go grab a seat."

Nicholas Panarello @nickpanarello   4 Apr
Every morning I wake up and can't decide what color neon to wear @nov_projectprob
🔁 Retweeted by Nov_Project Problems

A flurry of "good mornings" filled the air, though a few people were hunched over, catching their breath, only able to touch elbows with their own knees. Others shuffled back to the amphitheater, wiping sweat from foreheads and mouths.

"Guys, pay attention," Graham said. "It's cold and we want to get you outta here."

When all the rows were filled in, Graham continued.

"So when I raise my right foot, I want everyone on this side to say, 'Heeeyyyy . . .' And if I go real high, keep stretching it out: 'Heyyyyyyyyyyyyyyyyyyy.' You guys over on this side, you're going to say the word 'Nooooo' when I lift my left foot. Let's practice: Right foot: 'Hey.' Left foot: 'No.' Right, left. You gotta be sharp now."

And with that, Graham launched into a high-stepping, sumo-lunging, galloping-horse pose, and a cloud of call-and-response noise enveloped the courtyard.

"HeeeyyyyNoooHeyHeyHeyNo-NooooooHeyyyyyHeyNoNoNoNo-Heyyyyyyy . . ."

A few students stopped and stared as Graham picked up his pace, trying to fake out the group. Within moments, he'd become some kind of 6-foot-6 human instrument, a giant pipe organ being hammered by musicians at a remote keyboard. It was hard to tell if he was playing the crowd or the crowd was playing him. Ledin threw his head back in laughter, clapping. After a couple seconds, Graham was hopping like he was dancing on lava and the voices mashed into one joyful sound before the chorus collapsed into laughter with a dose of what-the-fuck-just-happened?

"It's not a cult," Mandaric deadpanned.

Graham held up a worn wooden stick and waved it in the air. It was carved with the November Project logo and a goat. No one knows why the goat.

"Okay, for you new cats, this is the Positivity Award. Hold on, whose first day is today?"

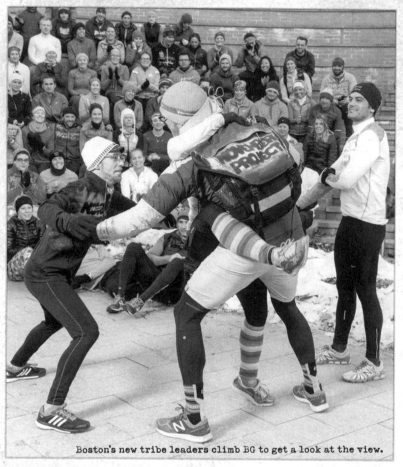

Boston's new tribe leaders climb BG to get a look at the view.

A couple hands shot up and were met with hoots and the muted claps of gloved hands.

"Look atchoo, checking us out on a sub-zero Monday," Graham said. "You are officially my motherfuckin' heroes. Welcome. Now put your hands back under your ass.

"This is an old oar handle from . . ."

Mandaric stepped over and whispered something into Graham's ear.

"Oh shit, right," Graham said, smiling. "Are there any birthdays in the house?"

"Does Saturday count?" a voice yelled out.

"Nope. But keep coming and in 2 years, we'll celebrate the shit out of your birthday. Does anyone have a birthday To. Day. This day, Monday of this day. No? Good. 'Cause I'm freezing my nuts off."

Normally, the birthday gal or dude is called to the

front after the workout and serenaded with the happy birthday song while they perform some silly routine like tossing one article of clothing in the air or twirling like a ballerina, log rolling, or slow-dancing with their birthday twins or getting crowd-surfed. Other times, they get birthday-boomed. You'll just have to show up to see what that is.

"OK, back to our regularly scheduled program. This is an old oar handle from our Northeastern rowing days.

"We give this award to somebody who drives the vibe in this group. Maybe they're super-fuckin' fast. Maybe they're super-fuckin' slow. But when they show up to train, which they'd do all the fuckin' time, members look at them and say, 'I'm glad they're here.' Today's PA is long overdue. It goes to a three-headed beast that's been driving all of you since early November. Make some noise for three of the most important people in NP in all 19 cities. Deniz, Emily, and Evan, come on up here."

Against a rainfall of applause, the three new Boston leaders bum-rushed Graham, all of them climbing his redwood-like frame like elementary school kids. No doubt, filling those size-16 shoes had been no easy task.

"Guys, for the group photo we're gonna change it up a bit," Mandaric smiled. "Straight face, straight back . . ."

The Serbian screwed the camera to his eye. Ledin, Katie, and the hundred others held their faces still like they were portraits hanging on a museum wall, the quad suddenly as mum as if a priest had farted.

"And just like those bus-driver mirrors, if you can't see my camera, I can't see you and you won't be in the picture," Mandaric shouted. "Okay, good posture, aaaand...HAVE A GREAT DAY!"

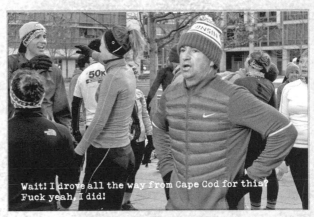

Wait! I drove all the way from Cape Cod for this? Fuck yeah, I did!

 ThePositivityAward @PositivityAward   Aug 29

Dear **@Nov_Project** **#NP17** leaders—I am tired of this "straight face" thing in photos with me. Please ask people to look happy!

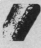 **ThePositivityAward** @PositivityAward   Aug 22

Without **@bmandaric** at **@Nov_Project** today it got DANGEROUS!!! Please come back soon Bojan!

 ThePositivityAward @PositivityAward   Aug 13

If **@Brogan_Graham** can put a bag on his cast for **@Nov_Project** the least he could do is unroll a **@TrojanBrand** (unlubricated) to keep me dry too.

 ThePositivityAward @PositivityAward   Aug 11

Hey **@Brogan_Graham** & **@bmandaric**- Was nobody sufficiently cheery this morning? Maybe some spareribs & egg rolls would have helped!

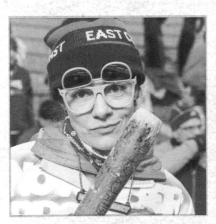
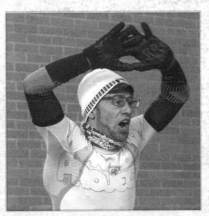
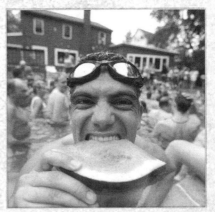

Ms. Pushups, Burpee Jesus, and Deniz. Love these people!

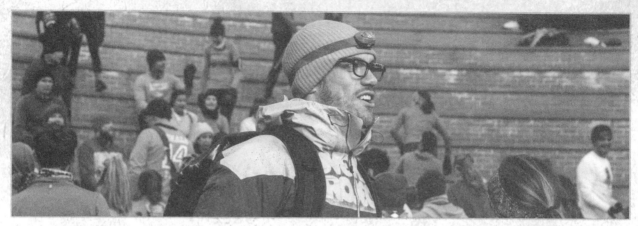

Homecoming for Bojan & BG at Today's Destination Deck (MIT)

🕐 23rd March 2015   👤 brogan   📁 Blog   💬 0 Comments

These days, both Bojan and I are lucky to travel North America to drop in on our current tribes, as well as launch new ones. Our life is on the road. He makes his way home to Boston while I make my way to my home base in SoCal. We lead this movement, without sleep or complaint, just like our fearless leaders, that's what we do. Rising and shining and connecting more and more with our leaders and members in each tribe has given us a better understanding of what this 19 city beast truly is. We've given up the stand-in-front leadership in trade for leading all tribes. In this trade we lurk in the back rows of countless group photos, introduce ourselves to unknowing newbies, wait quietly for the directions of the workout, and watch on with the rest of the members for exactly what to do. As we jump from one layover to the next, we cover ground, and connect the dots. What we don't get each Monday, Wednesday, and Friday each week is the feeling of being high, the feeling of owning the moment, and the feeling of having the entire group hanging on every word the way that we did back when we were both leading here in Boston. This feeling is one of the coolest benefits of being an NP leader. Leadership comes in countless shapes and roles, but leading in front is clearly a rush for those who do it best.

Today, Evan, Emily, & Deniz let us borrow their tribe back for one workout and take the NP Boston leadership role for a ride. The tribe with the hardest winter of all showed up proud on a frosty Monday morning to rip through 20 minutes of two-footed hop, dash, burpie, downhill dash, straightaway sprint, hoistee, dash, push-up circuit as the sun came up over MIT. The mean look of racing, the kind words of inclusion, and the warm embrace after we called "TIME!" were about as classic NP as it gets.

The truth is, being on the road gives us a point of view that makes the full NP picture much more clear and makes us proud of what this family has become. With that said, this morning, as the sun slowly made her way up over the frozen Charles River and onto the campus of some of the world's brightest minds (MIT students) and outfits (NP members) we were reminded of just how magic this Boston group is.

If you're reading this from outside of Boston and you've never experienced NP Boston, consider a trip here for at least a Wednesday and Friday. These leaders, athletes, and shared times are incredible. The tribe, now more than ever, is strong.

Flight leaves at 4PM today. See you at Mile 18 on Marathon Monday.

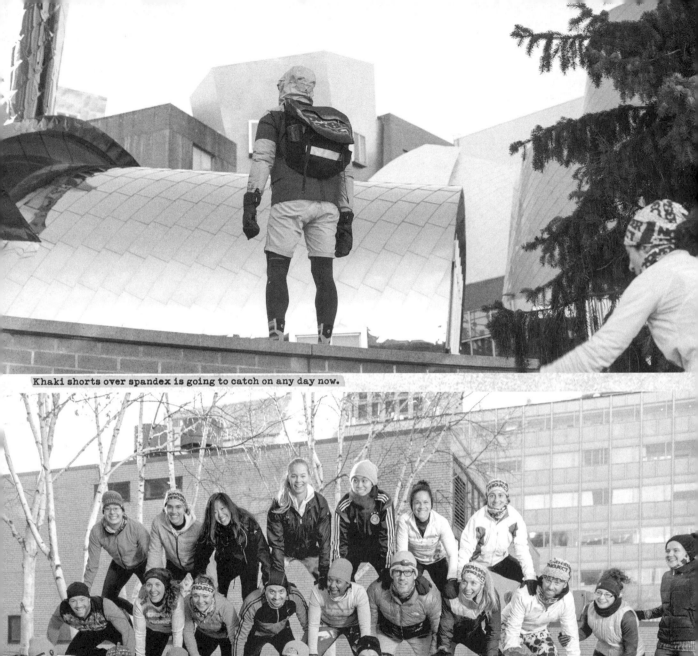

Khaki shorts over spandex is going to catch on any day now.

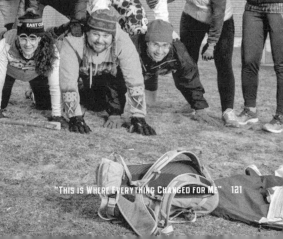

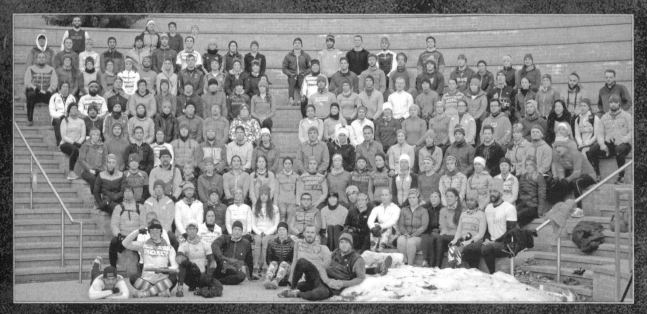

"THESE DUDES ARE HUGE. AND HILARIOUS. AND MOTIVATING. I FELT LIKE THEY WERE ALSO MANAGING A FINE BALANCE BETWEEN BG NEARLY KILLING US WITH CRAZY IDEAS OF WHAT WE COULD DO NEXT AND BOJAN KEEPING US ALIVE BY LENDING JUST A TINY OUNCE OF SANITY... BUT NEVER QUITE ENOUGH SANITY TO RUIN THE FUN. EVER. THEY'RE BOTH THE BEST KIND OF CRAZY."

—LAURA INGALLS, 36, HEALTH COACH AND DJ, NEWTON, MASS.

"I THOUGHT OF THEM KIND OF LIKE CELEBRITIES— OR YOUR FRIENDS' REALLY COOL OLDER BROTHER— THE KIND THAT IS IN HIGH SCHOOL WHEN YOU ARE IN MIDDLE SCHOOL AND YOU JUST KEEP THINKING, MAN I HOPE THEY NOTICE ME... AFTER A FEW MONTHS OF COMING TO NP REGULARLY, BG FRIENDED ME ON FACEBOOK. I INSTANTLY TEXTED ALL MY NP FRIENDS, I WAS SO PUMPED. BG AND BOJAN BOTH HAVE THIS QUALITY ABOUT THEM THAT IS EXTRA MOTIVATING TO ME. I AM HAVING TROUBLE PUTTING TO WORDS JUST WHY THAT IS, BUT WHEN THEY CHEERED FOR ME OR RAN BESIDE ME, I DUG DEEPER, SO MUCH DEEPER."

—ALICE NELSON, 28, GEOLOGIST, BROOKLINE, MASS.

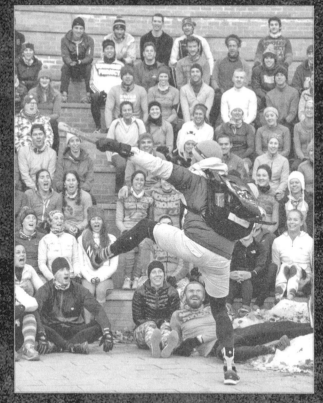

BG, the human orchestra conductor

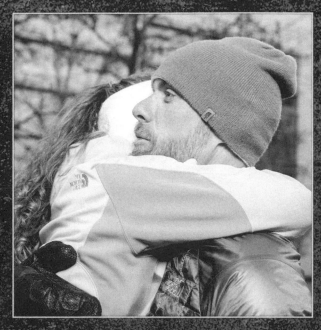

"I WILL ADMIT, THAT AT FIRST I FOUND THEIR PASSION TERRIFYING! I LEARNED QUICKLY THAT THERE ARE NO MISTAKES AND THE ONLY WAY TO DISAPPOINT IS BY BEING UNKIND, RUDE OR NOT BEING SUPPORTIVE OF OTHERS."

—KRISTIN CARLSON, 42, SPECIAL EDUCATION TEACHER, WATERTOWN, MASS.

"ONE MIGHT THINK BOJAN IS THE 'QUIET ONE' (COMPLETELY RELATIVE TERM IN THIS SITUATION,) OH BUT HE HAS OPINIONS, MANY OF THEM."

—REBECCA DANIELS A.K.A. RAD, 33, PHOTOGRAPHER, SAN FRANCISCO

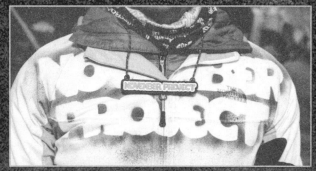

"WHEN I FIRST SAW BG, I ASSUMED HE WAS NOT HUMAN. NO ONE HAS THAT MUCH ENERGY, THAT MUCH ZEST FOR LIFE, OR IS THAT GIGANTIC."

—EMILY FAHERTY, 29, WEB EDITOR, HOBOKEN, N.J.

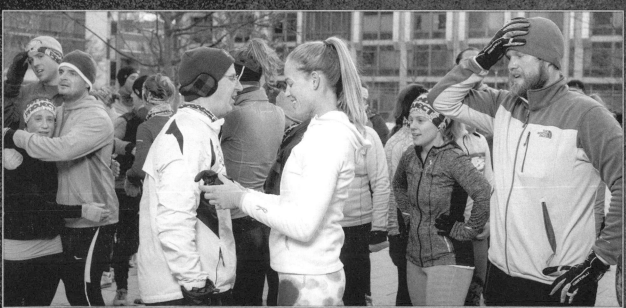

"I'm a Harvard researcher and a professional model. You review snacks and wear those funny finger toe shoes. At 6 a.m., we have a ton in common."

DESTINATION DECK

BY BROGAN GRAHAM

The Destination Deck (DD) was born from our first winter as a Tribe of Two. We'd meet somewhere on foot, running the miles to get there, hug, laugh, and stretch when we arrived. Then we'd hit the ground and flip cards until they were done. Once we got through the deck, we'd run back to our apartments and get ready for real life.

The deck, though many people do it in many ways, is done at NP like this: All black cards are pushups, all red cards are sit-ups. The value of each card gives you the total number of reps: 2 of Hearts = 2 sit-ups, 10 of Clubs = 10 pushups, and so on. The face cards are Jack (11), Queen (12), King (13), and Ace (14). This is simple. This is hard. Try it. Fuck it, try half a deck. Shuffle them up, put the deck down in a neat stack, get your ass on the ground, and one card at a time work your way through. Keep perfect form no matter how many breaks you need to take. Keep an eye on the clock. Take this workout to the sketchy floor of whatever hotel room your travels take you.

The most fun part of the Destination Deck almost right away became the locations. We wanted to make it colorful, interesting, and social. We also wanted to make the miles in favor of one neighborhood one week, and another the next. After the group began to build we did less and less cards and more and more weird shit instead. We always said, "Your dad told you never to go to certain neighborhoods and that's why we picked these locations [once the group was large enough to go wherever safely]."

We always felt it was silly that so many college students (ourselves included at one time) come to Boston for the same reason—"I can mix with all of the other students at all of the other [55+] colleges and universities"—and leave with a diploma and little understanding of the many neighborhoods inside Greater Boston. The Deck, especially after we started having to get creative, became a way to force ourselves and our members to

continue exploring the city. When someone says, "I've never run here before" or "I had no idea how to get here until today," we feel like we've won.

Below are a few of our most memorable DDs:

MFA Deck, October 8, 2012

We did a DD at the Museum of Fine Arts, or as us locals call it, the MFA. We used to get free admission as Northeastern students but rarely took advantage (I could actually see the MFA from my dorm room windows as a freshman). I always smile when I think of the MFA Destination Deck. For the first time with DDs, I'd come to Bojan with a super-excited idea and we took the group for a weird, wild ride, hoping it would work out.

This was back in 2012, when we didn't know if the number of athletes showing up would be a few dozen or a few hundred. In my memory, 74 folks were there for the MFA Deck. The MFA grounds are like most pristine lawns at museums...not for training on. Our workout that day was a combination of many things we liked: Run to the location on Huntington Ave. Gather. Explain the work. We split up into small groups, roughly 12 clusters, each getting their own deck of cards.

When the cowbell went off, the group rose to their feet, dashed to the driveway of the MFA, and sprinted directly to the preassigned "art space" where each athlete had his or her crayon (color chosen by the athlete) on top of a basic white piece of paper they'd each written their name on in all caps with a Sharpie before the workout began.

At the "art space," runners had an undetermined amount of time to draw the statue that stood proudly in front of the museum—a bare-chested Native American warrior leaning back on his horse, hands outstretched

Emily @jemily21 · 5 Oct 2013
@Nov_ProjectCAN @nov_projectprob **when a deck comes out for sociables but you think a work out is about to start...**

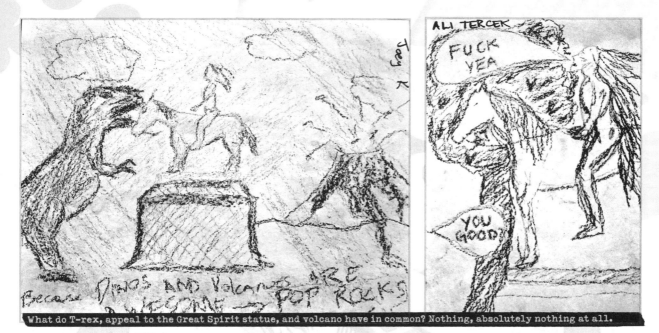

What do T-rex, appeal to the Great Spirit statue, and volcano have in common? Nothing, absolutely nothing at all.

toward the sky. When the bell went off again, they had to dash back to their decks and resume that work. Each art dash involved trading crayon colors with neighbors so that you never had the same color twice (this prompted social interactions). At the final bell, the art assignments were handed in, the group photo shot. Then the final run home. All before 7:15 a.m.

That day, we didn't post photos from the workout. Instead, we harnessed the power of social media. Each piece of art was put up in a full photo album, and the artist/athlete with the most LIKES won the prize of having their artwork as the November Project cover photo on Facebook for the week. If you go to the NP Facebook page now (we know your phone is within reach), you can scroll back in time and see the dude who won. While his drawing isn't exactly true to life, our online community seemed to love it the most.

Hurricane Deck, October 29, 2012

The Destination Deck on the Monday morning of Hurricane Sandy, in late October 2012, was epic and pretty stupid at the same time. It was warm and super dark. The rain was coming down hard, but the wind was ferocious. The group was small, in the 20 to 30 range I think, but we got down onto the ground and did a full session; no deck, but tons of work. As I remember it,

and my memory is at times as blurry as the visibility was, we did a Sebastian (7 minutes of straight-up burpees), hugged it out, and went our own way.

I clearly, CLEARLY, remember running into the wind upstream of the Eliot Bridge (as a rower would say). I looked at my mud-covered legs and thought, *"I've got 4 more miles to get home,"* but I settled into a nice pace and a huge smile. I like to remember that deck. That feeling of discovery, meeting a new set of people, a good deal of work under 20 minutes, and a prideful run home, is still there for many new folks on Monday mornings.

Kayak Deck, August 18, 2014

Every once in a while, when I think that I'm Mr. Creative and that Bojan is only in this to shut down my amazing ideas and fun...along comes something like the Kayak Deck. For months, Bojan had been working with Drew, a core member of NP Boston who worked at Charles River Canoe and Kayak, on the logistics of early-morning kayak racing with a group that could be as large as 250?! Waivers, a range of comfort on boats and in water, and many other variables...how long would it take? Is this even possible!?

On top of all of that, this was the Monday morning following our annual run-to-hidden-location social event

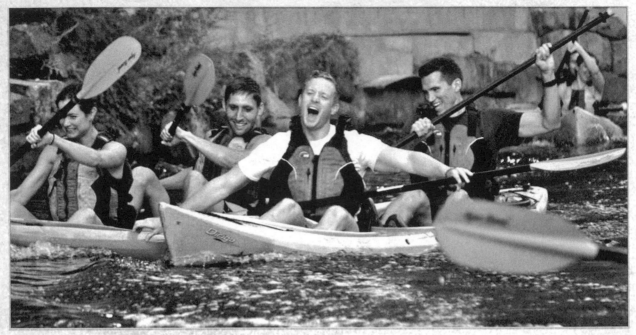

I'M HAVING ZERO FUN!

called Better Than Bedtime, where we paired up and dressed in matching outfits. The theme was Noah's Ark, They Came in Twos. Hungover, dark, Monday, kayaks, waivers, logistics, possible death via Charles River!?!? I was pumped that my man Bojan had come over to my side!! Fuck it, let's make this happen. The workout called for teams of four, with two runners and two paddlers. The running group would do laps and box jumps while their water-bound duo was paddling out-and-back from Kenmore to the main Charles River basin, passing under a bridge that the runners were running over. The sunrise, the vibe, the Speed Stack of waivers, and the zero death-count all combined to make this deck an outstanding hit!!

Bojan had dreamt it, built it, promoted it, photographed it, and didn't look back. To this day, I think this "deck" was one of our weirdest and most fun. And to you, Bojan—I assume you're reading this book, too (sorry if we didn't make a Serbian edition)—really great job. This workout was all you and all amazing. Onward, my dude.

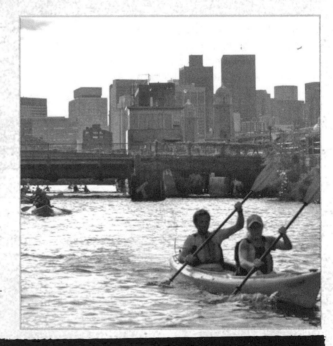

Nov_Project Problems @nov_projectprob · 8 Jul 2013
I have sand in my places #novemberprojectproblems #beachworkout
@Nov_Project

Egg Deck, May 12, 2014

I loaded maybe a hundred hollow plastic eggs with thin strips of paper. On each piece were typed directions: "bear crawl across the courtyard," "bray like a donkey for 30 seconds while spinning," "run back to your partner like a gorilla," "crab walk backwards." You get the picture. Silly shit. That morning at an outdoor courtyard on Boston University's campus along Comm Ave, we formed teams of two. While one partner held a plank, the other sprinted to one of a handful of elevated lawns planted with trees and shrubs and now scattered with eggs and started performing. It was happy chaos as everyone dashed, sang, chanted, crawled, and jumped their way across the yard while trying to avoid turning the workout into bumper cars. This was one of my favorite Destination Decks. People were having insane fun, eggs everywhere. And it wasn't even Easter. Just another regular Monday morning at NP. Boom.

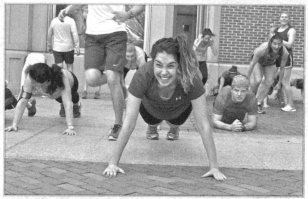

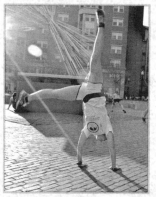

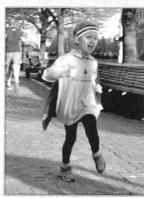

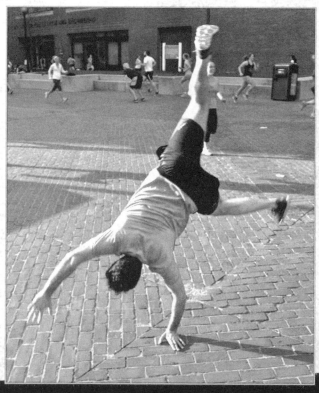

Oh, you didn't do cartwheels, monkey walks, giggling planks, and costumed sprints at your indoor workout this morning? That sucks...

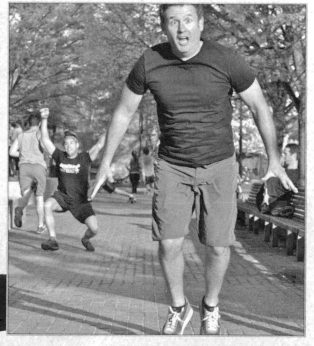

NOVEMBER PROJECT'S
DESTINATION DECK
FITNESS ELEMENTS

BY BROGAN GRAHAM

SEBASTIANS

Taken from the world of CrossFit. This jump-squat-push-up-jumping-jack mash-up was a no-brainer. No equipment, no resources, nothing; clothing optional. One of our most die-hard, core, badass-looking dudes at NP Boston is also an avid raver...I mean, CrossFitter...Okay, he raves too. Sebastian is the guy who will walk up to you and begin telling you all about his workout yesterday at CrossFit before you even know he's arrived. His intensity is what this workout is about. Seven minutes of burpees at November Project is called a "Sebastian." Women, men, kids, old folks. Try this. Burpees for 7 minutes. Know that our standard goal for men and women is to hit 100 total. Your bodyweight, your drive, your fitness. GO.

(Editor's note: The Sebastians record is currently held by Evan Dana a.k.a. Burpee Jesus from NP_BOS, who did 150 burpees in 7 minutes. "If I wasn't there counting each burpee, I'd call bullshit on Evan's 150 burpee effort," Bojan says. "That shit was impressive!")

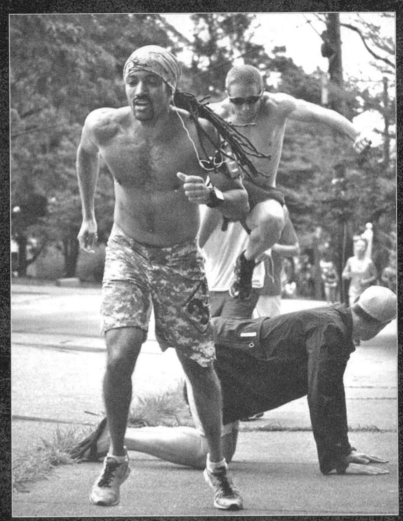

Sometimes we hurdle trash bins and benches, and sometimes we hurdle humans. #HurdleEverything

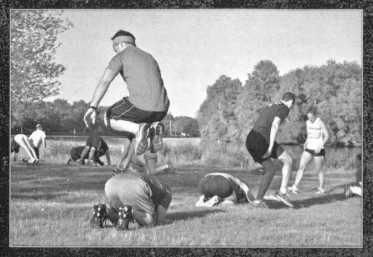

BOJANS

Partner workout. One person gets into a pike position with feet and hands outstretched on the ground...booty high in the air (my yogi women and men call this a downward facing dog). The other partner crawls under this space created, trying not to hit dangling boobs, dongs, or the cloud of morning breath. Once on the other side, the now-free crawler stands and turns around to face the downward dog partner who is now in a curled-up ball face down (namaste, my yogi friends; we call this a child's pose, or what BG does for 30 percent of every single heated yoga class he's been in). With both feet together the now-standing partner jumps this ball of human, landing on the other side. When the jumper turns around and gets down to crawl under, the piked dog is back up, booty high above the ground. Repeat 10 times, switch positions. We usually then have one partner sprint maybe a hundred yards or more while the other partner holds a plank. When partner one returns, it's back to Bojans. Repeat for 20 minutes. The idea is to work at anaerobic threshold, as the heart rate remains fairly high due to lack of rest between transitions of jumping, crawling, and sprinting. I think we named it Bojans because I was doing all of the talking, and I was pretty sure people were calling us both BG. Half kidding.

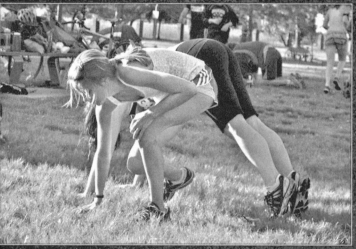

Two-legged jump, crawl under, repeat.

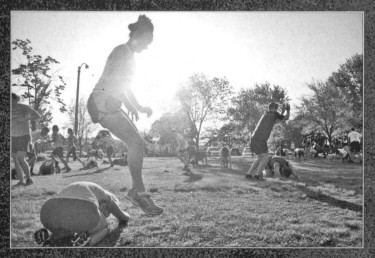

HOISTEES

These are a Dan Graham (we're related) special. During one of our breaks from meeting about World Takeover at the 2013 Summit in Edmonton, Alberta, the leaders started talking shop and exchanging ideas about workouts they loved. DG dropped "hoistees" on the group and pretty much every single city now uses them. Hoistees ended up on local San Diego TV news, demo'd by San Diego NP coleaders Jessie Craik and Lauren Padula, and were later mentioned in a 2015 *New York Times* article entitled, "The Early-Morning Workout Flashmob." I'm not going to give this one away. Just go to a week or two of NP and you'll end up doing some hoistees.

(Editor's note: Because you've paid good money for this book and expect plenty of prescriptive content, and because BG is much better at giving direction than taking it himself and has pretty much proved himself unmanageable, we've asked Bojan to jump in for further explanation.)

Bojan: A hoistee is a partner exercise where the movement of a squat jump is extended all the way down to a sitting position. Partners start by facing each other, holding hands, and touching toes. At the same time, both partners go down to a sitting position while their toes maintain contact. Once both partners' butts touch the ground, they spring back up by pulling on each other's hands and pushing against each other's toes to propel themselves up into the jump. At the top of every jump they yell out "HOISTEE!" The silliness of the exercise distracts the participants from the fact that each partner is completing a very hard and complex movement that involves a wide range of motion of the lower body, upper body, and core muscles.

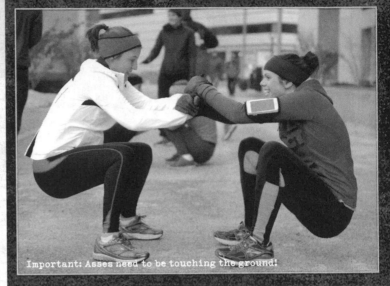

Important: Asses need to be touching the ground!

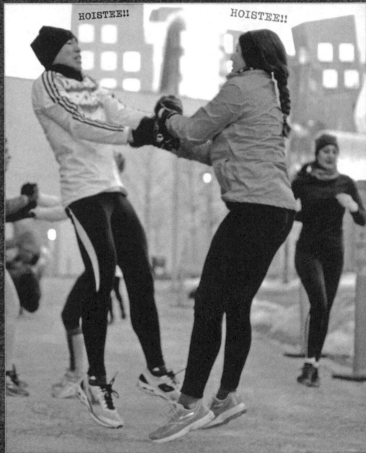

HOISTEE!!   HOISTEE!!

WALL JUMPS

We've found that runners, rowers, swimmers, and triathletes aren't using these explosive exercises enough. Wall jumps, also known as jump-ups or box jumps, are tiring. But they force athletes to relearn the explosiveness off the ground. We always say that you have to leave the ground with both feet, land on the wall/bench/whatever with both feet, then open your hips to the world to prove that you're really up there (a similar look to one powerful dry-hump thrust of the wide open world in front of you) before jumping back off and down. WARNING: This shit will make you fit and feel fierce. WARNING 2: Unless you do these somewhat regularly, you'll be mediocre at best.

(Editor's note: Here's Bojan again.)

Bojan: Wall jumps are an exercise that should be found in every trainer's toolbox. It is designed to increase the reaction speed of fast-twitch muscle fibers, increase the strength of leg muscles (specifically quads), and improve agility. To perform a wall jump, find a suitable obstacle (wall, ledge, park bench) that you can jump and land safely on without injury. Start with your feet at, or slightly wider than, shoulder width and place your hands next to your hips. From a quarter squat, propel yourself onto the obstacle by pushing your feet against the ground while simultaneously swinging your arms upward toward the shoulders. Make a soft landing onto an obstacle and extend your hips (like you're humping the world) before stepping down.

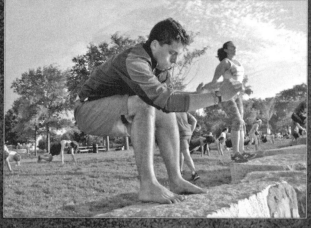

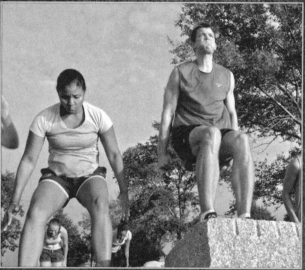

We'll be really good at pooping off cliffs.

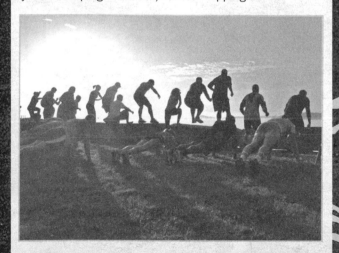

"FOR SCALABLE OPTIONS, FIND THE OBSTACLE HEIGHT THAT SUITS YOUR ATHLETIC ABILITY AND FITNESS LEVEL."
—GUY WITH SCRAPED-UP SHINS

BEAR CRAWLS

These are kinda boot-campy, but they're great. Butt up in the air, hands and feet crawling, head down. That's it. We don't act like animals enough during these adult days of ours. Try these in a circuit and your obliques, traps, and shoulders will wake up and join the riot against the unfitness that lazes around inside your body.

(Editor's note: Cue the Serb.)

Brojan: Bear crawls (bear walks) were designed by the bears of the Sierra Nevada mountains, and adopted by humans who tried to cross the distance from point A to point B while mimicking bear-like movement. Since most humans only have two legs, arms and hands are necessary to properly execute the exercise. The intent of the exercise is for people to recognize how weak their hips, shoulders, and core are, and how badass bears are for being able to hit 30 miles per hour while moving like this. I fucking hate bear crawls!

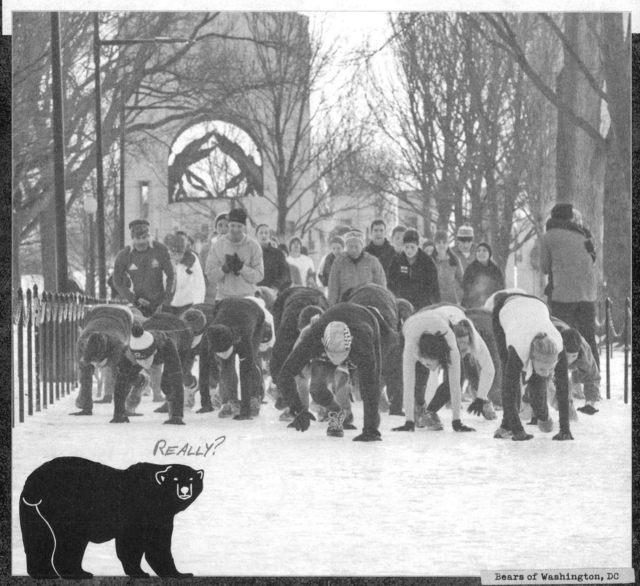

REALLY?

Bears of Washington, DC

SNOW PACK

Running on snow is great. Running on dry pavement or on trails is great. When you run on something between the two, or onto ice, that's when it sucks. Taking the tribe out into snow fields for workouts over the past few years, even after the most epic storms, has provided a good dose of "just fucking do this" and "stop trying to make sense out of all of this." Laps on the Harvard track in the snow, through snow-covered fields, and even laps around Harvard Stadium were just a few ways we got through 2015 and Boston's worst winter on record.

While the phrase "#weatherproof" was being dropped from the get-go, in the winter of 2014–2015 the Boston tribe took things to a whole new level. But the one problem with talking snow, ice, or how to be weatherproof, is that we now have tribes in Edmonton, Winnipeg, Calgary, and many other cities that are just as cold, if not way colder, than Boston. Edmonton gives out patches for anyone who shows up to train when it is −30°F. One 5-year-old girl approached Jenn Ference at a workout and asked for a patch on a day when it was only −29°F and was turned down. "Just keep coming back as the weather hopefully gets worse," Jenn said.

(Editor's note: Anyone seen Bojan?)

Bojan: The winter of 2015 was pretty hard on Boston. Record-breaking snowfall caused bunches of government officials to blame everyone but themselves for breakdowns in their shitty public transportation system. It also taught us that prison rules apply when someone moves a chair/trash barrel/whatever piece of furniture out into the street to save the parking space they worked so hard to shovel out, and then lay claim to it until the end of the summer. But the experience wasn't entirely negative. We learned that running in 2 feet of fresh snow is one of the hardest things in the world to do, and that running quickly turns into walking and shortly after that into crawling. Note to self: Invest in snowshoes. Also, Evan Dana, one of the fierce leaders of NP_BOS, taught us that you don't need to use free weights as long as you have some sturdy bags that you fill with snow. Any exercise that can be done with added resistance in the form of a free weight, we were doing with packed snow. And, depending on the quality of the

bags, sometimes the heft of our makeshift weights got progressively lighter as the workout went on. Eventually all that was left were some torn-up grocery bags floating in the air, like the scene from *American Beauty*.

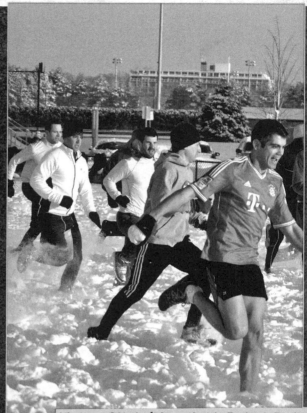

What snow? We don't have that in Turkey!—Deniz

"*I CAN'T WAIT FOR THE SUMMER!*"
—EVERYONE LIVING IN BOSTON IN MARCH

"*THIS HEAT IS UNBEARABLE, I CAN'T WAIT FOR THE SNOW!*"
—EVERYONE LIVING IN BOSTON IN JUNE, ALREADY FORGETTING HOW SHITTY THINGS WERE JUST THREE MONTHS AGO

THIS CITY IS YOUR GYM, DON'T WASTE IT!

BY BROGAN GRAHAM

Public spaces. Parks. Tennis and basketball courts. We look at the city differently than most. An architect looks at a cityscape and sees the world through concrete and glass and curves and height. A skateboarder looks at a city and sees rails and edges to grind on, slide down, and jump over. A cyclist commuting to work sees the street as a shared space and values every single block of bike lanes. November Project leaders look for "spaces." The phrase "The city is our gym" is kind of true. When we talk to prospective NP leaders in new cities, we show them how to look at central locations, parking, bike parking, proximity to public transit, and how each space would look with 20 people in it, and how it could still work with 220. Stadiums, hills, trails, and structures are the easy ones.

For example, so that they can express their creative visions for the rotating Fridays in DC, coleaders Danny Metcalf and Steve Christensen are always looking for grassy areas where people can hit the ground. They're looking for benches on which people can perform jump-ups and dips, and they're always paying attention to the legal risk factor. In DC, they have to deal with land and landmarks that are either totally fine or a huge f'ing deal. They have learned what we already know: Some security guards will warn you never to come back even as they let you wrap up all 35 minutes of the workout, and others simply shut the thing down. So, when scouting for locations, NP leaders are also on the lookout for a Plan B location.

The fun part is finding new locations and keeping it fresh. There's something awesome about the fact that if you miss a Friday workout, there's a good chance you'll never go back to that particular space with NP.

Races at November Project have always been a key

to drive athletes of all levels to train for something. What are you training for? This question is common in our world. Your answer doesn't have to be badass. In fact, you don't even need to have one. The conversation and the vibe of always having something coming up is what

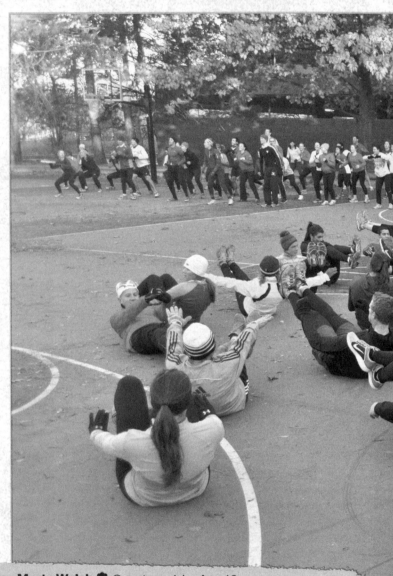

> **Mayor Marty Walsh** ✔ @marty_walsh · Aug 10
> Thank you @Nov_Project for letting me join you this morning. What a great workout!

makes all of this physical output and early-ass alarm clocks mean something.

In the early days, we'd cut deals to get tons of free bibs at local races, flooding the corrals with #GrassrootsGear. We'd take on certain races without paying (the running world calls this running "bandit"). Or we'd simply create our own. Some of our races were intense. Some were more about a theme/costume. Some were mostly about the beers at the finish line. And a few were a combination of all three. What we set out to do with our races and events was to make something new, fun, and creative, and to do it at zero cost to the participants. Here are a few of our favorites. Maybe they'll inspire some of your own.

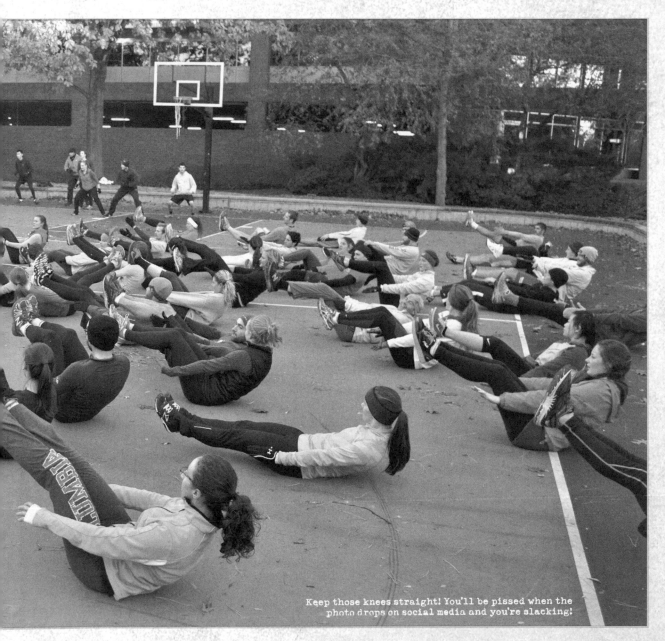

Keep those knees straight! You'll be pissed when the photo drops on social media and you're slacking!

NOVEMBER PROJECT RACES

BY BROGAN GRAHAM

The Running of the Bowls, November 1, 2012

The event was created to celebrate the first birthday of November Project. The unknown destination piece was taken from a set of annual events at Northeastern. It has its roots in something called Bike Gang, which was a creation of ours from back in our college days, where we put anywhere from 50 to 200 people on bikes, in matching gear, who had no idea where they were heading. Awaiting them, at the end of this super-slow traffic-stopping ride through Boston, was a house party with free beer and a DJ.

The Running of the Bowls was meant to have a certain look for those we passed. It was meant to be fun and funny, and the name just had a great ring to it. We met at the Boston Public Garden and led the group, which was dressed in all white and wearing matching red scarves that said NOVEMBER PROJECT on them (painted in the back alley garage connected to the Newbury Street Lululemon—total space hookup by our core member Leigh). The final part of the theme to this secret destination group run was that everyone had to bring a red bowl to drink out of when we reached our destination. We didn't know if the bartenders would approve of this or not...but it worked out in the end.

All of the running that night, almost 5-K, was done in the long dark alleys that lined the Back Bay. In between Tom Brady's house and Boylston Street, we looped, lapped, cheered, stopped, joked, and had a great time. The Running of the Bowls was good clean fun and was our first huge event that brought these fun/fit/outgoing people out at night. A special thanks to the Mass Ave Tavern for going with the bowl idea. I did call a few times that week and never got a call back about how that might work. Fortunately for us, and for everyone who participated, it worked.

Ninja Race, January 23, 2013

Okay, this was one that you were either AT or you will never really be able to understand it...but I'll try here. The Boston Ninja Race was something really awesome and harsh and a little bit dangerous. With the thermometer reading 12°C and a fierce wind, the members of November Project shook their heads inside subway trains and cabs as they made their way over to the starting line on the iconic Esplanade on Boston's Charles River. Fuck man, even just thinking about it now...chills.

Okay, so we picked a Wednesday night because it was a night when nobody ever went out. We picked the ninja theme, as in all black everything (some brought swords and throwing stars, NBD). We picked the race date of January 23rd because in the weeks leading up we needed something to train for that would act as a branch to swing for in December and January, in that odd time when there doesn't seem to be a light at the end of the wintry tunnel.

Anyway, we had 350 RSVPs for this free event, and our friends who did the official timing for this 8-mile out-and-back race (including 20 burpees at the turnaround) said that 254 bibs officially crossed the start line. The plan was to meet at the start line, start, and send everyone off into the dark. Racers would turn around over on

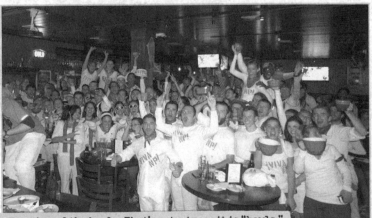

Running of the bowls. That's not a typo—it is "bowls."

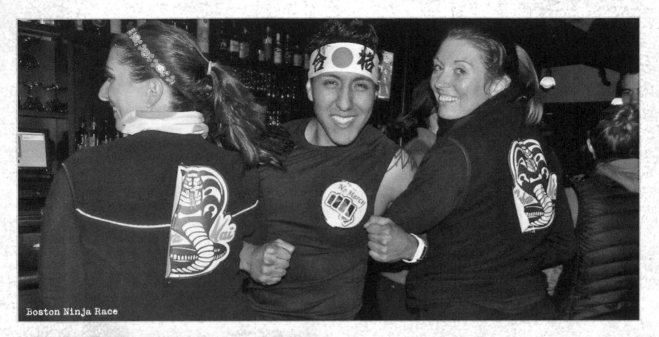

Boston Ninja Race

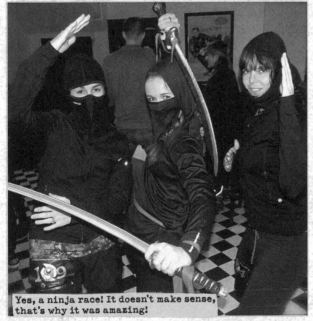

Yes, a ninja race! It doesn't make sense, that's why it was amazing!

the Cambridge side at Magazine Beach, where Bojan was waiting to oversee the burpees, and then come back home to the starting line. Bojan would ride his bike in with the final runner, and I'd hype the crowd at the beginning. We'd go to the bar and pass out one free beer ticket to each person who did the race (the winner, NP member Ian Nurse, also a 2:25 Boston Marathon dude, NBD, would be the only person who would be awarded a second free beer from November Project), thanks to our good friends at Harpoon Brewery.

The weather on race day went from bad to terrible. Temps dipped below −10°C. Many who knew us a little (but not well), assumed the race would be called off. But those who were close to the NP movement knew that the terrible weather was a gift, and that we couldn't have asked for better conditions for this event. Local cycling advocate and friend of NP, Greg Humm, brought his signature drum-bike and positioned himself in the dark, dressed head-to-toe in black, and went off banging on the full drum set attached to his handlebars. Runners would race by him on the Storrow Drive bike path and hear him, be drawn to him, but with his dark green and black ride, possibly never see him, as ninjas passed ninjas that night.

Ice formed on the eyelashes of many and seemed to freeze zippers and hands, making the process of thawing out at the after-party something to see. The Ninja Race was promoted the way we did everything else: blog, Facebook, Twitter, and word of mouth. The Ninja Race was by far Boston's harshest event to date. A badge of honor for all who ran.

Better Than Bedtime(s)

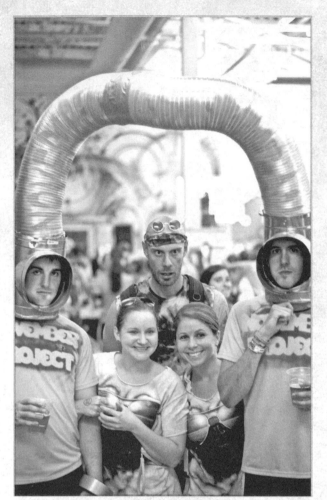

Better Than Bedtime was the first event we ever held. You see, back in 2012 we had almost a dozen members doing our Wednesday workout who worked for the almighty Harpoon Brewery. Like so many people who work for beer companies, they were proud, fun, and easy to talk to. The connection to an event was always something we'd hoped for, but it didn't happen until Jessie Cox, Harpoon's redheaded events/marketing outreach people-person, brought us into the conversation. She offered the Tasting Room at the Harpoon Brewery, which could accommodate a large number of us.

Meeting at Harvard Stadium (where else?), we made our way over to the Cambridge side, and then over to the Longfellow Bridge (this was before the construction, the single lane, and all the traffic backups). We then made our way to meet Jessie, who was waiting with tickets for "tasting" Harpoon brew right inside the brewery!

Like all of the events to come, none of our people knew where we were heading. And you had to be on the run to be at the party. If some of us were going to be sweaty and stanky...we were *all* going to be. Core dudes and gals made their way along with us—the faces of Neil Cronin, Alan Scherer, Jake Otto, and Kreg Pierless are all frozen in time in a certain photo that always comes to mind when I think about the first Better Than Bedtime. The sun was perfect, the summer was easy, life was uncertain, and we all believed in good, simple times. There was no theme. Just grassroots gear, beer, and laughs after a long, undetermined run.

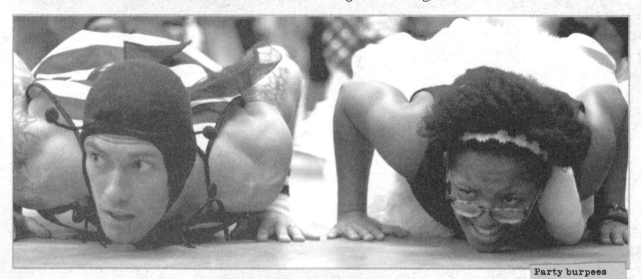

Party burpees

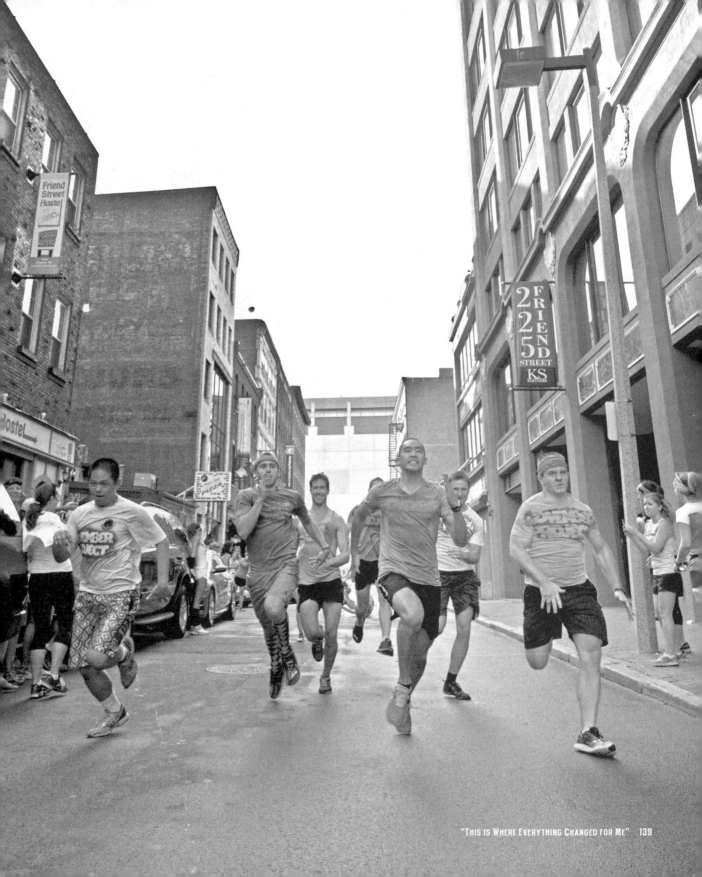

The next summer, Better Than Bedtime 2 went down in three cities, in three different time zones: Boston, San Francisco, and Madison. We were all running at the same time, and holding a glass to toast at the same time. Laura in San Francisco led the charge on her own, as did DG in Madison. I remember thinking of the connected feel that we had that night (afternoon out there in San Francisco—Sorry Laura and NPSF).

In the summer of 2014, we attempted the 17-city, "same-time" Better Than Bedtime event. It was a little bit of a mess, but still fun. The theme for Better Than Bedtime 3 was Noah's Ark, "They Came in Twos." Hoping not to offend any of the religious people out there, we promoted that "everything we know of must have been on that ark. You want to be a pair of T. rexes? Great. You want to be a pair of mimes? Great. If we know of it, it was on the ark." This time we met in Somerville (near Cambridge) and twisted and turned our way over the new climbing space (and arguably the coolest place in the Boston/Cambridge/Somerville area) called Brooklyn Boulders (the most badass climbing gym, yoga space, and training and event space). Again, free everything. It was amazing.

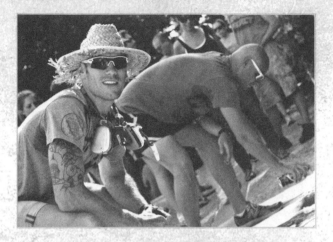

Scene Be Seen, November 18, 2013

Scene Be Seen was a name that Bojan and I bounced around and landed on via text. The theme was bright, blinking, neon, glowing, and visually stunning. As another night-racing event, we needed the visuals to be on point. Like the Boston Ninja Race, we had to consider what we were calling "unbroken miles," where at no point could our athletes have the option to dash in front of cars and kill themselves. We picked Pleasure Bay, which connected South Boston (Southie) and Castle Island with a giant seawall-like barrier that rises up out of the Boston Harbor (pretty much the Atlantic fucking Ocean). Being exposed to the conditions felt like the second surprise theme that night. Exposed. Another officially timed event, it would bring racers around two loops of the bay, creating a 5-miler—or was it a 5-K?...it really doesn't matter—the point was that it was cold and dark. There were costumes like we'd never seen. Real racing. Harpoon's new banquet hall was standing room only.

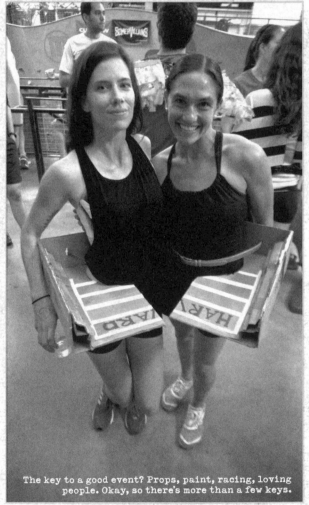

The key to a good event? Props, paint, racing, loving people. Okay, so there's more than a few keys.

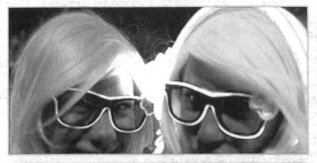

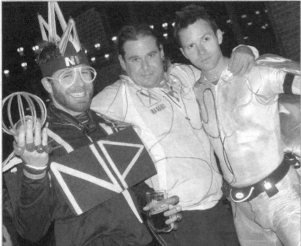

SUNRISE 6—Ks

DG took this one into his hands in Milwaukee. It was an event that was something to train for, fun to say, and would replace a workout. DG, like both of our parents, has always been great at taking something and making it not only a thing, but an important thing. THE Sunrise 6-K would award THE overall fastest runner with a giant summer sausage as long as a loaf of bread and as thick as a can of Coke. When he pulled this one-city event off and couldn't stop talking about it, I asked him if we could all go for it. He just kept saying, "I think this will work, I really do."

In February 2015 all 16 member-cities raced 6-K for time. Why 6-K (all you running dorks are thinking)!?!? Because it's fun to say. Because why 5-K? Why 26.2 miles? Why hurdles? Why *anything*? Everything is made up. DG made up the 6-K, and his people fucking loved it. They gave it to the entire family of NP tribes, and now we're all 6-K fans. 6-K!? Why NOT 6-K? And why not attend a full-on RACE before work? Workouts are great, but later in your normal day when you're at the water cooler talking to Karl-the-office-guy and he idly asks you "how's your day going?" and your answer is AMAZING!... well then. That's why we do what we do. Sunrise 6-Ks, join us for our next.

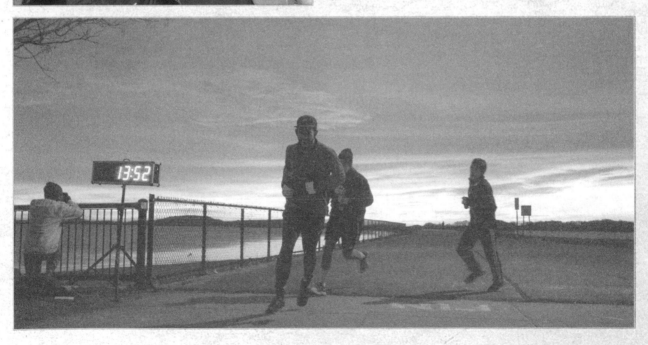

Simply Thank You! by Molly from NP_BOS

🕐 29th May 2014   👤 bojan   📁 Blog   💬 1 Comment

When I heard Molly's story, I had to share it with anyone who would listen. Molly is the girl who showed up to the workout a week after her apartment burned down. A few months later, Molly is settled in a new place where she decided to put the pen to the paper and share her story. Ladies and gentlemen, Molly Blumberg...

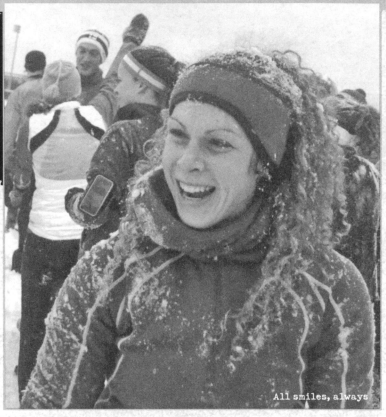

All smiles, always

I've been trying to write this for a while now. It took me some time to get started. I had thought that waiting until I moved into my new apartment, giving myself some time and space, would offer the right perspective. I've drafted my story a few times, but none of them felt quite right. I don't need to give all the specifics of my struggle to say what I really want to say to you all, which is simply, "thank you." What I want to talk about, what I really learned over the past few months, is the strength of community, of caring and love, of support and resiliency.

By now most of you know my story, or at least the most recent part of it. I went to work on a Thursday, my apartment caught fire around 2pm, and that was that. It was horrible, and upsetting, and unsettling, and it came with a whole set of issues I'd never had to deal with before. The truth is, there were things that I was struggling with well before my apartment burnt down. And while I like to think of myself as a pretty resilient person, I was really in over my head. I'm not good at asking for help—I had to enlist a chain of people in order to ask you all for help. I wanted to be able to take care of myself. I thought that the best way to come out on top was to shoulder this one alone. But I was running out of resources, running out of places to sleep, running out of options, and taking this one on solo was

just not going to be my reality. Up until that point, I would have said that the greatest thing I had learned through November Project was that I can always push myself a little further. I can fight through the pain, run faster, climb higher, than I had ever thought that I could. But that's only the first half. I now know just how much further I can go with the help and support of community. I can still push myself pretty far on my own, but when I reach my end, there will be people, hundreds of people, who will selflessly, and without second thought, pick me up and carry me the rest of the way.

It's been said many times before—there's something truly special about November Project. There's something a little magical that drags us out of bed on even the darkest and coldest mornings. It's more than the workout, the challenge of running the Harvard stadium, the desire to get fitter and faster. It's more than the smiles, the hugs, the fuck yeahs. I feel like it even extends beyond the general idea of community. For me, I think it's about the fierce consistency and the unconditional dedication to showing up together, no matter what. We're there to work together, to get each other moving, to achieve new goals and to share in that glory. What got me out of bed all winter was knowing that there were hundreds of other people who held the same core belief in just showing up despite everything else. It was knowing that there are few things better than being present in such a passionate community and pushing your limits with your peers. It was knowing that I could drop all the shit I was dealing with, give some hugs, challenge myself, and walk away feeling like my character was a little stronger because of the people I shared that all with.

For a few weeks, not many of you knew that my apartment had burnt down and I was sleeping on couches. From some conversations I've had with various members of the tribe and other stories that have been written, it's clear there are a lot of us out there dealing with a whole range of adversities. We don't always know everyone's story. I was personally lucky to be in a position to share mine and to receive the overwhelming support that I did. Regardless, for those few early hours in the morning, none of that matters, none of that defines us. We throw on our running shoes and we show up as equals, as supporters, as competitors, as racers, as empowerers.

We all have things that we carry with us—our unique combination of successes and struggles, our histories, our stories, our ambitions. We deal with these things and learn from them in different ways. Some of us carry them with us, or we set them aside, follow them, run from them. Everything we have experienced, the histories that precede us, the things we have yet to accomplish, all define the people we are, and they have led us to this place, this moment in time. But no matter where we are, or where we're going, what we carry, or what we've learned, we all show up. At 6:30 am on Mondays, Wednesdays, and Fridays we all show up. We show up for ourselves and we show up for each other. And we run.

VOICES OF NOVEMBER PROJECT

"NOVEMBER PROJECT IS BASICALLY LIKE ONE HUGE HALL OF MIRRORS WITH EVERYONE REFLECTING POSITIVITY BACK AND FORTH ON EACH OTHER FOREVER AND EVER."
—SARAH BUZOGANY, 29, FOOD ACCESS PLANNER FOR CITY OF BALTIMORE, BALTIMORE

"I HAD A JOB LOSS THAT CAUSED OVERWHELMING STRESS. IN A SEA OF THE UNKNOWN, NP WAS THE ONE THING I COULD COUNT ON THROUGH THE CHAOS. FOR A FEW HOURS EARLY IN THE MORNING, IT WAS MY THERAPY. I SWEAR I SWEATED THROUGH THE BULLSHIT. IT KEPT ME ALIVE AT A TIME WHEN KEY PEOPLE TURNED THEIR BACKS. I LEARNED TO KEEP MOVING."
—TARA MADIGAN, 42, NUTRITIONIST AND AUTHOR, BROOKLYN, N.Y.

"NP IS A SHAKE-UP OF THE OLD VERSION OF WORKING OUT, AND THE OLD VERSIONS OF OURSELVES. NO MATTER HOW INVOLVED YOU CHOOSE TO BE, FOR HOW LONG, JOINING NP WILL SHAKE-UP YOUR LIFE IN THE BEST POSSIBLE WAY, FOREVER."
—JENNIFER KELLY, 32, ATTORNEY, BOSTON

Neaera, NP's Original Bitch: In Her Own Words

My name is Neaera. My assistant/dad, James, was asked if we wanted to do a short writeup on how November Project changed my life. I am kind of a big deal, I get it. When my dad came to take me away from my dog family in exchange for currency (don't ask me how that works), the farm owner told him I was "the Bentley of hog-hunting dogs!"

From that day, everything changed. I landed in Boston—Commonwealth Avenue, to be exact. What the hell is this place all about—cars, trains, HARDWOOD FLOORS!!!! I was a fish out of water, but I knew I was destined for greatness, overflowing with cuteness. My dad takes me everywhere, exploring new sights and sounds, and it is awesome. He gives me everything I could possibly want, things that I didn't even know existed: 2-liter bottles, cardboard boxes, anything a Diva bitch could want, but something was missing.

I have the blood of a top-tier hunter coursing through my veins. I yearn to be moving. This thing called life seems to take my dad away from me every day, him grumbling about, "Someone's gotta buy the fucking kibble..." And I'm thinking, "Shit dude, no one's got a gun to your head, and when are we going hunting? I'll be here resting till you get back and will be ready for a full docket of activities upon your return."

My dad had been getting up very early a couple days a week. Although he is gone longer days with his job, he seems to be happier and more fulfilled. He is also creating a plush bed of fine synthetic fabrics with a damp but purely intoxicating aroma. Once a month, he comes back smelling like spray-paint. I wanted to know what was going on in the morning, but I am just not an early-riser kinda gal. One Friday morning, Dad not only woke me up, but demanded that I emerge from under the comforter and get ready to go. "Ready for what? Do I need to put my face on? What positive thing could possibly be going on at this hour of the morning? Are you just being a dick?"

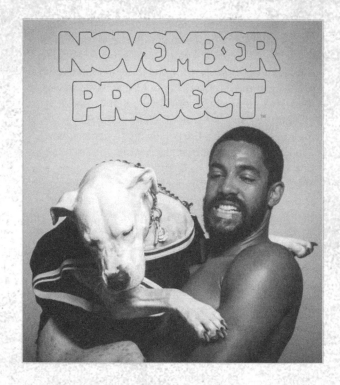

Could you imagine my surprise? There were other idiots awake. They were smiling and laughing and hugging and creating a group energy like I had never seen. After some bizarre chanting/tribal ritual the group started in motion. Running downhill quietly, what we were doing still was not clear to me. As we got to the bottom of the hill and made the turn, the energy level ramped up as we started to go uphill. We continued this a few times and then came to a big group at the top of the hill, where the energy is electric, everyone is glistening, they smell fantastic and taste perfectly salty. Talk about lick sticks!

We continued to do this for weeks, and I started to look forward to Friday morning. Sometimes, I would be waiting by the door ready to go. I think I am starting to figure this thing out. This is my pack, we are hunting, and they need practice. This is evident by the fact that we never catch anything. Dad knew I needed to hunt and connected us with the least productive pack this side of the Mississippi. Everyone stays positive and shows up next week to try again.

Not surprisingly, when some kind of satire hunting mag wanted to do an article on the group, they asked me to show up for the cover shoot. Dad came along also and managed to weasel his way into a couple of pics. But it was really my time to shine. After all, I am the Bentley in a land of recycled Hondas.

As my star started to shine, it became about more than the hunt. Dad's friends that drink beer and BBQ with him started showing up. They have a dog that didn't like me that much, but as we started hunting together, we became the best of friends. We started to do everything together—hiking, swimming, sniffing butts. Fenway quickly became my best friend, the most courageous hunter I know. He got sick, lost a leg, got some special stick with human words carved into it, and still came to do his part in the hunt. In the end, he had to move on to that great rabbit-chasing field in the sky. I love, respect, and miss him so much. And I realized that this had become less about the outcome of the hunt and more to do with the progress of the group and the personal connections we made through challenges and adversity.

I'm so grateful Dad seemed to realize that if he did not focus on moving his ass on the regs, he would lose his ability to hunt. He spends more time with me now outside and is super active. His energy level is much more positive, his stamina is top-notch, and his shorts have gotten a little shorter. He has all the moves of a fast and efficient hunter, although I am beginning to think the Northeast may be fresh out of hogs to chase. Regardless of the hunting outcome, we have found our pack, and I am honored to be their Bentley.

NOVEMBER PROJECT

Ever since I was an acorn, I had big dreams. Like being a flagpole on top of the Empire State Building. A mast on the USS Constitution. Forming the fuselage of the Spruce Goose. A baseball bat swung by David Ortiz.

But somewhere along the way, my lumber was hijacked and sent to a factory where I became an oar handle. Over the years, crew bros dripped sweat and wiped god knows what all over me. Not exactly what my mom had dreamed of. Then one night two freaky bald rowing dudes broke into the closet where my friends and I lived and took me away. I may never see those other oar handles again.

These days I get passed around among all sorts of different people. Big, tall, short, young, old, super fast, fast, and just plain super. Lots of camera flashes. They take me to restaurants and offices and everyone thinks they are doing something clever with me that nobody else has ever done. But the craziest thing is that all these people who kidnap me seem really happy. Really happy to be with me, tell their friends about me, and to give me to other people.

I'm still not sure what this is all about and when I'll go back to that closet at the Henderson Boathouse, but I'm trying not to overthink things and instead just roll with it.
@PositivityAward

"I had the unfortunate experience of losing my mother this past year. The Wednesday following her death at just age 60, 16 tribes from across the country supported me by wearing gray shirts, the color for brain cancer research. My heart swelled as I read the blog posts for that day dedicated to my mother, my family, and myself. Watching my dad in tears, telling me I have helped in creating something very special, was a point when I realized there is a very blurred line between the words November Project and Family."

ASHLEIGH VOYCHICK, 30, PHYSICAL THERAPIST, SAN DIEGO

NOVEMBER PROJECT HASHTAGS

#JustShowUp
#grassrootsgear
#HillsForBreakfast
#FuckYeah!
#freefitness
#raceeverything
#hashtageverything
#notacult
#verbal
#verbalharvest
#PrintMediaLives
#traverbal
#PaulLeak
#sunrise6K
#community
#weatherproof
#FOMO
#trainingforlife
#worldtakeover
#SteveNews
#stairsforbreakfast
#racingfit
#NP_Pledge
#JamesShorts
#PositivityAward
#NPSummit
#destinationdeck
#NP_TSA
#Dooster_Pledge
#Raceman
#recruiteveryone
#weekendearned
#weatherspoof
#itrainfor
#PRday
#BeBright
#thisshitisgood
#safetythird

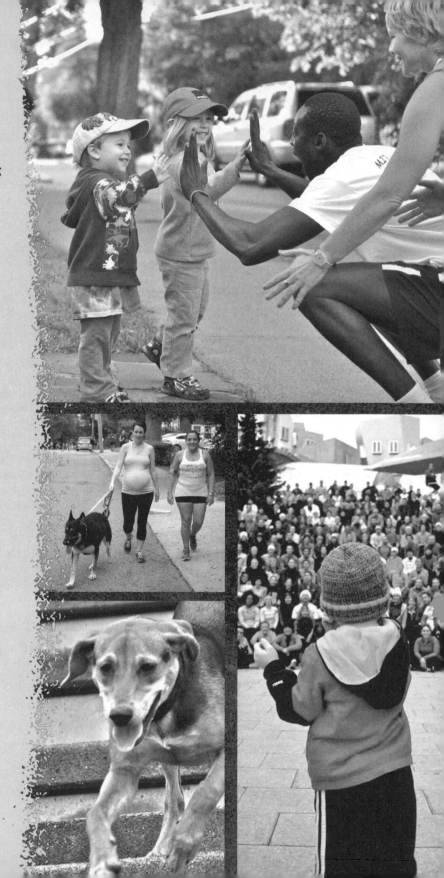

NOVEMBER PROJECT in a Word

Weirdaful
(Wonderful & Weird)
—Elin Flashman, 42,
Network and Systems Engineer, Boston

Happy
—Alice Nelson, 28, geologist, Brookline, Mass.

Badassery
—Alan Scherer, 42, photographer, Leominster, Mass.

Addictive
—Molly Rosignol, 46, family doctor, Madison, Wisc.

Life-changing.
(I know, that's a little bit cheating,
but the hyphen makes it ok.)
—Mary Anna Yram, 50, research compliance
coordinator, Medford, Mass.

Needed
—Goldie Graham, 31, yoga instructor, San Diego

Indispensable
—Tracy Davis, 28, event planner, New York City

Family
—Kristyn Kadala, 23, graduate student, Berkeley, Calif.

Solidarity
—Emily Faherty, 29, web editor, Hoboken, N.J.

Tribe
—Stewart Whitcomb, 33, architect, Indianapolis, Ind.

True
—Dylan Ladds, 26, filmmaker, Boston

Love
—Tory Dube, 28, holistic nutrition and lifestyle coach,
East Harlem, N.Y.

Authentic
—Jackie Madrigal, 37, business continuity vice
president, Brooklyn, N.Y.

fuckingawesome
—Gabrielle Light, 39, marketing consultant,
New York City

kindred
—Kat Ems, 35, IT professional, San Francisco

Positive
—Jean Tinnelly, 32, restaurant manager,
New York City

CONTAGIOUS
—Katie Date, 35, corporate outreach, Boston

game-changing
—Katherine Shea, 35, stage manager,
Brooklyn, N.Y.

LIFECHANGINGLYAWESOME
—Sarah Lindstrom, 22, student,
Madison, Wisc.

Community
—Julia Griffith, 26, project coordinator, Denver

Creative
—Kristin Carlson, 42, special education teacher,
Watertown, Mass.

Fantasticult
—Liysa Mendels, 29, research coordinator,
New York City

Fulfilling
—Sam Livermore, 26, freelance designer,
San Francisco

Happiness
—Rebecca Daniels a.k.a. RAD, 33, photographer,
San Francisco

hugs
—Malcolm Purinton, 35, beer historian,
Boston

NOV
PRO

PART II #WORLDTAKEOVER

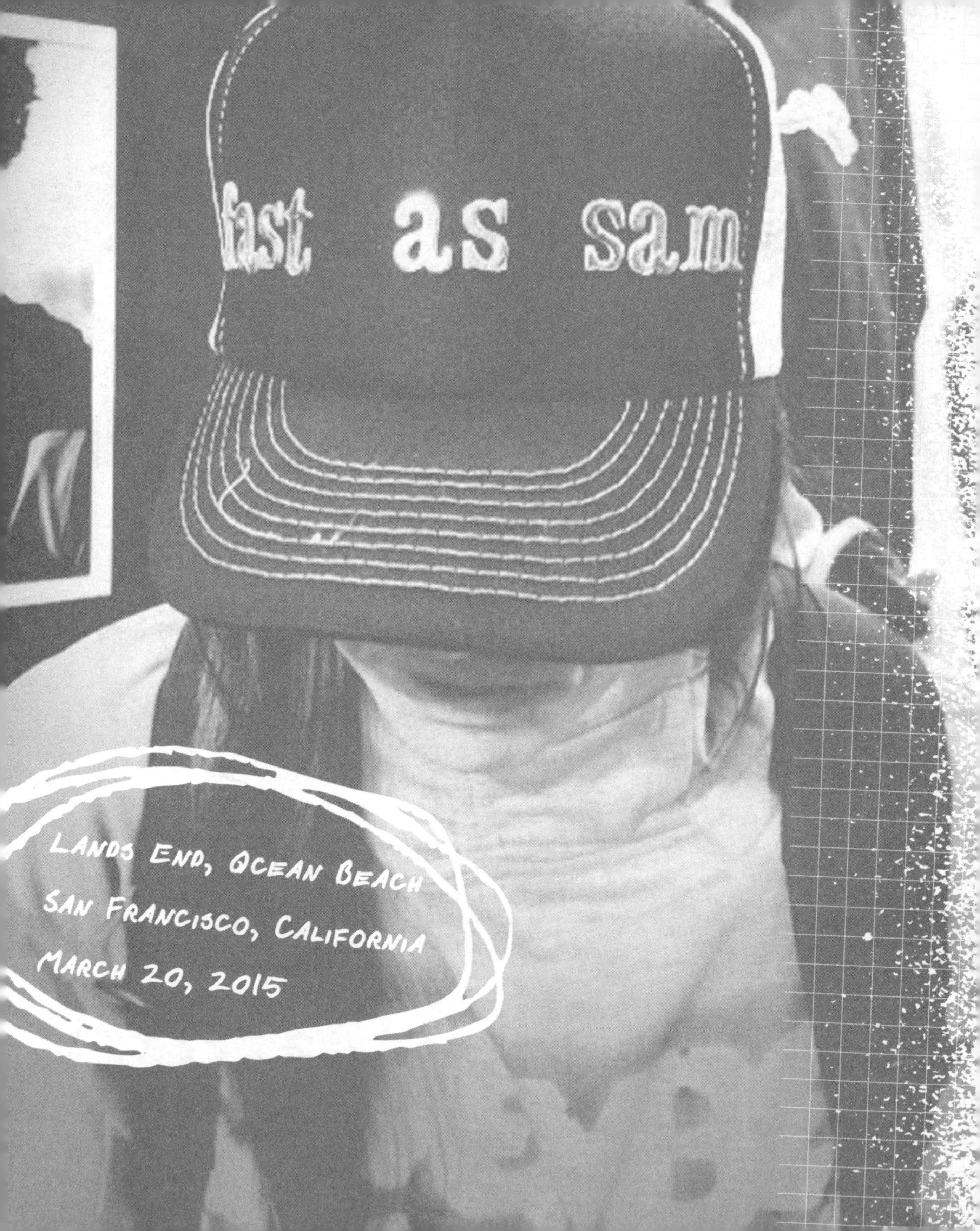

LANDS END, OCEAN BEACH
SAN FRANCISCO, CALIFORNIA
MARCH 20, 2015

CHAPTER 6

#FastAsSam #HalfAsCool

BY CALEB DANILOFF

Wisconsin Notes

- San Francisco blazed the trail for female leadership
- NP_SF members laugh at Summit Ave
- Karl can get a little foggy
- One of the tribe's most devoted members turns three
- Ethan Bookman makes an appearance
- Tragedy strikes
- Across the country, hats turn backward
- #WorldTakeover is real

A woman I'd never met pulled up in a rust-red Honda Element. I was staying on Geary Street at The Hotel California. (Yes, it's a lovely place; and yes, I checked out but am still here.) I hadn't been to San Francisco in 20-some years and wasn't sure about the best way to get to the workout. Friday was NP_SF's moveable-feast-of-hills, and that morning the tribe was gathering at Ocean Beach at the northwestern tip of the city, between Golden Gate Park and China Beach. I'd checked in with tribe leader Laura McCloskey when I landed, and within an hour a woman named Hilary Hayssen texted that she was looking forward to meeting me at 5:35 the next morning outside my hotel.

I climbed into the passenger's seat of Hilary's sporty vehicle, but couldn't quite make out her face. It was still dark. A splash of streetlamp glowed on one cheek. I buckled in. I had no idea how old she was, whether her hair was short or pulled into a ponytail. But somehow it felt like we knew each other and soon we began chatting like cousins. Turns out Hilary was 24, originally from Minneapolis, and had played Division 1 hockey at Harvard. The hockey rink sits across from the football stadium, and that's where she found herself after she peeled off her crimson uniform for the last time, hooking up with the crazy fitness group she'd heard ran the stairs on Wednesdays. "I missed having a team. I love working out with

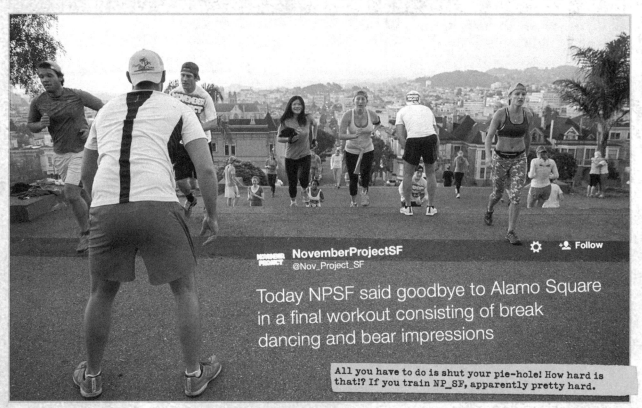

NovemberProjectSF
@Nov_Project_SF

⚙ +👤 Follow

Today NPSF said goodbye to Alamo Square in a final workout consisting of break dancing and bear impressions

All you have to do is shut your pie-hole! How hard is that!? If you train NP_SF, apparently pretty hard.

SPRING—SUMMER 2014

Talks begin on a November Project book. A proposal is written. And rewritten.

SEPTEMBER 2014

The Second Annual November Project Summit in Madison, Wisconsin. BG and Bojan see, for the first time, that the tribe could—and would—travel. These thrifty, free fitness junkies save the dates, save the dough, and field teams in BG's hometown (one that not many people on the East and West Coast pay much attention to). At the North Face Endurance Challenge Series marathon relay, November Project sweeps the podium and most of the top-20 spots.

MADISON★

others, pushing each other, having fun, sharing the experience, and for the first time in 18 years, I didn't have that."

Hilary moved to the Bay Area to pursue clinical research and chase adventure in her free time. I asked her about the differences between the Best Coast and the Beast Coast. "Boston is massive and loud," she said. "You are constantly surrounded by people. They're yelling at you, motivating you. It's such a rush. San Francisco is smaller and less intense—not workout intensity, but social-vibe intensity. We let people fall into us like a feather bed while Boston yanks you into the cold water."

We stopped to pick up another tribe member and then headed for Fulton Street, rolling past Alamo Square, the *Full House* neighborhood. With its sloped paths, steps, ample green space, and postcard views of the city, the park was a natural choice for NP workouts. But despite their best efforts to keep the early-morning sweats quiet, too many neighbors complained too many times, and the tribe had to find a new spot. It wouldn't be the last time.

"SF's workouts are more scattered," Hilary continued. "I don't mean less organized, but they're designed with a lot of chance and change of direction. We have 'dice rolls' thrown in—random workouts based on rock-paper-scissors or Boggle, for example. There's less yelling to go harder, faster. More high fives and stops for hugs. We get distracted frequently. The vibe is quirky family."

A lot of that has to do with leader McCloskey, a 29-year-old former Division 1 track standout.

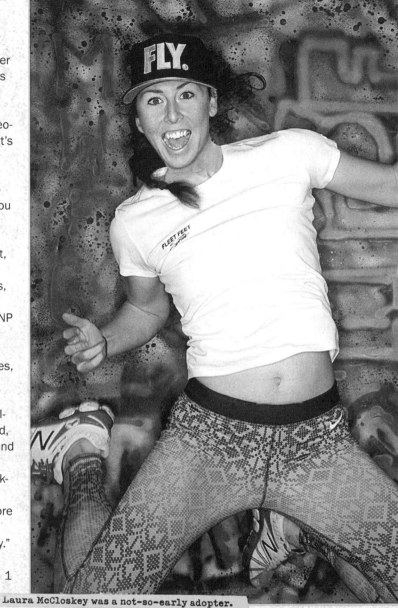

Laura McCloskey was a not-so-early adopter.

3,014? FUCK YEAH!

SEPTEMBER 2014

The challenge of hitting a goal of 3,014 people in a single workout at a combined 16 cities is issued.

WEDNESDAY, OCTOBER 29, 2014

Bojan and BG hand over the reins to the Boston tribe to Emily Saul, Deniz Karakoyunlu, and Evan Dana, the first full leadership transition. For the Mother Ship tribe, the beat goes on, proving that the movement is bigger than just the individual leaders. The music is clearly now playing the band.

> **"Also, being a chick running the show, it was like NP is not just for big, tall dudes. So it was less intimidating for San Diego to start or for any of the female leaders. NP could have totally continued as this Big Dudes thing forever. I was like, you know, fuck that shit."**
>
> —LAURA McCLOSKEY

"Laura makes a point to meet every new person," Hilary said. "I was intimidated at first because she's very much the matriarch of the tribe, but I now know how approachable she is. And knowing her outside of NP, she leads how she lives: carefree but head-on."

San Francisco was the third tribe to join the NP family, with McCloskey posting her first blog post in May of 2013. The second chapter to come on board was Madison, Wisconsin, a tribe driven by BG's older brother, Dan, a 6-foot-5 swim instructor.

"This is kind of arrogant of me to say," McCloskey later told me, "but when the Madison tribe came on, that's family. This works because it's BG's brother. It made sense and at that point, I don't think anyone was thinking, 'Let's do this all over the world.' But when San Francisco, this little West Coast tribe, started to grow, and Madison got big, too, people were like, 'Hmm, maybe we can do this in other places and it will actually work.'

"Also, being a chick running the show, it was like NP is not just for big, tall dudes. So it was less intimidating for San Diego to start or for any of the female leaders. NP could have totally continued as this Big Dudes thing forever. I was like, you know, fuck that shit."

Since then, November Project had grown to 19 tribes, three in Canada and 16 in the continental United States. (*Editor's note: At the time this book went to press, those numbers have swelled to 30 cities.*) A week earlier, I'd joined BG for the official launch of the Virginia Beach

tribe. After 2 months of pledging, they got a Founding Father's Fuck Yeah! in a dark parking lot off South Boulevard. BG addressed some 30 eager faces, presented the new leaders with their own engraved Positivity Award and a set of official NP stencils, tagged a bunch of shirts, and brought his bellowing hype to the predawn sweat fest. Bojan was doing the same thing up in Winnipeg. The Virginians put on an ass-kicker, packed with hoistees, partner pushups, triceps dips, stair climbs, and capped it with frenzied sprints up a 60-foot hill at a landfill-turned-park aptly named Mount Trashmore. A week later, on the other side of the country, that hill was still echoing in my quads.

When we pulled up to the parking lot at the bottom of the hill, the light was a royal blue. More than a hundred souls milling about, chatting and hugging and snapping cheek-to-cheek selfies. Bikes leaned against a long wall that snaked in both directions. We were hidden behind a curtain of mist, a wide stretch of sand, and the Pacific Ocean. "Karl the Fog loves to crash this spot," Hilary said. Dozens of shirts and shorts were laid flat on the pavement, wrinkled and empty, like we'd just missed the Rapture. I saw one woman in cowboy boots and denim shorts and, for a split second, wondered how far she thought she'd be running in those, but then I smiled. Nothing was strange at November Project.

I was a little anxious about this morning's workout, not knowing exactly what the rituals would be (I heard there might be dancing, something I relished after a couple of

NOVEMBER 2014

BG leaves his digital marketing and events marketing role at New Balance to take on NP full time with Bojan. The movement is now set on taking flight, with the help of The North Face to begin in 2015.

BG is walked out of the New Balance HQ building with a few boxes of size 16 890v4's, with Josh Rowe and Andy Downin by his side. All three laugh, shake hands, and know that they'll all be sharing some kind of space in the people-in-motion industry.

WEDNESDAY, NOVEMBER 5, 2014 — 3,014!!!!

The goal of 3,014 members across the country in a single workout is hit, with 1,500 alone showing up at Harvard Stadium. A far cry from the three runners they had just 2½ years earlier.

forties, but my last drink was 16 years earlier). Or how hard I'd have to push myself (SF had a super-speedy rep, built on hundreds of tightly coiled twentysomething legs). And being from Boston, the Mother Ship, I felt extra pressure to represent, perhaps more than my *Runner's World* credentials or working on the November Project book did.

In the dim light, McCloskey was easy to spot—tall in bright pink leggings, a blue long sleeve, and a lime-green trucker hat under her bike helmet. Seven years earlier, she was clocking 2:10s in the 800m. These days, she ran sub-3:10 marathons. She'd known Graham from college. "BG thought he was a track athlete, and he ran with the women's track team in the off season."

The light shifted a few more degrees as if being turned by hand crank, revealing the vague outlines of the

NovemberProjectSF @Nov_Project_SF · 30 Dec 2013
2014 is coming. Time to join a gym, **eat healthy for 3 days and buy over priced sneakers, right?**

Wrong. So wrong.

#NPSF #PUTDOWNTHEWALLET

cliffs, the mish-mash geometry of ruins of the Sutro Baths, and beyond those, parkland threaded with trails, cedar veins disappearing into the tree line. A couple people I knew only from Facebook materialized as if stepping out of my newsfeed. "In our house, you're known as the guy who lives in the stadium and writes books," said Nathaniel Fisher, a marketing and communications professional. *Great, the stadium golem.* Clearly I'd been breaking my "I'm-still-a-professional" rule of only two NP Facebook posts a week.

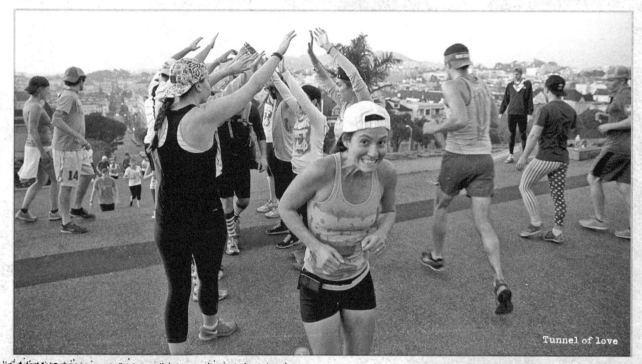

Tunnel of love

WEDNESDAY, NOVEMBER 12, 2014

To mark NP's third birthday, a giant purple bag of thank-you letters and gifts of appreciation is delivered to BG and Bojan from the Boston tribe at a Harvard Stadium workout. The boys, for once, are left speechless. The contents fill Bojan's basement, and it takes them a month to read every letter and open each gift.

THANK YOU. THANK YOU. THANK YOU

JANUARY 2015

Ethan Bookman types the first words of this book.

FEBRUARY 2015

Boston faces record-shattering and soul-crushing snowfall without a single canceled workout. Led by Boston leader Emily Saul, tribe members shovel out stadium sections on Tuesday evenings.

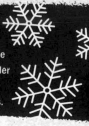

While Fisher was in his early forties, most of the San Francisco tribe was dew-covered and known for a particular brand of high-grade zaniness—dance-off circles, schoolyard games, leapfrogging. In fact, one of SF's most core members was Fisher's 3-year-old son, Tommy. His pint-sized tee was laid out with the rest, awaiting the weight of the stencils, the hiss of black spray paint, and the pungent reveal of a fresh NP logo. Tommy's mom, Katy Davis, a 38-year-old pediatrician, was buckling him into a red jogger stroller. I took in the towhead for a moment, his dimpled cheeks and pudgy hands. *No way is he beating me.*

The tribe threw Tommy a birthday bash the month before. He dressed as his favorite flying creature—a pterodactyl—while "the adults" wore a variety of wings, greeting him with dance, cake, and song as the sun rose over Corona Heights, above the city. "It was pretty incredible," Fisher said. "He couldn't stop talking about it. He's an only child, and here, he's the only child of a 100-plus-person family." McCloskey, who is also the tribe's interpreter of hard-to-understand people (one of her coleaders is an excitable Irish ex-pat named Paddy O'Leary), recapped Tommy's experience that morning in a blog post (at right).

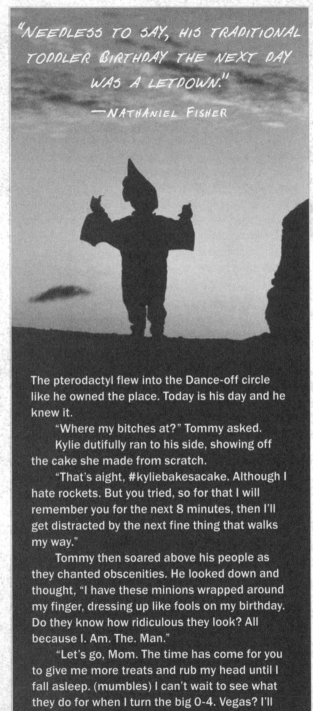

"NEEDLESS TO SAY, HIS TRADITIONAL TODDLER BIRTHDAY THE NEXT DAY WAS A LETDOWN."
—NATHANIEL FISHER

The pterodactyl flew into the Dance-off circle like he owned the place. Today is his day and he knew it.

"Where my bitches at?" Tommy asked.

Kylie dutifully ran to his side, showing off the cake she made from scratch.

"That's aight, #kyliebakesacake. Although I hate rockets. But you tried, so for that I will remember you for the next 8 minutes, then I'll get distracted by the next fine thing that walks my way."

Tommy then soared above his people as they chanted obscenities. He looked down and thought, "I have these minions wrapped around my finger, dressing up like fools on my birthday. Do they know how ridiculous they look? All because I. Am. The. Man."

"Let's go, Mom. The time has come for you to give me more treats and rub my head until I fall asleep. (mumbles) I can't wait to see what they do for when I turn the big 0-4. Vegas? I'll get Sunish on the planning now."

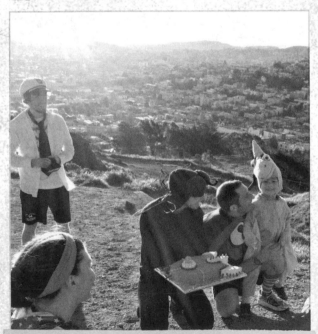

San Francisco's most popular member is 3 years old and part pterodactyl. Don't fuck with him.

The crowd started tightening around McCloskey. Many of the eyes fixed on her belonged to transplants, several time zones from home, many for the first time. "Good morning," she shouted. "Raise your hand if today is your first day."

A smattering of arms shot up.

"Welcome. Anybody visiting from another tribe?"

I raised my hand, along with a few others.

"Okay, we've got Canada, New York City, Boston. Great."

"Anybody here writing a book about November Project?"

I raised my hand again and stepped forward. *Don't make me dance. Please. All I got is a couple Axl Rose snake moves that always morph into the zombie shuffle from Michael Jackson's* Thriller *video.*

"Everyone, this is Ethan Bookman. He's from Boston. Welcome to San Francisco, Bookman . . . Okay, a couple of announcements . . ."

I stepped back, unclenching my sphincter. And then chuckled. Over the past several months, I'd been operating under a pseudonym, thanks to BG's mom. When we met last fall in Madison, she had trouble with my name and decided Ethan Bookman was easier to remember. Apparently, this path of least resistance was common with Ann Doody, a 6-foot-1 ski instructor and artist who more or less raised a pair of oversized rambunctious boys on her own, the original Mother of Dragons. I wasn't the first friend she'd renamed.

But on one level, this existential outgrowth was fitting. Before NP, as a sober runner with over a decade of clean living under my belt, I figured I had changed enough for one lifetime. I'd already done the impossible, plus written a book about it. I was good, thanks. But I kept showing up to NP after my *Runner's World* story hit recycling bins. Partly because it was a hard workout, partly because I'd met some interesting people, and partly because I just wanted to see what the hell BG

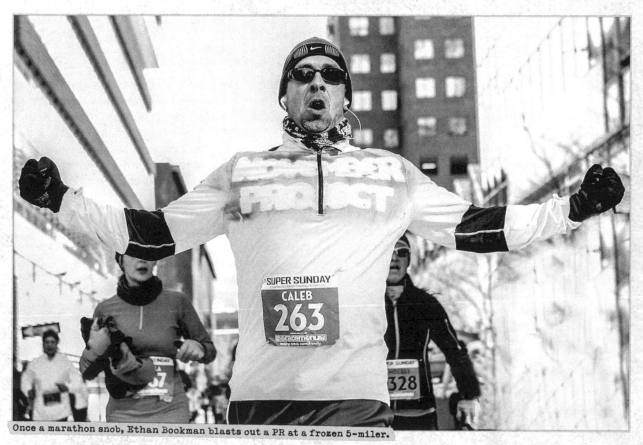

Once a marathon snob, Ethan Bookman blasts out a PR at a frozen 5-miler.

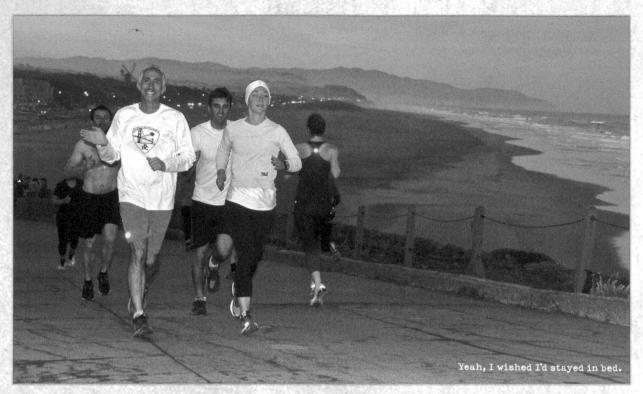

Yeah, I wished I'd stayed in bed.

would say next. Also, at the time, I was dealing with some tough family issues, which often left me depressed, angry, feeling stuck. I forced myself to the stadium, just for the change of head space. Tapping into all that positive energy, even as I mostly kept to myself, I often returned home softened and recharged. Being around so many young athletes somehow energized me, prevented me from becoming that crusty codger yelling down at kids cutting across my lawn. I pushed myself more—*Sure, I'll run across the Grand Canyon. Pikes Peak Marathon, why not? A hundred sections at the stadium, what day?* I wore colors. Took out my headphones (most of the time). Put down my car keys and climbed on a bike after 25 years. NP was about redefining the borders, first in fitness, then in life.

"Something softened in you at NP—an anxiety, a worry, perhaps," my wife Chris told me. "I see photos of you on their FB page and there's a lightness about you that didn't used to come out very often. But the biggest thing I noticed was that this was a group of people you didn't mind socializing with on your own. And the day I

saw you spend an afternoon getting your costume ready for a themed workout was the day I knew you'd leaped headfirst into the Kool-Aid. Just kidding about the Kool-Aid. Well, kinda."

"You all ready?" McCloskey began. "Because we don't have to worry about noise this morning, we're gonna do all the warm-ups and all the chants we've ever done at one time. Get your basketball stance on. Bring in your football feet."

McCloskey bent her knees and began stuttering her legs in place, arms swinging and slicing at her hips.

"Get your butt down. Lower than that. Now slap the ground and say, 'Hey!'"

A resounding collective slap. "HEY!"

"Now get your hands up and jump . . . MAKES ME WANNA . . ."

"SHOUT!" came the response.

McCloskey picked up the pace, pounding the ground, leaping into the air, belting out more song fragments, the crowd popping like a giant bag of Orville Redenbacher. "Everyone get closer. Keep moving. Closer. Butts-in-faces close." Coleaders O'Leary and Daniel Clayton, standing on the wall, joined in, trading turns shouting at throat-scorching pitches: "GOOOOOOOOOOD MORNING!" and "YOU GOOOOOOOOD?" From a hundred-some variety of responses crowding the air, a sonic ball of energy rose overhead like a joyous thundercloud. You could almost touch it.

"AND STOP!"

McCloskey explained the workout: quarter-mile hill repeats along Point Lobos Avenue. When we reached a pair of lion statues at the Lands End visitor center, she said, we were to touch their heads and turn back down. As many as we could in 30 minutes. Fastest male and female would win a bib for the Rock N' Roll Half-Marathon in 2 weeks donated by race ambassador and tribe regular Brian Kelley "That's it, that's all the instructions we have for you today."

And off they went, like a string of beads snipped loose. Tommy, in his stroller, was pushed by Davis.

I kept one eye on him and the other on McCloskey, who headed over to the wall. She cinched a black bandanna across her face, pulled on rubber gloves, and grabbed a can of Krylon spray paint. McCloskey admits that when she lived in Boston she was super-skeptical of NP. Too campy, too much repetitive lingo, too much BG worship. "I'd show up every once in a while, with my headphones. I was like, this is cool but . . . I've already got friends."

Everything changed when she was planning a trip to Uganda to volunteer her physical therapy services. McCloskey decided to collect used running shoes to donate, as well. BG helped out by posting her cause on the November Project blog. "Within 24 hours, I had an apartment full of sneakers. People were showing up at my doorstep. I was overwhelmed. I mean, people didn't know me at all. I didn't talk to anyone. But seeing how willing people were to deliver these sneakers,

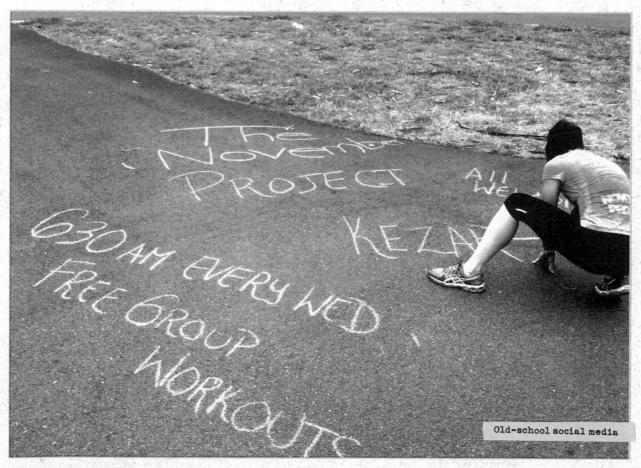

Old-school social media

I was like okay, this is actually something incredible they built."

Back in the Bay Area, McCloskey spread the word by chalking sidewalks with "JUST SHOW UP" and workout details, while posting on free activities sites. "There was no pledge process back then. I just started a Facebook group. I didn't really ask Bojan and Brogan."

Bojan remembers it a little differently.

"We had a lot of back and forth trying to talk her out of starting a tribe, knowing that she's ADD, always looking for her next adventure. We didn't want her to start it and then move to New Zealand, or the moon, and leave it all behind. We had our doubts. Laura would attend the Bos-

ton workouts, but she'd rarely do the prescribed work. She'd stand around with her arms crossed, most of the time doing her own thing, and then leaving early 'for work.' But after she mobilized the whole Boston tribe to donate running shoes and workout clothes tagged 'November Project' for children in Uganda, and then hand-delivered three giant totes with 200 pounds of gear after sweet-talking the airline into waiving the baggage fees, we knew she understood what NP really stood for. And we knew that we had to do whatever we could to keep her around."

However it went down, the sassy physical therapist has since built the San Francisco tribe to an average showing of 200 a pop, and brought on two coleaders, O'Leary and Clayton, both 27-year-old sub-2:45 marathoners. While McCloskey wants to keep the numbers manageable and her core folks intact, her vision has always extended beyond the morning Bounce.

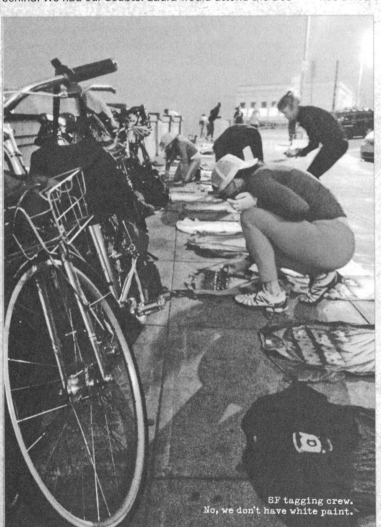

SF tagging crew.
No, we don't have white paint.

"It's not from six-thirty to seven-thirty in the morning that you get to know people, but from all the side stuff. And that's something Dan, Paddy, and I have worked very hard at building. We set up cheer stations for all the marathons and half-marathons in the area. Every weekend, the tribe is putting out: 'Who wants to go on a trail run? Who's up for an overnight camping trip?' San Francisco is a playground for outdoor activities. Here—it's we get up at six and hike into the woods, where we'll rappel down a mountain to where our kayaks are and then paddle over to our surfboards, that kind of thing. We're not all road racers training for Boston."

As the first wave of runners came streaking down the hill, McCloskey squatted over the first shirt and turned her hat backward, revealing a piece of duct tape with the words "Fast As Sam" scrawled across it. She positioned the silver stencils and went to work. I joined the line heading up the winding path, the Tommymobile a few clicks ahead. I turned on my jets. "Have a great workout," McCloskey yelled, and then turned back to her task.

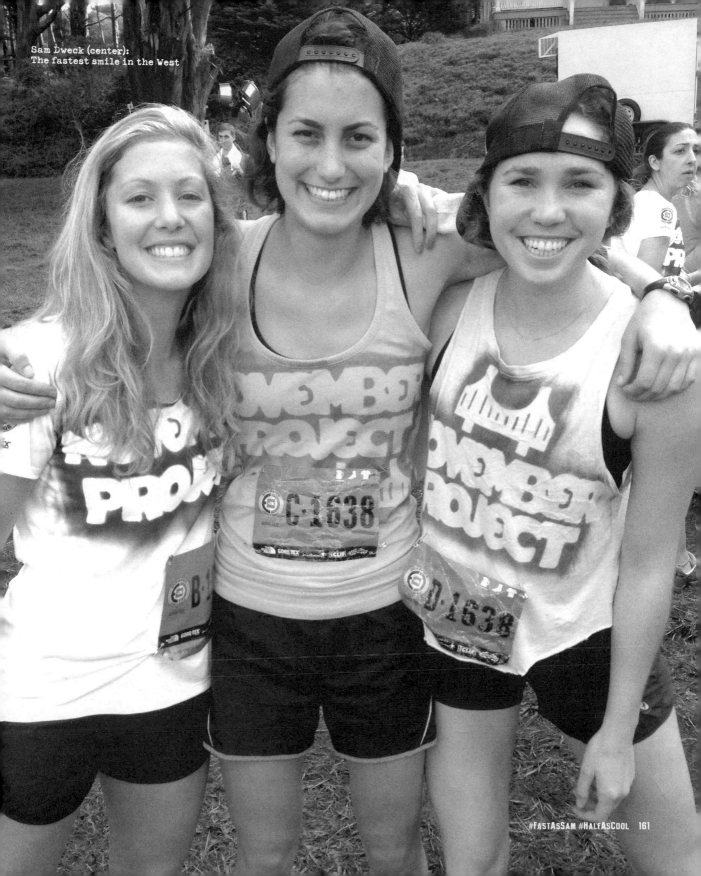

Sam Dweck (center):
The fastest smile in the West

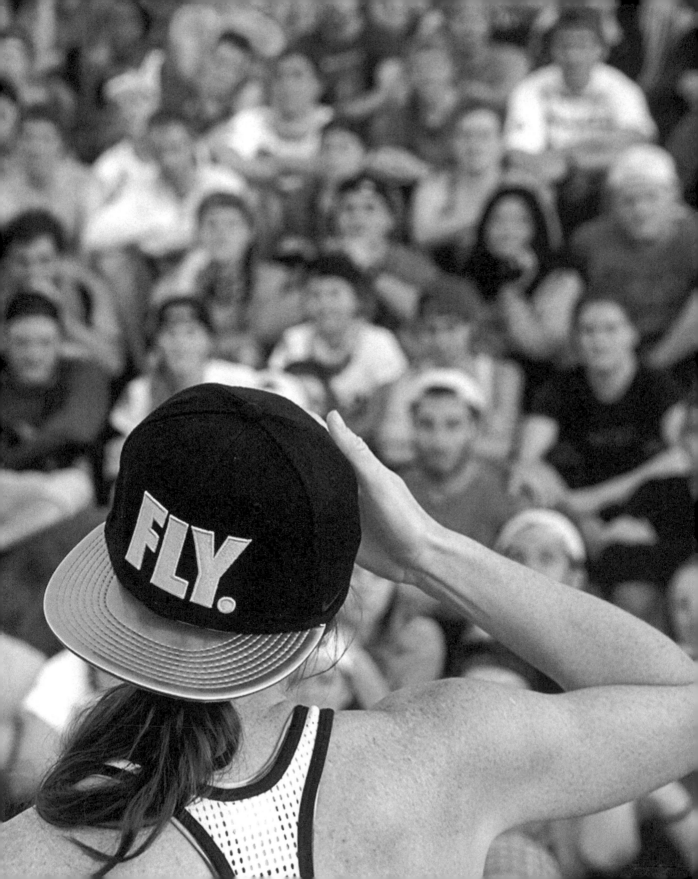

The Sam on McCloskey's hat was Samantha Dweck, a beloved tribe member who would have been there that day battling for that half-marathon bib, her brown curls tucked beneath a backward ball cap, a smile cutting through the fog. Two months earlier, the radiant 24-year-old drowned while kayaking on the Eel River some 5 hours north in Humboldt County. It happened during a camping expedition with a bunch of friends from NP. Passing beneath a bridge near a river bend, the current had flipped her kayak and sucked it against a pylon, trapping her beneath the water. Twenty-three other tribe members were part of the flotilla, some in the kayaks ahead of hers, some behind watching in horror, many of them there this day, grazing the lion's head with their fingers at the top of the hill. One of them was O'Leary.

"That accident, losing that always-upbeat, beautiful girl was by far one of the worst things I've ever experienced in my life," he said. "When the kayak turned over, we just expected it to pop up straight away. But it didn't. We paddled to shore as quick as possible. Three of us got underneath the bridge, on top of the pylon, to see if we could free the boat. We all really thought we'd be able to resolve the situation. But the water was just too powerful, thousands of gallons of pressure. We couldn't budge it. It took Rescue 3 hours to free Sam."

Because of the anemic cell phone reception in the area, it took multiple broken-up calls and dropped voice mails from O'Leary for McCloskey, back in San Francisco, to piece together the tragedy. "My brain immediately went into *what's NP's role and how can we fix this*, which obviously you can't," she said. "I felt this acute responsibility. A lot of these people are younger than me, early twenties, babies. I felt this very strong need to pull everyone together and hold them close."

Dweck had been one of those babies, initially homesick when she first moved here. Back in Carlisle, Massachusetts, she'd been a state champion pole vaulter and competitive gymnast. After graduating from Brown University in 2012, she moved west to pursue her interest in sustainable local food systems and engage in her love of nature and recreation. Once she stumbled on NP, home didn't seem so far away anymore, McCloskey said. "She found a whole new friend base and never missed a workout.

McCloskey about to deliver the devastating news

"Sam was your adventure girl, just down for everything, would say no to nothing," McCloskey continued. "She had this incredible presence and self-confidence about her that everyone was envious about. She just had life figured out, at least it seemed that way. She was 5 years younger than me, but I wanted to be her when I grew up."

The accident happened on a Sunday, and the tribe's Monday workout was scheduled to take place in less than 12 hours. They decided to go ahead as planned. "We tried to keep it as light as possible," McCloskey said. "It's a smaller crew, but it's usually when the most newbies show up, so for us to get heavy on a Monday would have been a little funny."

By the next workout, on Wednesday, word had spread across all 16 (at the time) tribes.

"Sam was always known for wearing her hat backward," McCloskey said. "It was adorable. She always kept her curls back with a hat. To see two-hundred-plus people in front of me with their hats on backward was one of the most powerful things that has ever happened in my life. But then to see photos of it happening among tribes at all the workouts across the United States almost brought me to my knees."

Before the workout, McCloskey said a few words, told a few anecdotes about Sam, and underlined that the SF tribe wasn't built on burpees or pushups, but on human interactions. "We're a family that happens to do fitness on the side," she said. It took everything in her to hold it together. Dweck's father, Richard, who lives in Mountain View, about an hour away, was in the crowd. He was wearing his hat backward, too.

"Rich got up and said something beautiful, that he'd never seen her happier in the last few months than when she was with her NP people. He said something incredibly healing for the people who were on the trip. He went up to the river where the accident happened and said he's never seen a more beautiful place in his life, and 'I know you guys did everything you could.' I think it took a lot of heaviness off the shoulders of the people on that trip. There wasn't a dry eye in that crowd. There were like 10 newbies that morning and I can just imagine them like, 'What is going on here?' But it was probably the best day to walk into this group of people which is so much more than just a workout group."

McCloskey and O'Leary, who was also tagging shirts, began calling time. As sweat-covered runners pumped the brakes and came to a stop, they lined up and grasped hands above their heads, creating a human cheer tunnel. Each person took his or her spot at the end, locking hands with a fellow member, sometimes a friend, sometimes a friend they hadn't met yet. I clasped fingers with the woman in the cowboy boots. Her name is Krissi Polentz and she, along with several others, was dressed Western-style because one of their favorite tribe members was moving to Dallas that day. Signaling the official end to the workout, the last NPers to streak through were Tommy and Davis. I could only imagine how Tommy will look back on this part of his childhood, and how it will help shape his path forward. Seeing the glee in his eyes, I'd never wanted to relive my single digits more badly. I was jealous of a 3-year-old.

McCloskey and O'Leary corralled everyone down to the beach. "Okay, human NP, start assembling," O'Leary said, standing on a graffitied retaining wall as McCloskey unscrewed the lens cap on her camera. Karl the Fog had cleared out, and a funnel of golden sun spread across the ocean like an oil painting, the whites of the waves curling just before the shore. O'Leary directed people until everyone, including Tommy, was positioned in place. Below him stood a colorful, living, breathing, sweat-glistening pair of letters: NP. For a moment, there was only the sound of the water. Then McCloskey lowered her camera. "Have the best day," she shouted. Then she and O'Leary packed up their gear and, along with about 40 other tribe members, headed up to Louise's Diner to linger over coffee and eggs before they had to switch the cords and plug back into their 9-5 lives.

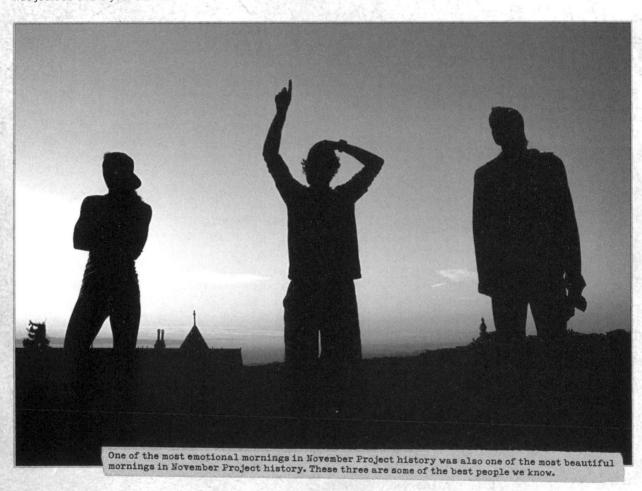

One of the most emotional mornings in November Project history was also one of the most beautiful mornings in November Project history. These three are some of the best people we know.

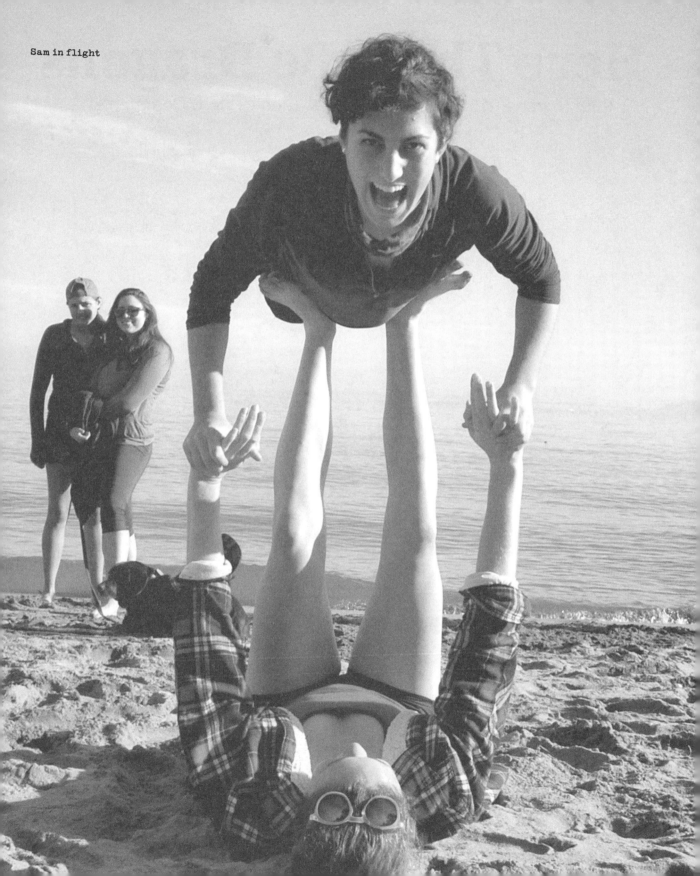

Sam in flight

Here There Be Dragons

🕐 20th March 2015   👤 Clayton   📁 Blog   💬 0 Comments

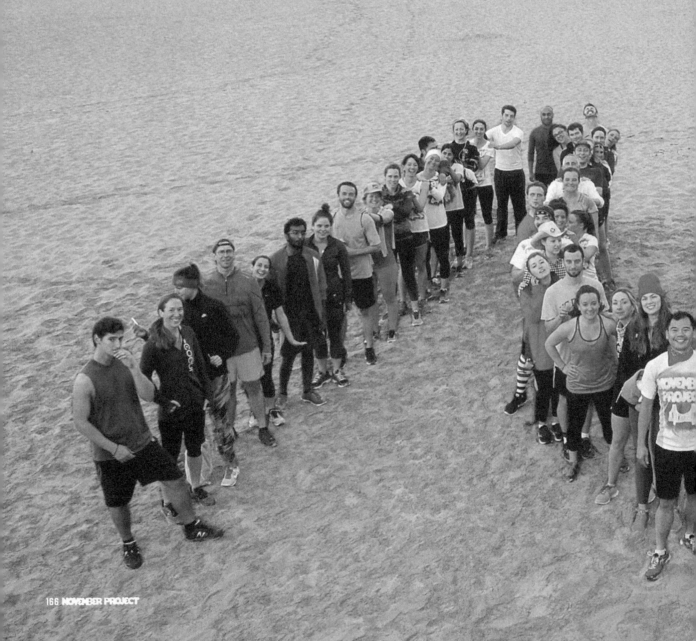

Lands End. The place where land LITERALLY ends. The world is flat. Well . . . not flat, you spent all morning running up a giant hill at the end of the universe, so . . . no, not flat. But don't you kind of feel that way when you stand at Lands End? Like, if you started swimming out into the Pacific you'd eventually go off the page? And then who knows if you'll ever resurface at the right side of the page!? I mean, like, what the heck is out there, right?

I don't know, maybe you don't feel this way . . . maybe you're not terrible at geography. Maybe you understand basic physics . . . Show off.

Anyways.

This morning was pretty freaking cool. About 100 people showed up to CRUSH hills and get their #GRASSROOTSGEAR tagged. We were loud. We were SO loud and it felt really freaking good. Paddy, Laura and I unleashed all of the chants we've ever done all at once to take advantage of the rare opportunity. It was wonderful.

Thank you ALL for coming out. Cheer on your fellow tribe-members this weekend as they race in Oakland. Kadala is taking it easy this weekend and ONLY running a full marathon. (*Slacker*)

Peace.

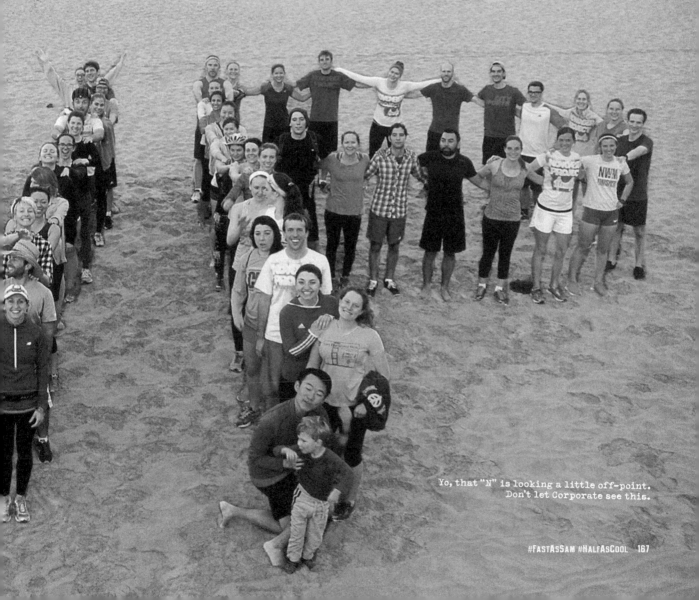

Yo, that "N" is looking a little off-point.
Don't let Corporate see this.

A Father's Grief—And Solace: In His Own Words

Richard Dweck, 59, Mountain View, California

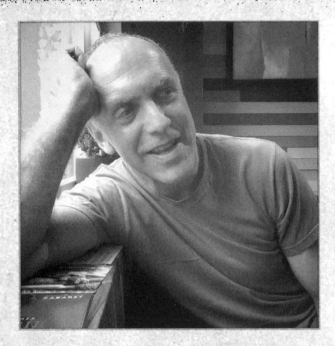

Richard Dweck loves one particular photo of his daughter, Sam. It shows her leapfrogging over another girl crouched on the sidewalk. She is suspended mid-flight, her blue hat turned backward, her legs split in the air, pink shoelaces flying. It's dark out, but you can see the joy in her eyes, framed beneath a pair of brows that are arched almost in wonder. She's sticking her tongue out at the camera yet somehow still flashing a smile. But this isn't some childhood photo Richard keeps in his wallet. Rather, it's one of the last Facebook images of 24-year-old Sam before she drowned. Three days after the tragedy, a crushed Richard found his way to Alta Plaza Park, compelled to commune with the fitness group that had meant so much to Sam as she launched her new life in San Francisco—and where that photo was taken. —CD

My daughter died on a Sunday, and I went for my first November Project meeting on that Wednesday. There were at least two-hundred people there—to embrace me, comfort me, and tell me how much they loved my daughter. Of the two-hundred people, at least a hundred came up and hugged me and we cried together. I don't know how I would have gotten through it otherwise if I hadn't gone to NP that day. It was the biggest, warmest safety net I could have imagined, because I was sinking like a brick.

I just felt like this was her group and they had given her so much in the short amount of time she'd been in San Francisco. I just wanted to be with them. I knew the people who were on the kayaking trip with her were going to be there and I wanted to see them, feel their energy. They were the last people to see her alive.

Some people from November Project called me right away, maybe Tuesday, after I found out and seeing my daughter and dealing with her remains. They said, "We want you know we've already come up with all this funding for anything you need, any costs incurred." They paid her rent for several months so the two roommates had a chance to decide what to do. They ended up having this woman move in, who was always over there with the three of them anyway. So this home got to be preserved. It was because of them.

Then that weekend, this one guy, Sunish, organized a run-walk-bike where they spelled out "Fast As Sam" on Strava [a popular app with runners and bikers that among other features details routes on a map]. My ex-wife and son were there for that and we walked the "Sam" part. Afterward, we had a wonderful lunch with everyone. It was very meaningful. Before that, we went to a tagging ceremony, where they spray-painted hundreds of items with a "Fast As Sam" stencil someone made. It was amazing just to see all the other NP tribes that didn't even know her doing things, too. In Boston,

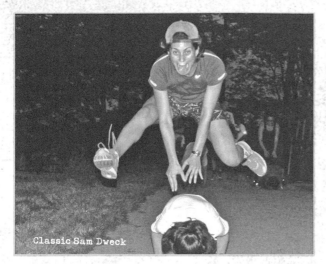
Classic Sam Dweck

they had a whole workout dedicated to her. I think they said they had one thousand people around the country running with their hats on backward.

Samantha and I were very close. Three or four times a week, she'd tell me about something that had happened at November Project. It sounded like a great group of people who got up early and worked out crazy-hard together and then enjoyed socializing at night and on these weekend trips. For no profit, for no reason other than the love of the game. It was the most positive thing I could imagine. I told her I wished I had something like that when I was her age.

I knew. But now the world knew, I guess, that she was the most optimistic, loving, upbeat, positive person that many of them had ever met. Some people from NP said, "I felt like she loved me before I even opened my mouth." She was all positive energy. Even when a person did something horrible to her, she never said a negative word. She'd be crushed and depressed, but would never say a bad word. Her energy really resonated with them. She was also a role model. She worked hard at things, and I think people were impressed and inspired by that as well.

These are kids having the time of their life. They're on their own, establishing their own life and the meaning of it. So I didn't want to go back every week and make it about Sam, and have it be sad. But I did want to see them again. So I waited a few months. They were so happy to see me and said, "You should come every week." They really are open to me attending things. They have a good, supportive memory of my daughter.

On a lot of levels, Sam was as happy as she had ever been in her life as she started her career and adult life, post-college. She and I were very connected. We talked a lot. I instilled in her a desire to do great things in life. She had the intelligence, the drive, the personality and enthusiasm to do big and meaningful things. She was just in the beginning of figuring out what those things were. There was so much more to come. **NP**

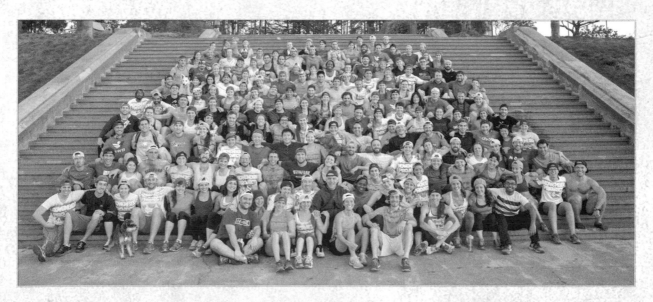

THE VORTEX

The tribe runs around in a circle continuously while the leaders take turns yelling out categories. If that category applies to you, you run into the middle of the circle and perform the stated exercise then return to the vortex. Example categories could be anything from simply "If you are married" to the more complex "If you are afraid of spiders, snakes and/or ducks." We really feel like we get to know the tribe with this workout.

CHAOS LAP

Can be screamed at any point throughout the workout. When yelled, everyone stops what they are doing and sprints out of the park. When you hit the sidewalk, you can take either a left or right and run a full lap around, giving every person you see a high five. Enter the park the way you came and resume the regularly scheduled workout.

COMPLIMENT SQUATS

While facing a fellow tribesman and performing squats, you compliment your partner with a straight face in an effort to make him or her laugh. If you are successful, you continue running up the steps to your next opponent, and the laughing loser of the two returns to the bottom step to start again. Some of our favorite compliments have been "I bet you look sexy eating corn" and "You make Kegel exercises look so easy."

ROCK, PAPER, SCISSORS

A workout widely used today in the NP world originated in SF. Challenge your opponent to a simple game of rock, paper, scissors while performing squats. The winner gets to direct the loser to which corner of the park they have to run. Each corner has a different challenging exercise, along with a hill or stair climb that returns the runner to the central workout site. Once there, they challenge a new opponent.

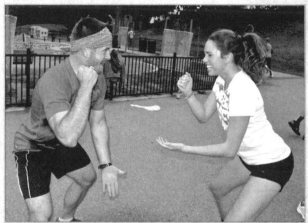

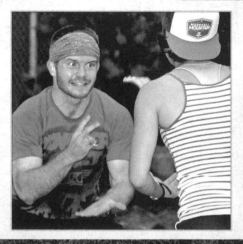

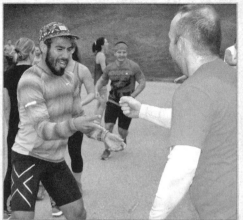

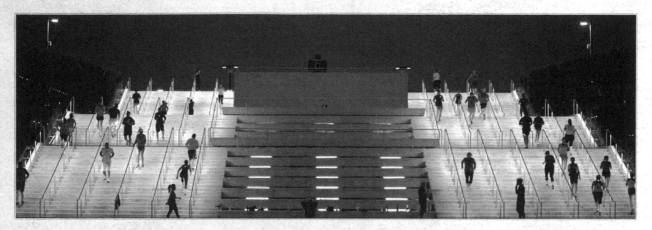

TAKING NOVEMBER PROJECT BEYOND BOSTON

BY BOJAN MANDARIC

Long before DG (Dan Graham) called me one day and said, "All right, I want to talk to you and not my idiot brother because I think what you guys are doing is okay, and I would love to do it in Madison, but I don't want to give BG the satisfaction of knowing that his loud ass is doing something right." Brogan and I had been talking about World Takeover. People laughed at this notion, thinking that it was just BG overhyping everything, and that my lack of English comprehension prevented me from understanding the concept of "world."

But we were serious. We wanted to bring NP to more cities than Boston. But we didn't know how that would look. DG was a trendsetter. Laura was a friend who we tried to scare off. We didn't have the balls to tell Andrew (Ference) that starting with three workouts a week wasn't the best idea, but Danny (Metcalf) in DC was the real test case for how to work with someone we didn't know, who had no connections to Boston. And that tribe is now the second largest after Boston; they're absolutely killing it on every level.

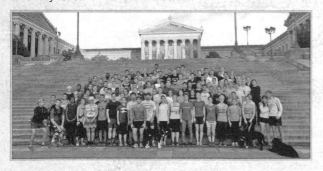

With our full-time jobs, families, and management of 15-plus cities, we realized things were moving WAY too fast. The first time we met the leaders of NP Chicago and New Orleans was at the November Project Summit in September 2014, 4 or 5 months after they both became official tribes. We were expecting them to put their heart and soul into something we're so passionate about, but we'd never exchanged bear hugs. Something had to change. We needed to slow down. So instead of pursuing quantity, we decided to pump the brakes at the start of 2014 and suspend the pledge process. We wanted to focus on the quality of the existing workouts, get culturally aligned across all the tribes, and encourage collaboration between all the different leaders.

We like to say that the November Project experience is the same across all of our locations. Workouts are always hard yet scalable and designed for all fitness levels. The community is welcoming and encourages breaking free from uptight social norms. One thing that makes each location different, however, is the amazing personalities of their leaders. From Bobby in Indianapolis to Pat, Sydney, and Nick in Baltimore to the four-headed beast of the South: Cameron, Preston, Kate, and Will from New Orleans, our leaders range from college students to Stanley Cup champions. They are the movers and the shakers of their respective communities, and BG and I are the luckiest dudes alive because we get to call them friends.

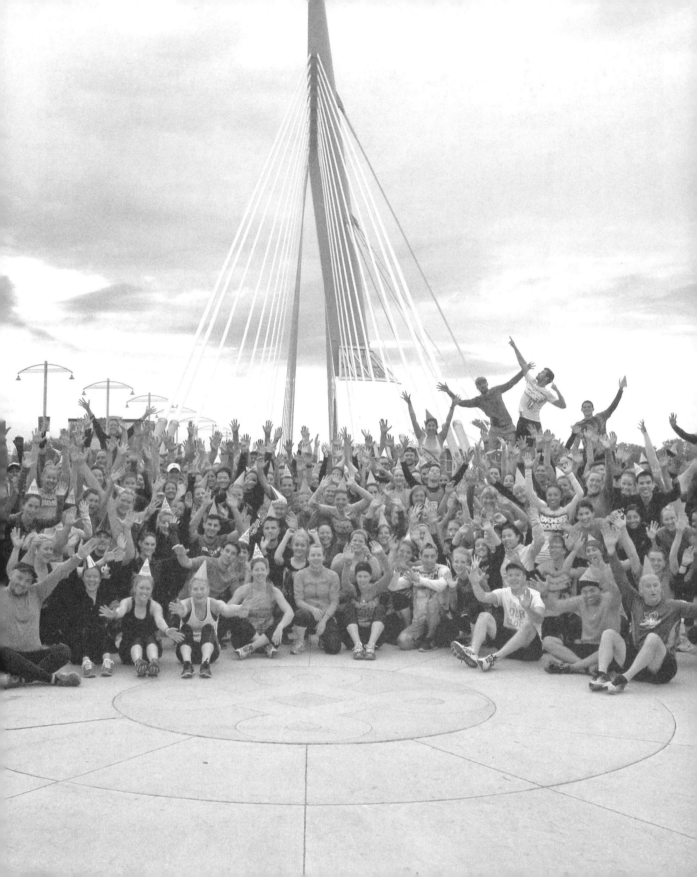

HOW TO START NOVEMBER PROJECT IN YOUR CITY
Read the whole document before making a move.

WHY THIS PLEDGE/APPLICATION?

We've worked hard to create a community that we can be proud to put our name on. This is a community that brings people together to work out for FREE regardless of age, athletic level, ethnicity, social status, or occupation. This is a community that grows and strives through the love for your city/town/neighborhood and the people in it. We know that will is not enough in order to lead a November Project tribe, and that's why we created this application/pledge document that every applicant should fill out to be considered for a position of a tribe leader in his or her city/town. Application submission does not grant you the right to start a November Project chapter in your area. It just announces your interest in starting one. Your application will be considered and, after the trial period, granted or rejected depending on the quality and competency of the candidate. If you are a trainer looking to expand your clientele, or a business owner looking to promote your business, stop right now. Your application will not be granted. The number one goal and mission of what we're doing is to drive people out of bed to get fit and build a better world to live in.

We own all rights to the product names, company names, trade names, logos, current and future product packaging and designs (trademarks) of November Project, LLC. Unauthorized use of any such trademarks, including reproduction, imitation, dilution, or confusing or misleading uses, is prohibited under the trademark laws of the United States and other countries. You are expressly prohibited from using or misusing any trademarks or names except as expressly provided in this Agreement, and nothing otherwise stated or implied in the Services confers on you any license or right to do so.

Everyone can start and run a free fitness community. Not everyone can start and run November Project.

What you are getting yourselves into:

1. TIME COMMITMENT

Understand that being the leader of your November Project branch may begin with the simple 60-minute workout you first host but will be guaranteed to grow into many hours of dedication each week. This is a part-time job that some weeks can fill enough hours to be seen as a second, completely unpaid, full-time job. You will start with only one workout per week, and that will fall on Wednesday. Once your Wednesday group grows large enough to add a Friday you will . . . and eventually a Monday . . . and then eventually you'll become connected to the nationwide fun in multicity events, races, and parties.

Understand that the preparation for each session, the blogging, the photos, the events, social media outreach, face-to-face connections in the community, and traditional media interactions will be some of the many things that will enhance your life as you take on this opportunity with November Project. All tribe leaders have found that they no longer have time to be a part of their own November Project workouts once they grow beyond the first handful of members. Hosting a workout becomes your role at NP as you quickly become a coach, inspirational speaker, photographer, matchmaker, social media expert, and professional stunt-daydreamer for all things community. If you are not willing to commit yourself fully to this role and to your tribe, your application will not be granted.

2. ATTENDANCE COMMITMENT

You have to be at every single workout. Finding a partner to colead your branch of November Project is key to starting the process. As leaders, we plan our lives, vacations, and EVERYTHING WE DO around November Project.

This is not for you if you:

- Have a job that requires a lot of travel that could take you away from the tribe you're thinking of starting.

- Are a student or a professional associated with late-night hours or unpredictable schedules that could keep you in bed in the morning hours.

- Are not comfortable working out in the rain, snow, humid weather, or scorching heat.

- Are not comfortable with public speaking or hugging strangers.

- Are not willing to pull unusual flash-mob type stunts and be, as we say at November Project, "respectively disruptive," from time to time.

3. OUR #WEATHERPROOF CONCEPT

NP is going to happen rain or shine and you have to be there! We are #weatherproof and let everyone know it. Sometimes this borders on insanity, but usually those workouts and adventures that take us to the edge in harsh weather conditions are the ones that make us feel the best (or simply most badass). Remember, people at your local tribe will know that you're going to be there to train with them at 6:30 a.m. because November Project ALWAYS DOES. You're creating something that the community knows they can count on and will be far more reliable than the train schedule in Japan.

4. WHY 6:30 A.M.?

November Project ALWAYS trains in the morning on weekdays. The early time stems from our predawn rowing days when you definitely needed lights for your boat and a sharp-eyed coxswain. But around us, apartment windows were dark, it was quiet, and it felt like the world was ours. In other words, no one's busy at 6:30 a.m. It's the perfect time to work out. Weekends and afternoons are reserved for socializing. It's that simple.

5. LEADER DESCRIPTION

- Being one of the fittest members of the tribe is a must. Leaders must lead by example. This means being in front of the pack at all times. "The quality of the team is based on the speed of the leader." Who do we consider fit? A person that can do one or all of the following: run a sub-3:25 marathon or sub-1:30 half-marathon; do a 3-minute plank finishing with 10 pushups; do 90+ burpees in 7 minutes. If you don't know what burpees are, this is not for you!

- Outgoing personality: You may talk to a waitress, a trucker, a banker, and a bank-robber while recruiting for NP in a single afternoon—your word of mouth when recruiting is HUGE. Honestly, how are you at interacting with complete strangers?

- Sense of humor: Our workouts are physically intense yet fun and funny.

- Local: You must be familiar with your city/town/neighborhood because you will eventually have to come up with different workouts and mixing up the locations is the key. Know your landmarks, public parks, stairs, and hills like the back of your hands and the tops of your feet.

- Creative: NP workouts have a standard to them that members can shoot for, but many times they have to be adjusted before the start of the session due to the unpredictable nature of outdoor training in urban environments. Having a background in coaching is a huge help.

- Connected: You must already be involved in local community. Being the new guy in town makes starting an NP tribe pretty much impossible.

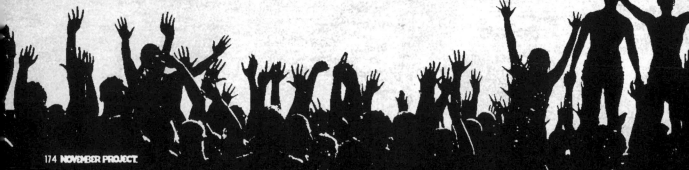

- Social media skills: New to social media?! This will be an education that you'll have to jump into immediately. All coleaders and attempting pledges must be well versed in Twitter/Facebook/Instagram and must own a camera to capture legit images at all workouts.

- Familiar with WordPress blog platform.

- Must be a hugger, not a shaker.

- Punctual/reliable.

- Competitive and supportive.

- Really good at pretending to be a morning person ("morning people" don't really exist; it was a made up term back in the 1600s that has recently been proven incorrect by scientists in labs who were holding beakers).

HOW TO APPLY?

If you think that you fit the description and are willing to commit to everything that's laid out above, please:

1. Send us a 500-word email describing who you are, what you do, and why you want this (please include your photo).

2. Get on a Google Hangout/Skype with us so we can see you and hear your passion in person. We'll respond to your initial email to set this up. If you don't hear from us within 48 hours, we're probably in the woods, so please be patient.

If we decided that you are the right personality, we want you and your coleader to begin to build your community without any help and without dropping the name "November Project." We want you to build your group to prove you're the right person/people from the outreach standpoint. Start with your friends, family, and anyone you can recruit. Pick a park, or a run loop, or some hills/stairs. Use YOUR social media network (no association to November Project) to organize your 6:30 a.m., sub-60-minute workout. Starting exactly on time is key—none of that "I was only 2 minutes late" bullshit.

Each workout should be photographed at the end, with your group staring into the camera with completely straight faces (because that shit is funny, scary, badass, and so on). Share this photo through your personal social media channel with the caption: [city name], pledging to November Project, [the workout], [location], and use the hashtag "#NP_Pledge." Tweet this from your personal account to @Nov_Project and post the same photo to the November Project wall on Facebook.

DECISION

After eight or more Wednesdays (New Orleans pledged for 11 weeks), if we think that you are worthy of proudly displaying #GrassrootsGear on your chest, we'll add your location to the family of worldwide tribes on our rapidly growing site and create official November Project Facebook and Twitter pages. Once you're in, you're in. We'll mail you the "N0V3MB3R PR0J3CT" stencils and a few rounds of Krylon black flat paint, grant you access to the weekly blog, our social media streams, and all of the additional nationwide and worldwide attention that will come in our bright future.

Essentially you're going to be a fucking leader in your community, and it will be by far the best feeling you could ever have. You'll hug strangers, kiss babies, and take photos (don't try and do all three at the same time—we had a guy in Boston go to the hospital and jail for attempting this move). You'll lead workouts that will be the best part of many people's day/week/life. You'll watch people get faster, fall in love with fitness, see improvements, find friends, fall in love, create real connections, and generally bring this small world even closer together. This is serious stuff we're dealing with. Please don't step up unless you're committed to the many items above.

Love and thanks,
November Project
You think you have what it takes? Apply now!

Dude, Don't Tell Me How to Social Media

BY BROGAN GRAHAM

Social media was getting big when Bojan and I were in college. As rowers on the Charles River in Boston, each spring we'd line up against the Aussie rowers at Boston University, the slow, smart dudes at MIT, and the Harvard twins who were super-pissed at Zuckerberg (shit, did they fucking row with white-hot anger). Yes, we were in the era when Facebook was getting its first baby breaths and many of the real-life characters from *The Social Network* movie were our competition. Off the water, we watched Facebook start as a block of simple info and a face pic: who you are and your best, square profile image. When Facebook opened up and you could use non-Ivy League email addresses to start an account, Bojan and I were some of the first ones in.

I remember "Friending" whoever I could—at the University of Miami, Yale, random schools where I didn't know anyone—in a quest to see who could rack up the most friends, hot girls in particular. (This was a contest I dominated over my teammate Brian Baraty who, to be fair, set up my account.)

Love or hate Harvard, love or hate social media these days, whatever. Just know this. We watched Facebook go from some kind of directory to some kind of show-and-tell to some kind of way to motivate, and further, as some kind of way to create a community. But that last bit, the part about community, would be a dangerous line to read too much into. Let's be clear: Bojan and I didn't start NP to disrupt any major cities, to meet new people, or as a way to drive good vibes for thousands of people. That just happened. Our goals were much simpler. We just wanted to (first) gather good/crazy athletes to train with us under our name and (later) reach more and more folks who needed a push and (lastly) create a great entry point for new or lapsed athletes who needed a safe place to start or restart.

In the spring of 2012, it was my weird idea (without talking to Bojan) to paint shirts and bring them to the workout when there were just a few of us. But before that had happened, it was his idea (without talking to me) to start a WordPress blog and a Twitter account. Facebook, though the driver of so much of what we've accidentally built, came third in our four-way social media attack.

The blog that Bojan built was simple. It had the ability to hype upcoming workouts, recap what had just taken place, and show a few of the best images of our friends in motion. For those out there who don't know about WordPress or even what a blog is . . . that's fucking awesome. Basically—and Bojan, please jump in—a blog is a website of your own making where you can say whatever you want. You can post images, tell stories, and go on and on about important things or nothing at all. FREEDOM lives in blogging because you're always right. Even when you're waaaaaaaaay off on something and your words get people pissed or confused, you've at least gathered an audience, and that in itself is a win. Bojan thought we needed a website, so he made that happen. But how do you get these recaps and inspirational nothings OUT to the world? That is where Twitter comes in.

Twitter. I have a good friend who does social media consulting (I always crack up at that job description, picturing dozens of bald suits in a boardroom learning to attach photos and drop hashtags and how to act cool with smartphones, paying top dollar for . . . #Indoors #FaxMe #CC_Everyone). He told me that unlike Facebook or Instagram, Twitter is like a cocktail party where chatter and conversation are nonstop and layered with varying levels of education, topic value, and (my favorite) levels/kinds of humor. On Twitter, you get to choose your

November Project @Nov_Project · Aug 31
Say more brilliant shit on the internet today. By Friday we can return to simple fart jokes. #Monday

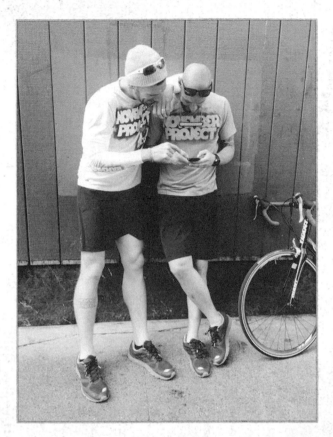

"UNLIKE FACEBOOK OR INSTAGRAM, TWITTER IS LIKE A COCKTAIL PARTY WHERE CHATTER AND CONVERSATION ARE NONSTOP AND LAYERED WITH VARYING LEVELS OF EDUCATION, TOPIC VALUE, AND (MY FAVORITE) LEVELS/KINDS OF HUMOR. ON TWITTER, YOU GET TO CHOOSE YOUR AUDIENCE. WHO YOU FOLLOW IS BASICALLY ALL THE PEOPLE WHO ARE IN THAT ROOM WITH YOU. BUT LISTENING IS OPTIONAL."

—BG

audience. Who you FOLLOW is basically all the people who are in that room with you. But listening is optional. No one will notice you looking over someone's shoulder for a more interesting dinner companion. You can get into it with anyone, or you can hear what they're spitting into their world and then attempt to derail the conversation into your direction (our game).

Others, like yours truly, end up being the loud one at the party. We don't really care who's listening, and we don't pay attention to what time the host wants us to all go home (we're never going home, by the way). We're just fine over at the bar, talking to whoever will listen. The tweets we send out into the world may sound insane, silly, or insensitive at times. But we know that if we keep at it, with enough time our audience will grow. I've gotten a little better at listening over the years, and now I liken our Twitter style to a guy on a low-rider bicycle cruising through the party at a pretty good clip, glancing around for gems and large gatherings to check out. We don't stop often. We think we're cool. We may actually be giant dorks, but no matter what, we're getting noticed.

But for starters, NP would probably never have happened the way it has without social media. That timing was critical to our growth. But we also use social in a super-active, engaging way. We are not passive. It's not about interacting with the world from afar. Social media just feathers the bed for real-world exchanges. Our dude Andrew Ference, who started tweeting out our workouts, was one of our largest recruiters via social. It wasn't about how many Favorites those tweets got, but how many bodies showed up. We rally and hype in 140 characters, but the movement is built in person. Our social media work actually makes people go be social: hug three strangers, share sweat with a group. And then tribe members go back behind the keyboard and wait for some high-quality workout photos to go up so they can tag the hell out of it, change their profile pic, and get people asking, "What the hell is this November Project I keep seeing in your feed?" Sure, you can pay to have more followers and look really popular. We're always interested in quality engagements that go beyond hitting the Like button. For us, conversations and engagements are god when it comes to social media.

But let's spin the dial back to the early days. November Project and social media. We had our blog and Twitter and that was it. Tweets could reach out into the world, and those who followed us could hear what we had to say. The problem was that when you're new to the party, nobody really cares to listen to you. We opened an account like anyone else on Twitter, with 0 followers. But unlike basketball superstar Kevin Garnett, we didn't have tens of thousands of followers after our first dozen or so tweets. But we did have about a dozen. It took some time to build our audience. In fact, it wasn't until we asked a friend at the local run-specialty store in town to retweet (RT) our call for athletes that anyone at the party noticed us over there in the corner, picking our noses. That's right, Marathon Sports, and our good friend and former teammate Nick Littlefield retweeted our call to "Come one, come all #novemberproject is in full swing. Next meeting @ Harvard Stadium 05/09 @6:30 am."

For the uninitiated, this retweet thing is actually simple to figure out. Let's just take it back to the cocktail party for a second. You want people to hear your thoughts or jokes or whatever it is you have on your mind, but nobody cares to listen to what you're saying because they don't know you exist. That is, until a more influential person—let's say the host or hostess of this party, someone who has been around for longer and who is well-known among the party guests—repeats (RT's) your exact words to their much larger audience. BOOM, you're alive! Instant credibility.

Never mind that I was once fired from a weekly Sunday morning gig I had at Marathon Sports for being in New York City during a shift or for being hungover 85 percent of the time I worked there or because I was too awesome. It doesn't matter now. When Marathon Sports sent out that historic retweet, they helped us reach more like-minded runner types, people who might actually take this "November Project" thing seriously. That is where our very first recruit, young Sara Wild, came from. She saw the tweet . . . and well . . . go back and read about her in Chapter 1.

But here's the HOW-TO section, the part you might actually use to improve your own social media game. Facebook, Instagram, Snapchat, and whatever else comes next . . . it all comes down to this . . . ready? The secret sauce is made from a mix of confidence, voice, and consistency. Those three things are far more important than anything else.

Yes, having badass photos in our Facebook albums of our sun-soaked men and women running up and down the Harvard Stadium stairs is important, especially since the posts hype the location for the next workout. Yes, having Dooster film company, a two-man team of twenty-somethings, shooting all of our biggest moments at no charge and telling our story like none other, is amazing. But more than anything else—and it bears repeating—the first three pieces of the puzzle are confidence in what you're saying, a voice worth listening to, and consistency that is on point.

CONFIDENCE

There's this Asian American woman in her thirties who races up and down hills and stairs just like everyone else. She does the workout in her authentic San Diego style, yet she lives and, pretty much, owns Boston. This doesn't mean that she's loud or comes off as a know-it-all. She's just confident. We ended up calling her "Ashley Fierce" and eventually we just shortened it to "Fierce." Guys love her, gals love her, and nobody can really put their finger on what it is that she has. But she has it. An X-factor. Confidence. Fierce's confidence makes her cool, smart, hip. So be confident. Join and own conversations that you can add to, and learn from the ones you can't. Be like Fierce. Be confident online and in life.

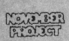

November Project @Nov_Project · 23 Nov 2015
Get your frozen ass to @Nov_Project_YWG this week.
Bring your hugging arms, racing legs, and $0 in cash. #iron26
👤 November Project WPG

VOICE

Voice. The style in which words are tossed into the pan. The pace. The cadence. The rhythm. The slang. The person behind the words that can be felt through the blog, through the title of the Facebook album, through the exact photos picked. Voice is fun and funny.

When I had the opportunity to do the social media outreach for Hubway (Boston's bike share program that popped up in 2011), we had to use a more mature, smarter voice than the one we use for November Project. Transportation nerds, city officials, cyclists, and commuters in and outside of Boston were all paying attention to this voice. You can't tweet out "Get on a fucking bike or you're soft. #RealTransportation" from an account like that. No way! You'd have officials from the City of Cambridge on the phone within minutes. No. You have to use a smarter voice that says things like, "Did you know that Boston, Brookline, Cambridge, and Somerville are now leading the charge for bike share commuters in the US? #Hubway." And in case you're struggling with the whole hashtag (#) thing, just let me say this: You'll never understand it. If you don't get it by now, just stop asking. Even those of us who DO know what they're about don't really know what we're doing with it. Everything in this world is made up. (Dad, I know you're reading this, forget trying to keep up with hashtags.)

Voice is everything. You're already far too familiar with my voice, your boss's voice, your best friend's voice, and those of the famous people you love to know about. Think about your voice, the phrases that are "soooooo you," and then build yourself as you. Social media or not, our voices set us apart from each other. Figure that shit out. It is important.

> "WE ALL KNOW THE VALUE SOCIAL MEDIA PLAYS IN THE RECRUITING GAME, BUT WE NEVER THOUGHT THAT DATING APPS COULD HELP BRING PEOPLE TO THE WORKOUTS (BECAUSE WE'RE FAITHFUL MARRIED HUSBANDS). LUCKILY, WE HAVE A BUNCH OF CREATIVE, SINGLE LEADERS WHO WON'T STOP AT ANYTHING TO SPREAD THE GOOD WORD OF FREE FITNESS."
> —BOJAN

CONSISTENCY

Bojan is the one who's in charge of this. He's the reason that our blog posts go up the same day, usually before noon. Social media, like current NEWS, yes NEWS, has an expiration date . . . and it is usually a few hours before it is old news. Bojan insisted that we get our posts up and out there so that people in their real life could connect November Project with their social media life, when the energy from the workout was still peaking. We have always aimed for "before lunch" for our full social media plan: Write a blog post that recaps and jokes about everything that went down that morning, and that also hypes what's coming next.

That piece should also include a few of the best photos of the day. Those photos, along with the other 10 to 300 images shot each morning, go into a Facebook album. In that album, the location is marked as November Project (hyperlinked so that people can click to see what the heck kind of crazy group their friends are training with early in the morning). The explanation of the album, the info, the details, or whatever it is they call it, is the link to the blog, which in turn gives the full story to new or regular members. This takes them to our site and OH, WHAT'S THAT? NP IS IN HOW MANY CITIES!? And the next thing you know, somebody's cousin is on their way to November Project Minneapolis all because someone was tagged in an epic Bojan photo that was shot at sunrise. The bragging is all done for you on Facebook. The biggest trick is to get it all written, edited, and posted while your legs are still on fire.

Twitter is simpler. A "This morning was awesome! [link to post] #community #RacingFit" along with up to four of the best photos is enough for a tweet. We tweet after every workout. Tons of our Canadian tribes are all

November Project @Nov_Project · 23 Nov 2015
Some wise guy once said "#BeTheWeirdYouWantToSeeInTheWorld," we might be making this up.
http://november-project.com/be-the-weird-you-want-to-see-in-the-world-gandhi/
👤 Janji, The North Face, Christopher and 2 others

"VOICE IS EVERYTHING. YOU'RE ALREADY FAR TOO FAMILIAR WITH MY VOICE, YOUR BOSS'S VOICE, YOUR BEST FRIEND'S VOICE, AND THOSE OF THE FAMOUS PEOPLE YOU LOVE TO KNOW ABOUT. THINK ABOUT YOUR VOICE, THE PHRASES THAT ARE 'SOOOOOO YOU,' AND THEN BUILD YOURSELF AS YOU."

—BG

about Twitter, while some of our Midwestern tribes are barely in that game at all. I'm sure you have friends who ask about Instagram or the next thing that is coming up. All I can say is that new technologies are always waving their hands and older ones are dropping into the abyss. Whatever works for you is what will work for you. Just keep your trains running on time. Consistency, remember? Keep your posting times, days, and weekly pace on point—just like NP workouts that go on regardless of the weather conditions.

The only workout we've ever canceled was on the Friday of the manhunt that followed the Boston Marathon bombing. We tweeted out that we were not going to have a hill session in Brookline that morning, and that everyone should stay home. For many in our network, in this real AND digital community, this was the first sign that something was VERY wrong. Many saw this tweet and turned on their TV for more news. Even more checked Twitter, saw the STAY HOME notice, and then got the minute-by-minute updates via local news-media accounts.

Like the revolution in Cairo a few years earlier, real NEWS, actual unfiltered images and words, was accessible via Twitter without it first being filtered through the "real media." NEWS has changed, and people need it quicker than what can be pumped out from vans full of cameras and perfect haircuts that arrive late on the scene. Users of Twitter, Facebook, Instagram, Snapchat, and a zillion other social media platforms, deliver news information with flash-fierce confidence, voice, and consistency. They are now beating traditional news to the punch and have themselves become the "hot leads" that establishment media sources troll for their next breaking story.

Bojan wasn't getting his hands into social media in the same way that I was. I love that shit. I love doing it for my 5–9 and my 9–5. I just love it. You open an account for New York City's bike share system, Citi Bike, then sit back and watch 10,000 followers step up to hear the gems you're going to toss out into the party. It's powerful stuff.

Again, confidence, voice, and consistency are the three pillars upon which your social media success depends. Now, if you have to go one step further, if you have to drive a car that has a nice shiny polish on it, then you'd do well to also add some QUALITY. Quality images and videos that tell a story will separate your social media accounts from the pack. People want more than just content. They want good, QUALITY writing. Good, QUALITY images. Good, QUALITY films and videos that move at a pace that keeps them engaged and entertained, but uncertain of where the ride is going. Our attention span has grown shorter as our eyes have become more (and ever more) attuned to our screens. Your audience is savvy. Believe it. Even 15-second videos on Instagram can seem to run for an eternity if they don't exhibit quality or confidence, or if they're simply filler (lack a voice). You can't fake QUALITY.

So get out there, get vertical, get virtual, GET MOVING!

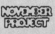
November Project @Nov_Project · 18 Dec 2015
Yeah, but did your tribe have PRINTED bibs for your #Sunrise6k?!
NP NYC **did...** #printmedialives
👤 John Honerkamp, Paul Leak and November Project NYC

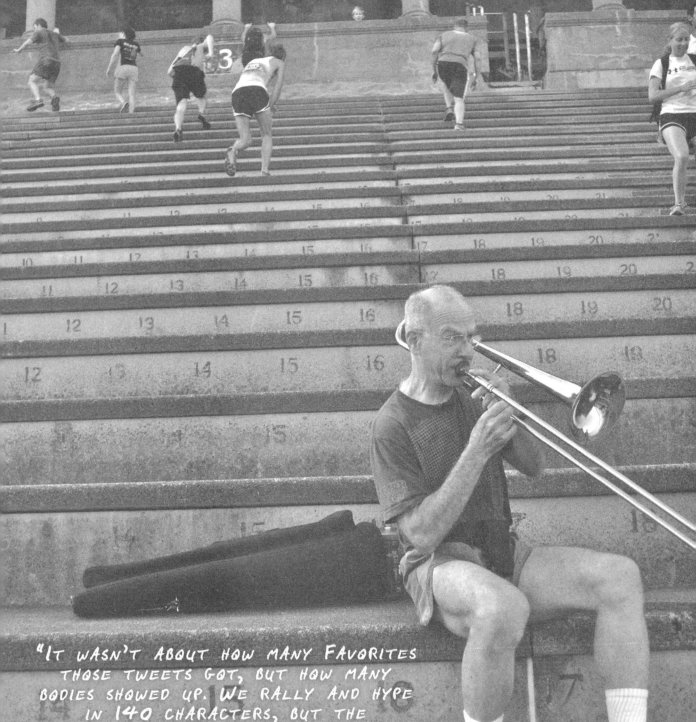

"It wasn't about how many favorites those tweets got, but how many bodies showed up. We rally and hype in 140 characters, but the movement is built in person."

—BG

PHILADELPHIA, PA

INDIANAPOLIS, IN

BALTIMORE, MD

MINNEAPOLIS, MN

LOS ANGELES, CA

NEW YORK, NY

MILWAUKEE, WI

CHAPTER 7

How to Change the World in 4 Easy Steps

A.K.A. Finally A Short Chapter

BY BOJAN MANDARIC AND BROGAN GRAHAM

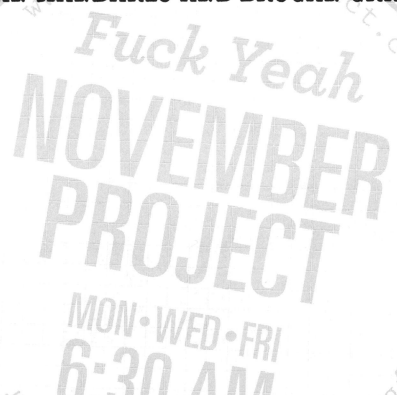

This is the part where you're expecting us to drop some seriously enlightening knowledge that will splatter your brain all over the wall, but most of the things that you will read below came about not by taking some fancy movement-starting classes or from reading books by guys who initial their first name, go by their middle name, and suffix the last name with some Roman numerals. No, we're not that smart. We are just two dudes who wanted to surround ourselves with other like-minded dudes and gals, and as shit started blowing up, we paid more attention to things that worked well while trying to do more of them while staying away from things that didn't go so hot. For example, we understand that just because we think a locked gate means access to a well-manicured field is allowed to those who can clear the 8-foot-tall fence, doesn't necessarily mean that everyone else has the same interpretation. So after a well-balanced diet of praise and ~~angry emails~~ constructive criticism we recognized that to start a #FREE fitness movement, or any kind of grassroots community, we had to nail down the following:

INCLUSIVENESS

Our members range in age and fitness levels, so all of our workouts need to be scalable so both the elite athlete and the recovering couch potato can work together and still walk away feeling like they worked up a pretty intense sweat. We always pick locations that keep the group together or in a loop so that there's always overlapping and overtaking. However, we encourage support and motivation, so as members pass each other, no one is made to feel like they're underperforming. Focus is on one's personal effort, and that focus is encouraged by the group. We design exercises to cater to all athletic abilities. If you can't do a pushup from your toes, drop to your knees. If you're struggling with 20 air-squats, we'll put 40 seconds on the clock and see how many you can do, then the next time you try to beat that number. No matter how fit you are, you can always improve.

Take Harvard Stadium. The fastest and slowest members are contained in the same space, a 37-section horseshoe. Everyone remains within sight of everyone else. As the lead dogs double-back and pass the slower ones, they push and encourage. And all of a sudden everyone is working much harder than if they were running alone. The slower end of the group strives to catch the middle of the pack, while the mid-packers are chasing down the top guns. The elites are always working hard to stay there, as it feels like everyone is breathing down their necks. By the sheer power of the mass working off of each other, everyone is going faster.

STRONG CULTURE

We, as leaders, are built into the community and are always there when you show up. Not late, not weather dependent. We are weatherproof, and our commitment is unwavering. Rain, sleet, high winds, extreme humidity, hurricanes, and the countless Boston snowstorms that crippled traffic and public transportation systems could not stop November Project from training outdoors. In our 3-year history, we've NEVER canceled a single workout for weather. As a matter of fact, some of our frigid Canadian tribes give out a "Badge of Honor" to everyone who comes out when the wind chill drops temperatures to −30°C. Not only do they not complain about the conditions, they look forward to the opportunity to earn bragging rights. That's strong culture.

When members of November Project ask, "Will you be at the next workout?" they're not looking for a wishy-washy, half-assed, "maybe." They want a goddamn ver-

FEBRUARY 2015
Started by Dan Graham in Milwaukee. Sunrise 6-Ks are held throughout the November Project nation. The flames of inter-tribe competition are fanned.

SUNDAY, MARCH 8, 2015
Edmonton is not the only Canadian tribe anymore! Winnipeg, MB (Rick Duha, Thomas Hall), and Calgary, AB (Tammara Francis) are now part of the family. Shortly after, Virginia Beach, VA (John DeBoer) gets the green light. #NewsCh19

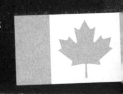

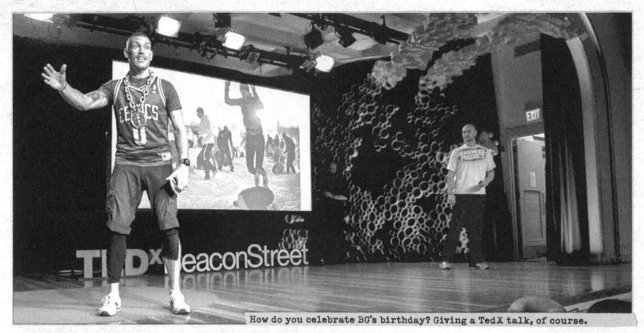

How do you celebrate BG's birthday? Giving a TedX talk, of course.

bal commitment. By saying "yes," you've made, or "dropped" (if you really want to get technical), what we call a VERBAL. We want you there and we want you to feel accountable about being there. So what if you don't show up? Well, if you break a verbal, your photo (believe me, we will troll your social media feed for just the right one) and details of your no-show will end up on the We Missed You section of our website. Essentially, this gives our members the ability to throw one another under the bus by highlighting broken promises. We didn't build the We Missed You page to torment anybody; we built it to drive accountability. Yep, strong culture.

We say we're huggers not shakers, and we practice that at all of our workouts. We made sure that we gave each other a giant hug each morning when it was just the two of us, and we keep up the tradition to this day: Before we jump into logistics, travel, or upcoming things,

a giant hug. If you come to any November Project, you should expect to hug the person standing next to you, but not because we're trying to create uncomfortable situations. Instead, we're hoping to take relationships that are often instigated online (through our social media outreach) and realize them off-line through real human interaction. People spend too much time avoiding each other, looking at screens, looking away. Hugging is not touchy-feely, new-age, Kumbaya corniness. If it's good enough for your mom, it's good enough for you. Hugging is human, always has been. Plus, huggers lead better lives. Huggers risk more; they live more; they put themselves out there. Shakers, on the other hand (motherfuckin' pun intended!), play life safe, they follow the norms, and they don't shake (not intended) things up. Shake shit up and don't shake hands. Hug with your real human self. Try it. Live it. And . . . say it with us now: strong culture.

WEDNESDAY, JULY 8, 2015

Phoenix, AZ (Jackie Knoll), and Vancouver, BC (Graham Snowden and Richard Hortness) are now official. #21HumpBeat

AUGUST–SEPTEMBER 2015

August marks the addition of Toronto, ON (Claire Hutchinson and Sam Hirons), and Seattle, WA (Casey Winkler), shortly followed by the Kenary brothers leading Worcester, MA.

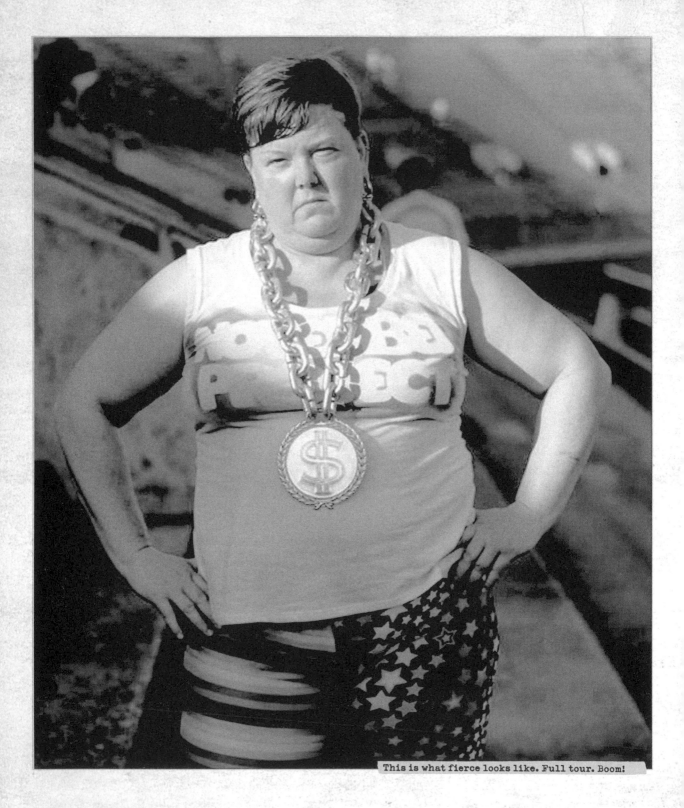

This is what fierce looks like. Full tour. Boom!

FIERCENESS

The definition of "fierce" is showing a heartfelt and powerful intensity. Fierce doesn't always describe the fastest or strongest person. Fierce is the person who pushes toward their goal with undeniable intensity. Fierce people lead by example and don't look for excuses. A fierce person sees a challenge and tries to systematically overcome it regardless of how long it takes. Ashley Brow is a sight-impaired woman in the Boston area who became a runner with November Project. Her walk turned into an assisted jog, and then a run without taking any breaks. Was she faster than our hill beasts Smooth, Derrick, or Morgan Brown? No way. Was she as, if not far more, fierce (you walked into this one . . .)? FUCK YEAH! When presented with an obstacle, a fierce person looks for a way around it. With the intention of not missing out, injured athletes still attend NP workouts to do core work and whatever else they can do. We call this the "Injury Deck" (see page 96). Fierce is what gets these folks, now with even more excuses, out of bed. Fierce gets them out the door. Not every person who comes to November Project is fierce, but the ones who are, or who evolve toward it over a period of months, are nothing short of pure inspiration, no matter their speed or strength.

FUN, NEW, CREATIVE

In a world where everyone's eyes, ears, and emotions are dominated by phones, tablets, and screens of all kinds, you must be fun, new, and creative if you want to stay relevant. Sliding a fake bright-orange parking ticket under someone's windshield wiper with a heartfelt note encouraging the long lost art of kindness not only attracts attention but provokes a wide range of emo-

tions. This rollercoaster usually starts with spotting the neon paper on your windshield: "AH FUCK, I GOT A TICKET!" After readying for the offense but then finding only a kind note of encouragement, annoyance and stress turn into relief and a pleasant "You got me" moment, which ends with approaching the next interaction of the day with a giant grin. This is just one of the many nontraditional ways we try to engage our community, encouraging them not only to get fit with us but to be kind to one another, to really and truly "see" their fellow citizens. Look on our site and you'll see a place where you can print your own decoy tickets. Use them to grab someone's attention away from technology and their stress of life. Use them to make someone smile and enjoy a moment that would have otherwise been lost. Use these tickets to feel badass as you lurk for the cause of good. Just get out and be creative . . . be new, be fun. Hurry up and join the fun/new/creative side of life—we all need these three characteristics because we're all almost dead.

Finally, it's important to note that a well-established balance between these four ingredients is a key. If you were to focus too much on one while not paying as much attention to the rest, it will not work. So take this recipe, add it to whatever you're trying to accomplish, and build your own movement. There's really nothing to it, as they say—but to do it!

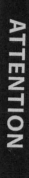

Name _____
Address _____
City/Town _____

NOVEMBER PROJECT

TO THE RECIPIENT OF THIS NOTE:

This is NOT a parking ticket! Someone wants to get your attention and remind you that instead of being pissed at a ticket you should use that energy and do something nice for a stranger. Holding a door, or saying a thank you does not count. Those are the things that you should be doing anyway. Think about something simple and kind or maybe funny that would make YOUR day. Now channel those ideas and go interact and be amazing!

If you want to share this note with someone else in your life, go to november-project.com/ticket and print out as many as you want and go make your city a better place.

Disrupt someone's day by giving them a fake parking ticket.

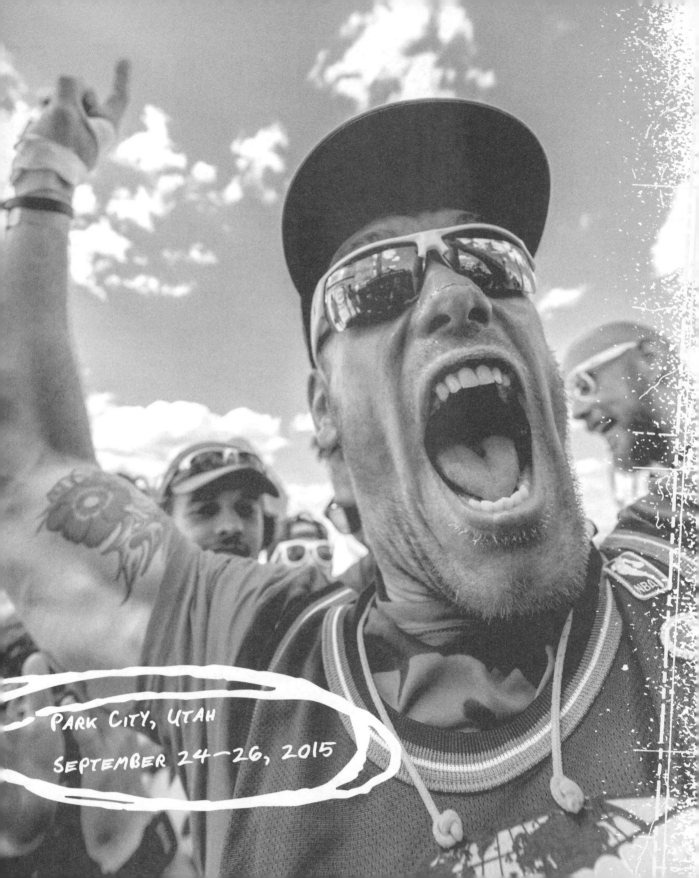

PARK CITY, UTAH
SEPTEMBER 24-26, 2015

CHAPTER 8

#NPSummit3.0: Leadership

BY CALEB DANILOFF

Wisconsin Notes

- Whose body is this? That thin air ain't no joke!
- Airport bar/hotel/race/world takeover
- We woke up the sun at the state capitol
- 57 leaders under the hood
- November Project goes into the world chest—first
- All eyes on the podium
- A poolside striptease
- The tribe is strong

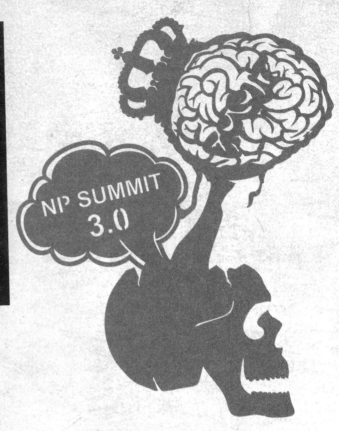

NP SUMMIT 3.0

From: Janel
To: November Project Coleaders
Re: Summit Itinerary
Thursday, September 24, 2015
12:42 p.m. Leaders begin arriving SLC airport
[most arrive at 2:57 p.m.—last flight comes in
at 7:06 p.m.]
7:20 p.m. Load bus
7:30 p.m. Depart for Park City Peaks Hotel
8:10 p.m. Arrive at hotel
8:15 p.m. Check in to hotel rooms
8:45 p.m. Start Gear & Beer
10:00 p.m. End Gear & Beer—Go to bed!

8:57 P.M.

If you were staying in a room on the north side of the
Park City Peaks Hotel one Thursday night in late September of 2015, you might have heard a commotion
outside your window: voices, laughter, music seeping
through speakers. If you pulled back the curtains to
investigate, you would have at first seen only a variety of
rental cars parked in the lot, along with several long
white vans with matching logos on the doors. But
beyond all that metal and rubber, in a grassy field
marked with two wooden tables and several hackberry
trees, your attention would have been drawn to a swarm
of silhouettes and shadows. Flashlight beams bouncing
about. Murmurings, clapping. Were there a dozen
voices? Thirty? Fifty? It would have been hard to tell
from indoors.

If you made your way to the parking lot, taking up
position between the cars, you'd be able to tell that
some of the people knew each other, but that many
seemed to be meeting for the first time. You'd hear cans
cracking open as small groups circulated like moths
around two of the tallest figures. Occasionally, the skit-
tering light would catch a wooden carving shaped like a
world map hanging like a necklace against a chest. You
might expect the police to show up at any moment.

If you skirted the crowd and climbed one of the trees
overhead, you would have observed an odd sight. An
inflatable ball, a blue globe, being tossed from hand to
hand as, one by one, each figure stepped into the circle.
Washed over by multiple flashlight beams, you would
have heard each announce a home city and a name.
"Winnipeg, Richard. New Orleans, Kate. Indianapolis,
Bobbie. San Diego, Angelo. Denver, Dan. Seattle, Casey.
Los Angeles, Steve . . ."

**THURSDAY–SATURDAY,
SEPTEMBER 24–26, 2015**

The third annual summit in Park City, Utah.
There are twice as many leaders, twice as many
tribe members, and four hundred times the fun.

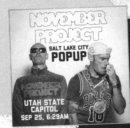

THURSDAY, SEPTEMBER 24, 2015

After the pop-up workout on the steps of the Utah State Capitol
building, the cities of Kansas City and Kelowna, BC, join the tribe,
bringing the number to 26 and changing the hashtag to #Iron26.
So long #Oceans23, we hardly knew you!

The group held tight as 59 names and 26 cities from around North America were issued into the thin, cooling air. Among the group were three nephews of a renowned craft-beer brewer; an aspiring actress; a lawyer; a man with a brain disorder; an assistant principal; an online marathon coach; a graduate student; a speech pathologist.

You would have then witnessed the largest of the men, dressed in several colored tops, present small hammers to three of the participants. "These represent brute force, perseverance, and grit. We're giving these to you, Laura; to you, Paddy; and to you, Dan, for handling one of the toughest things any of us have had to face over the last year, for showing incredible leadership, and growing your group into one of the tightest and fiercest on offer." You would have seen light cut across the faces of the chosen, slightly downcast eyes. Even during this upbeat moment they seemed to feel an emo-tional pain that lingered below the surface. But its source would have been a mystery to you.

Then the other tall figure, the one with the bald head and scruffy beard, commanded everyone to place arms around shoulders and tighten the circle. In the inky night, bodies merged, arms and hands moving like phalanges. The creature then started swaying and making noise, *Ohhhh, Heyyy, Ohh, Heyyy,* getting faster and louder, faster and louder, louder, louDER, LOUDER, LOUDDDEERRRR! *Are you good? FUCK YEAH! Are you good? FUCK YEAH!!! Are. You. Good? Fuuuuck Yeah!!!!* Then the mass broke apart, amid claps and hollers and whistles, and individual pieces began clinging to each other, separating and attaching to new pieces. Ones becoming twos. Twos becoming threes. Fifty-nine becoming one.

You still have no clue what you just fuckin' witnessed.

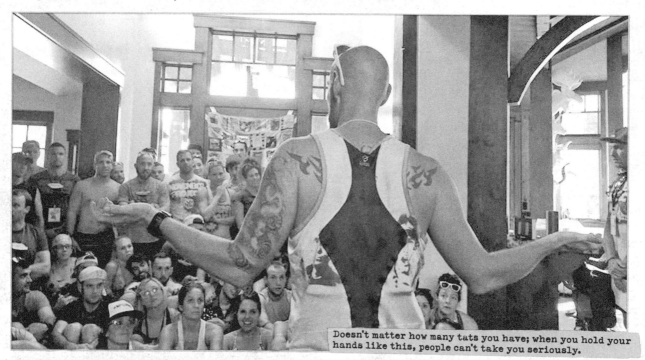

Doesn't matter how many tats you have; when you hold your hands like this, people can't take you seriously.

SATURDAY, OCTOBER 3, 2015

The future of NP is literally born when baby Marli Zdenka Mandaric enters the world. At 6 days old, Marli becomes the youngest attendee of a November Project workout. Bojan and baby Marli are both crapping their pants on the regular.

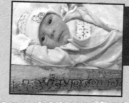

SATURDAY, OCTOBER 24, 2015

The last word of this book is written. **The End.**

NOVEMBER PROJECT
TRIBE LEADERS

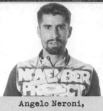
Angelo Neroni,
San Diego

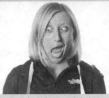
Ashleigh Voychick,
San Diego

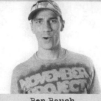
Ben Bauch,
Minneapolis

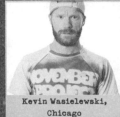
Ben Otto,
Los Angeles

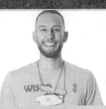
Ben Schwabe,
Milwaukee, Wisc.

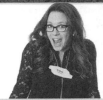
Bobbie Werbe,
Indianapolis

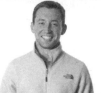
Brendan Scully,
Chicago

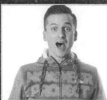
Casey Winkler,
Seattle

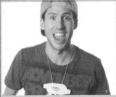
Chris Capozzi,
Boston

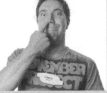
Chris Payne,
Boston

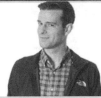
Dan Clayton,
San Francisco

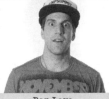
Dan Layo,
Philadelphia

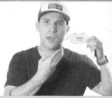
Danny Metcalf,
Washington, D.C.

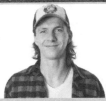
Hank Kenary,
Worcester, Mass.

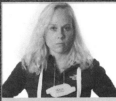
Holly Reiland,
Minneapolis

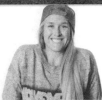
Jackie Knoll,
Phoenix

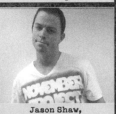
Jason Shaw,
Indianapolis

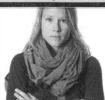
Jennifer Ference,
Edmonton, Alberta

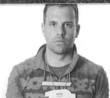
John "Coach" Honerkamp,
New York City

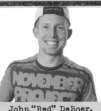
John "Red" DeBoer,
Virginia Beach

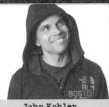
John Kohler,
Kansas City

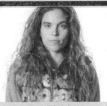
Kaelan Dickinson,
Washington D.C.

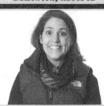
Kate Gilly,
New Orleans

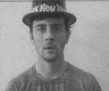
Kevin Wasielewski,
Chicago

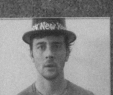
Kristopher Utt,
Virginia Beach

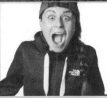
Lauren Padula,
San Diego

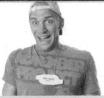
Matthew Sellen,
Denver

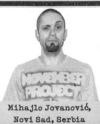
Mihajlo Jovanović,
Novi Sad, Serbia

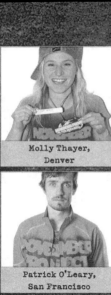

Molly Thayer,
Denver

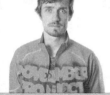

Nadim Chin, Edmonton,
Alberta

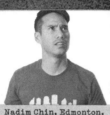

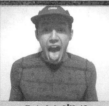

Nicholas Rodricks,
Baltimore

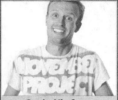

Orrin Whalen,
Los Angeles

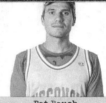

Pat Bauch,
Madison, Wisc.

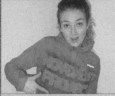

Patrick O'Leary,
San Francisco

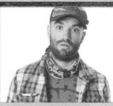

Patrick O'Neil,
Baltimore

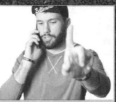

Paul Leak,
New York City

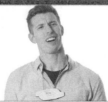

Peter Nazarewycz,
Calgary, Alberta

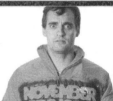

Preston Reeder,
New Orleans

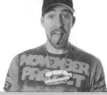

Rakel Eva Sævarsdóttir,
Reykjavik, Iceland

Richard Hortness,
Vancouver, B.C.

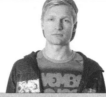

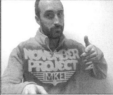

Rick Duha,
Winnipeg, Manitoba

Roger Huffman,
Milwaukee, Wisc.

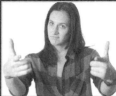

Roz Huber,
Kelowna, B.C.

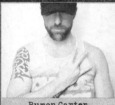

Rumon Carter,
Victoria, B.C.

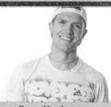

Ryan Wooderson,
Denver

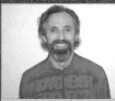

Sævar Þór Guðmundsson,
Reykjavik, Iceland

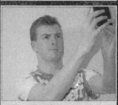

Sam Hirons,
Toronto

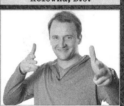

Sam Kenary,
Worcester, Mass.

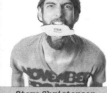

Steve Christensen,
Washington, D.C.

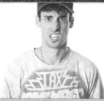

Steve Selnick,
Los Angeles

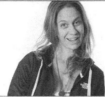

Suzanne Allaire,
Philadelphia

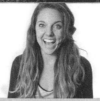

Sydney Van Horn,
Baltimore

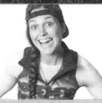

Tammara Francis,
Calgary, Alberta

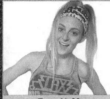

Tara Wall,
Los Angeles

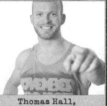

Thomas Hall,
Winnipeg, Manitoba

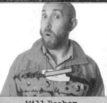

Will Booher,
New Orleans

11.

Friday, September 25, 2015

5:15 a.m. *Meet in lobby*
5:20 a.m. *Load bus*
5:30 a.m. *Leave hotel for pop-up in SLC*
6:30 a.m. *Start SLC Pop-Up*
7:40 a.m. *Bagels delivered*
7:45 a.m. *Load bus*
7:50 a.m. *Depart for hotel*
8:30 a.m. *Arrive at hotel*

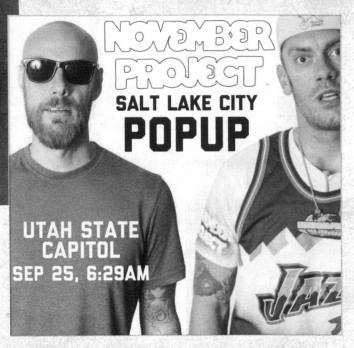

"DRIVING THROUGH DARK CANYONS TO A WORKOUT WITH TWO PEOPLE WHO WERE COMPLETE STRANGERS A MERE SEVEN HOURS PRIOR WAS EXCITING ENOUGH. AS WE NEARED THE CAPITOL BUILDING, IT WAS LIKE COMING UP TO AN UNKNOWN LOCATION FOR A MUSIC FESTIVAL. A FEW BLOCKS OUT, YOU SEE PEOPLE WALKING TOWARD THE VENUE. AND YOU START TO GET EXCITED, 'THESE PEOPLE MUST BE GOING TOO... YEAH, DEFINITELY THAT'S A LOT OF NEON.' WE HAD NO IDEA HOW MANY PEOPLE WOULD BE THERE, SO MAKING THAT RIGHT TURN AT THE CAPITOL BUILDING INTO A POOL OF NEON, GO-PROS, DRONES, GRASSROOTS EVERYTHING, AND HUNDREDS OF INSANELY EXCITED HUGGING STRANGERS AS DAY WAS BREAKING...THAT WAS FUCKING COOL."

—EMILY LERMAN, 32, RESEARCHER, CENTER FOR REFUGEE AND DISASTER RESPONSE, BALTIMORE

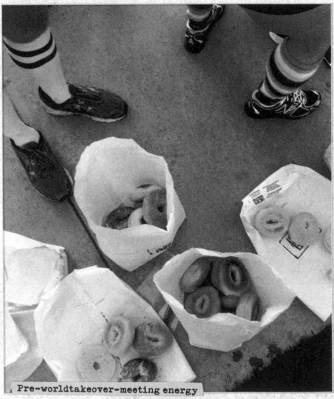

Pre-worldtakeover-meeting energy

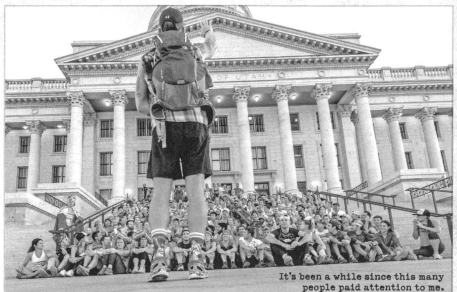

It's been a while since this many people paid attention to me.

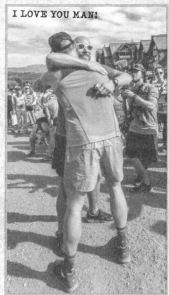

I LOVE YOU MAN!

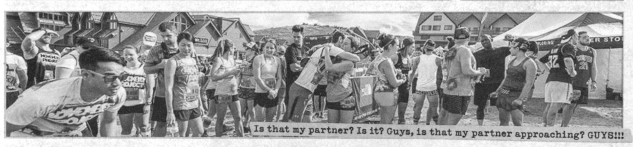

Is that my partner? Is it? Guys, is that my partner approaching? GUYS!!!

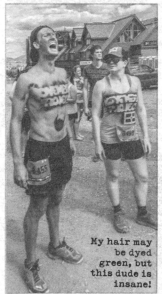

My hair may be dyed green, but this dude is insane!

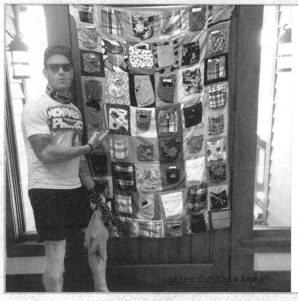

Caption for this image.

brogan_graham
Park City, Utah

FOLLOW

189 likes   7w

brogan_graham Thank you again @erinroselarsen - This "cell phone locker quilt" was a total hit this fall in Utah. #NPSUMMIT #nophones #lockers #handmade #GrassrootsGear

liv.to.run This is very cool..!

sasha.teninty Whoooop @erinroselarsen! ♥🙏

bradford_smith I'm calling you later.

erinroselarsen You guys are nice. 😑

novemberprojectsf He must have heard about your verbal, @erinroselarsen

novemberprojectsf #theverbalheardaround theworld

erinroselarsen #DOUBLEVERBAL

tinyenormous I'm confused and scared. And happy. Fine sewing tho Erin!

Add a comment...   ○○○

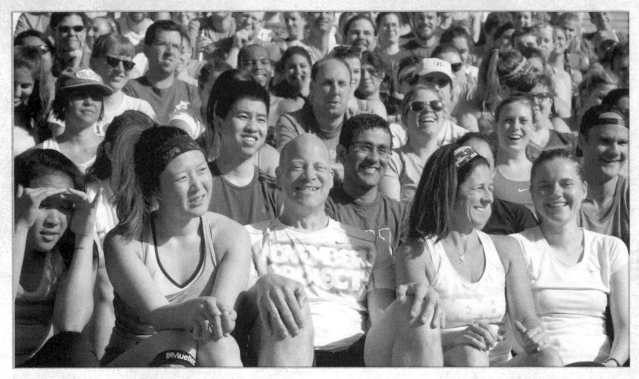

"MY FIRST EN MASSE TRIBE EXPERIENCE. TO FEEL THE ENERGY, LOVE, AND ACCEPTANCE IN SUCH A HUGE WAY WAS SO OVERPOWERING IT BROUGHT ME TO TEARS. IT WAS HARD. BUT I RAN, AND ROLLED, BURPEED, AND HOISTIED TO THE BEST OF MY ABILITY. AND HAD A TON OF FUN. WHILE WE WILL ALWAYS CONSIDER OURSELVES 'BOSTON SOUTH WEST,' IT DAWNED ON ME THAT IT'S NOT THAT I DON'T BELONG TO ANY TRIBE, IT'S THAT I BELONG TO ALL OF THEM!"

—TERESA ECCLES, 50, HOMEMAKER, BOONEVILLE, ARKANSAS, NOMAD TRIBE

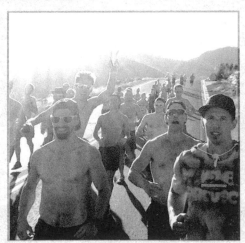
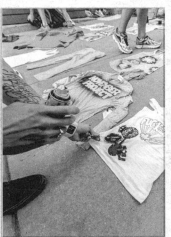
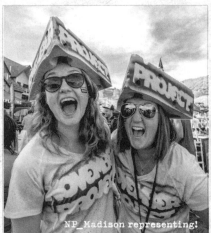

NP_Madison representing!

Passport Stamps:
Have Grassroots Gear, Will Travel

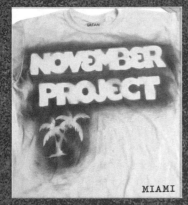

MIAMI

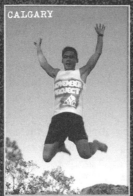

CALGARY

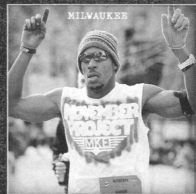

MILWAUKEE

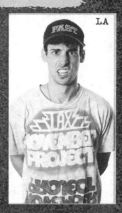

LA

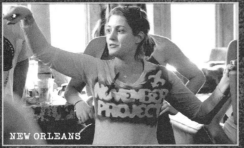

NEW ORLEANS

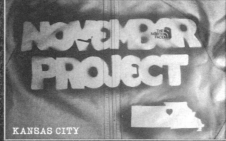

KANSAS CITY

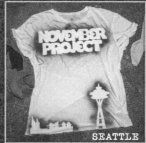

SEATTLE

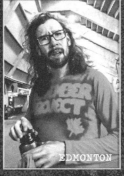

EDMONTON

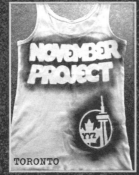

TORONTO

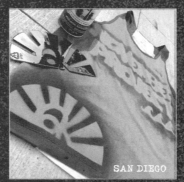

SAN DIEGO

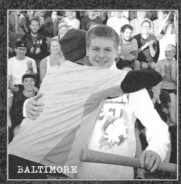

BALTIMORE

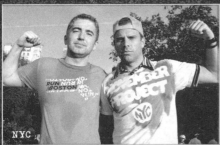

NYC

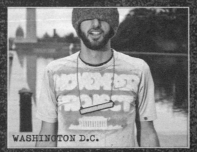

WASHINGTON D.C.

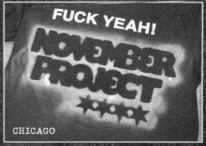

CHICAGO

**Friday, September 25, 2015
(cont'd)**

9:00 a.m. Load bus
9:15 a.m. Depart for the lodge
9:30 a.m. Summit Session 1
12:30 p.m. Lunch
1:35 p.m. Summit Session 2
5:30 p.m. End Summit
5:40 p.m. Run from the lodge to hotel
6:00 p.m. Free time: shower, nap, eat, swim
7:00 p.m. Dinner in hotel restaurant
[hotel catering]

Janel Kozlowski Fink stood at the glass door on the first-floor landing, taking a photo of two deer grazing on the rocky slope behind the mountain lodge. A tall red-head with a shaved undercut and a warm smile, Fink had been a D-1 high-jumper at Northeastern University when Graham and Mandaric were pulling oars in Husky unitards. Now living in Seattle, the 34-year-old had a stone-cold head for organization, and she operated her own event-planning outfit. So last year when Graham and Mandaric started plotting out the second leader Summit in Madison, Wisconsin, she stepped in to help, handling details large, small, and in-between. For free, naturally. This year she's agreed to do the same, though it had proven to be three times the work.

"Last year, three vans were enough for all the coleaders," she said. "This year, it's two vans plus a coach bus. It's insane how much this thing has grown over just 1 year. I had to start planning this one 6 months ago."

Fink snapped a couple more shots of the deer, heads bowed, sipping from the ground. "NP has had such a big impact on my life and I wanted to give back. I was in a car accident in 2013 and got bad whiplash. I credit NP with keeping me motivated to fight to recover. I honestly think that without it, I would had fallen into a deep depression and stopped working out altogether."

The lodge where Fink was standing belonged to a relative of Graham's. An in-law once-removed is how he put it. In any case, it was Hollywood huge: soaring ceilings, slate fireplaces, multiple patios, mountain views everywhere you looked, a marble-topped bar with saddles for stool seats, and big-game trophy heads—elk, moose, antelope—studding the walls. On the deck outside the front door sat a colorful pile of dirty, untied running shoes of various sizes.

Inside, the owners of those kicks, some 55 November Project coleaders from across North America, had gathered, some of them (Kansas City, Kelowna, British Columbia) inducted into the family just 90 minutes earlier at the Salt Lake City Pop-Up. Most of them were still in sweaty workout gear. According to the tightly scheduled itinerary, after getting back to the hotel post-pop-up, they had only 10 minutes to get ready for the day-long gathering that would be held a few miles away. "About enough time to dunk your balls in a cup of water," Baltimore coleader Nick Rodricks joked as the bus pulled up to the hotel. "Better make it a cup of coffee," quipped Dan Layo, a lawyer from Philadelphia.

In the corner of an adjacent sitting room, wrapping

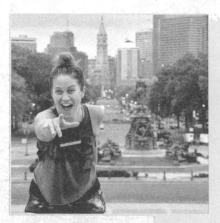

*"The hugs, man. The city of brotherly love can't get enough of the hugs—as well as the community. Philadelphia has a lot of born-and-raised residents. If you're from Philly and you grow up here, you have your tight-knit circle of friends and it's a hard group to crack. You move here from anywhere else and it's harder to find friends. NP breaks down those walls for people. It broke them down for me."
—Suzanne Allaire, co-leader, NP Philadelphia*

paper and ribbons filled black garbage bags as if a family's Christmas morning ritual had just taken place. The vibe wasn't far off from that, actually. The day had started with a gift exchange between cities that had been randomly chosen by Mandaric and Graham before the Summit. Among the presents were gag pillow cases, Old Bay seasoning, maple syrup, bedazzled vests, wall hangings, a set of military challenge pins. There were backstories, jokes, and hugs. A warm-up for the business ahead: an agenda that would include liability waivers, changes to the online fitness tracker, workout design and execution, recruiting and retention, shirt-tagging technique, and visions for what 2016 would hold for the movement. Welcome to November Project's Leadership Retreat/Management Conference/State of the Union/War Room.

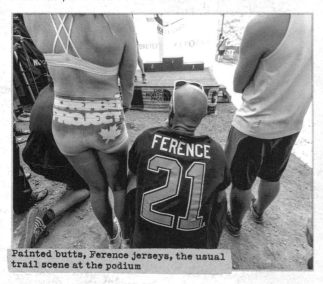
Painted butts, Ference jerseys, the usual trail scene at the podium

The Accidental Summit

Like a lot of milestones in the movement, the idea to gather tribe leaders for a fitness brain dump, assorted antics, and beers started with Andrew Ference. At least indirectly. After the scrappy NHL defenseman left the Boston Bruins for the Edmonton Oilers in 2013, Graham and Mandaric had been talking about visiting their old pal up north the next time the Bruins visited Edmonton. It was early December, 2013, and three more cities were signing on, and would soon turn the #Powerful7 into the #Power10 (*Note: For the etymology, see the timeline entry for Wednesday, January 29, 2014.*)

"We have had people who move here and the first thing they do is come to a November Project workout. They found it was the best way to get immersed in the city and meet people. To me, that's one of the biggest successes for us. People from outside the city hear about what we're doing and see us as a place where they can feel safe and meet people. And then we have people in the tribe who will do everything to make that person feel like Edmonton is their home. It amazes me every time. We're Canadian. We're the nicest tribe you'll find, and we love to travel to other tribes so we can thaw out."

—Nadim Chin,
Co-leader, NP Edmonton

"As many of our conversations go," Mandaric recalled, "we started on one subject and ended up God knows where. The discussion about us going to watch the game turned into 'What if we brought a bunch of leaders to the game?' to a 'Let's have ALL the leaders at the game!'"

Mandaric and Graham had actually only met half of their coleaders in person. Skype and Google Hangout had to suffice for the rest. "It was a great opportunity to get everyone introduced to each other, to talk about challenges, share wins, and start friendships. Doing it in December in Edmonton at minus-30 degrees? Fuck yeah!"

The duo scraped their bank accounts, scored some free rooms at the Westin, booked a van, and sent out the invites. "From a planning and budgeting perspective, it was overwhelming and stressful. But it was worth every cent as we realized the value in connecting our leaders and developing November Project culture. Once we got everybody in the same room, we knew this needed to be an annual event."

CHANGE AGENTS

After a lunch of baked potatoes with meat and veggie toppings, the group drifted back to the living room for part two of the day's Summit work. A handmade quilt with numerous pockets the size of iPhones hung on the back of the front door. Graham reminded everyone to put their online lives on pause. After depositing their cell phones, the leaders then squeezed into chairs and couches and took places on the floor, clutching "Face Books," notebooks with a photo of a tribe leader on each page (whipped up just 48 hours earlier by Boston tribe member and printer speed demon Scott Champagne). Each cover displayed the FB "Like" button. Despite their social media focus, Graham and Mandaric had a soft spot for printed materials (#PrintMediaLives)—and for #Irony.

A few minutes later, Graham's older brother, Dan, also known as DG, took the floor. He was dressed in a gray T-shirt with a blue buff around his head, sunglasses perched on his temple. He was a fit and towering figure, though 1 inch shorter than his younger bro. ("Dan still hasn't forgiven Brogan for growing taller than him," their mom, Ann Doody, said.) The former swim instructor is the only member of November Project to have started two tribes—the first in Madison in 2013 and the second in Milwaukee, where he had moved with his wife, Meggie (also a tribe member). But just because DG was BG's older brother didn't mean he got a pass on the 8-week pledge process. "I think it was payback for all those times in high school when I made him pay like everyone else to get into my parties," DG said.

In many ways, DG had become a de facto leader alongside Graham and Mandaric, an elder statesman of sorts. DG cleared his bearded throat, and with a razor-quick wit and that familiar, zany Graham sensibility told his tale. "I was super fat for a lot of years," he said. "I did the really classic out-of-high-school-didn't-do-anything-ate-everything thing and I got really, really big. I'm telling you this because a lot of you don't know that version of me, just like a lot of people don't know that version of you, your struggles, your past that might be weird. My brother helped me a lot with my fitness. He was the fittest person I'd ever seen and I wanted something like that, needed something like that.

"So as you look around this room," DG continued, "know that you're all doing an amazing thing, and an amazing job at it, but also know that you're not like anyone else near you right now and that's pretty fucked up, actually. When we had 16 cities, I told my brother and Bojan that if you lined everybody up and listed their attributes—she's an ultra runner, he's Irish, he's enormous, he's a charming mofo from Canada—everyone was different. I mean, what are we looking for in Miami? What do we need in Atlanta? What are these leaders going to look like?

"So I've been thinking about this a lot: What is it that we all share? In my opinion, it's two things. One: an absolute, genuine desire to help others and to be an active leader. Desire is the big one. And two: pride of your city. And everyone has that. These new people coming on, they can't *wear* enough shit that blasts out their city. They want you to know where they're from. That is pride. You have the pride to rebuild a community. You're showing up to connect, to build something special."

DG then called on Jackie Knoll, the coleader from Phoenix, which had come on board in the summer of 2015.

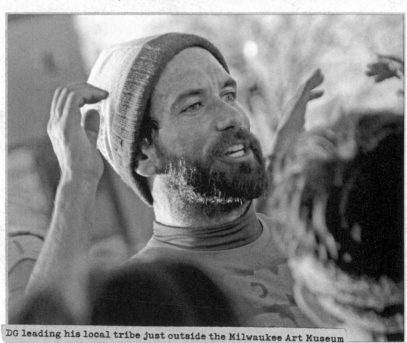

DG leading his local tribe just outside the Milwaukee Art Museum

"NO MATTER WHO YOU ARE, WHATEVER YOU ASSOCIATE WITH, THIS COMMUNITY IS FOR YOU. ALL WALKS OF LIFE FROM BELIEVERS TO YOUNGSTERS TO SIX-FIGURE MAKERS TO GOVERNMENT OFFICIALS TO DRAG QUEENS BOND OVER THE SIMPLE ACTIVITY OF MOVEMENT. REGARDLESS OF THE LABEL THAT WE DO OR DON'T HAVE, WE ARE ALL COMPLETE PEOPLE, BUT HOW DO YOU CELEBRATE THIS COMPLETENESS? WE'RE IN THIS AS ONE, WITH NO TYPES, LABELS, STEREOTYPES, OR TAILS. CONTINUE TO INCLUDE WITHOUT JUDGMENT AND WE'LL CONTINUE TO BUILD THIS TRIBE AND THIS WORLD AS A BETTER, SMARTER PLACE TO BE. THIS TRIBE IS EVERYWHERE. THE TRIBE IS STRONG."

—ORRIN WHALEN, CO-LEADER, NP LOS ANGELES

"Phoenix is an incredibly transient town," said Knoll, a 31-year-old speech pathologist, her long blond hair spilling out of a trucker cap. "Almost no one there is native, except for me. I love Phoenix and I wanted to bring that same sense of community that I experienced at NP-DC with me when I moved back to Arizona. I give some Phoenix history at every single session or tie it into the workout. I know all the different areas to explore. I'll always give people tips on cool places to go."

Nick Rodricks nodded his head in agreement.

"Most people think about Baltimore and they think *The Wire* TV series and maybe the riots that took place this spring after Freddie Gray [was killed while in police custody]," the 25-year-old environmental consultant said. "The reason I wanted to start NP there was because I was tired of that shit and there's so much stuff I love about Baltimore. I wanted to stop the 22-year-old who came to Baltimore and said, 'This sucks, I'm moving to New York.' If you lead with a fuckin' love of something, it's going to rub off on others. So don't think of yourself as a fitness leader but as an agent of change in your city."

"Exactly," DG added. "Which brings up another point. Be yourself. People want to follow genuine leadership. They want to follow a genuine person. They want to see a genuine relationship between coleaders. The opposite is just as true. When you go somewhere to get fit and see someone up there and they're putting on a good show but you can tell they're just there for the paycheck, you probably don't go back. That's not just athletic stuff but everywhere. Don't try to change into something you're not. It happened to me when I started Madison. I tried to be these guys," he said while pointing at BG and Bojan, "and it didn't work. My coleader Ben Schwabe started and he

tried to be me and I had to shut that shit down. So now he's the quiet guy and we make silly videos before the workout and it works."

For the next half hour talk circled around handling leadership transitions (there had been several), nurturing coleader relationships, and describing a workout to the crowd ("Keep it short, use vivid words, be loud, shut down hecklers, and leave no time for questions," said Pat Bauch of Madison). Mandaric would later give leaders 10 minutes to design a workout using only the outside stairs, driveway, and part of the road.

"Okay, let's talk about recruiting," DG said, switching gears. "Every conversation you ever have might lead to NP, so you need to be ready. You need an escalator pitch for the red light, an elevator pitch for the elevator, and a 1-minute pitch when you actually have people's attention. You need to prepare yourself for the excuses—I'm not a runner; I'm too old; it's too early. Okay, where's my man Danny Metcalf?"

Metcalf, the 24-year-old cofounder of the DC tribe, waved his hand, and DG lit up.

"I just love this guy. I met him at the first Summit and I called him the week after. When he picked up, he said, 'Hey man, I'm on a 10-mile training run.' And I could hear his breathing. Then he said, 'Check this out: On the move, I'm going to recruit this guy up ahead of me.' So he runs up next to the dude and I get to hear Danny recruiting this guy at probably a 6:30-pace. It was just a perfect pitch of NP: how you play with all your friends, make the city your playground, have the most fun you'll have all week, you should definitely come be part of it, give it a try. In that moment, I was just blown away. I'm thinking I've been doing this shit all wrong."

Metcalf smiled at the memory, his eyes glistening under a yellow bike cap. The young marketer and granola bar entrepreneur (shout out: Mission: Bars) holds the distinction of being the first tribe leader with no ties to Boston or to Graham and Mandaric. An outsider. But the badass triathlete with national team aspirations was an instant hit, raising the Bounce to the level of an art form while brimming with the same gleeful enthusiasm as Graham, though Metcalf probably only comes up to his nipples. "Mini BG" and "BG Lite" are some of the nicknames that get tossed around. Together with coleader Steve Christensen, Metcalf, at the time just 22 years old, built the DC tribe into the largest one after Boston, with hundreds showing up every Wednesday at the steps of the Lincoln Memorial to sweat it out against a backdrop of marble bathed in rising sunlight.

Although Metcalf has been the heart of the DC tribe, and last spring delivered a TedX talk on the movement, he has had to step away and yield to another leader. A year ago, doctors discovered a brain tumor. It was benign, but the surgery to remove it triggered a condition known as postural orthostatic tachycardia syndrome, or POTS, in which an excessively reduced volume of blood returns to his heart after he stands from a reclining position. Exercise, in particular, can bring on dizziness and fainting. There is no known cure for this condition, and long-term treatments have yet to be developed, though POTS sometimes recedes on its own. For now, though,

> "NP INDY WAS BORN AS PART OF THE #POWER10. I CAN IMAGINE SOME PEOPLE WERE LIKE, 'INDIANAPOLIS, INDIANA, HAS A TRIBE? BEFORE CHICAGO, LA OR NYC?' YES. INDIANAPOLIS, INDIANA, HAD A TRIBE BEFORE CHICAGO, LA OR NYC. SORRY BOYS. I'M NOT SO SECRETLY PROUD OF THAT."
>
> —BOBBIE WERBE,
> CO-LEADER NP INDIANAPOLIS

Metcalf's fitness future has, cruelly, been paused. He still shows up to workouts when he can and has become more of a spiritual leader to the DC tribe.

A lot of people in the room didn't know that version of Metcalf.

"To wrap up my portion of the program," DG said, "this is the coolest thing we'll ever get to do. And we all need to be able to help each other out. If I need your help, raise your hand if I can give you call?"

Suddenly, everyone was shaded by a canopy of hands.

CULTURE CLUB

And with that, Graham (BG, that is) and Laura McCloskey of NP San Francisco led a group of the newer leaders down to the driveway for a dose of NP Culture 101, from social media to social events to workout rituals. "This is a movement," Graham said, as the group gathered in front of the garage. "There are a bunch of common threads to connect us, and if we do these small things together, we can freestyle the rest of it."

Most tribes have done just that, injecting city and personal flavors into their workout culture. Sometimes it bubbles to the top. Events like the Sunrise 6-K, a twice-yearly 3.7-mile race that DG started in Milwaukee, now takes place in every NP city. But mostly the flavor is decidedly local. In San Francisco, with its swaths of parkland, trail systems, and waterways, a lot of weekend camping trips are organized by tribe members. In New York City you can expect the epic, the latest being a workout conducted on the Staten Island Ferry.

Dressed in black shorts, classic white grassroots gear, and a red running cap, Graham slapped a Positivity Award against his sizable palm. He asked several leaders to show the group how they present the oar handle to a high-vibe tribe member.

"That's great," Graham said after one speech. "The only thing I'd say is it has even more impact if you tease it out a little, you know. Describe the person, but maybe don't even say 'he' or 'she' right away. Say why you're giving it to them, but don't say their name until the last possible second. Everyone will be locked in. Make it a real fuckin' moment."

"And you don't have to give it out every week," McCloskey added. "We only do it once a month. Shit, actually, I think our last one was 8 weeks ago . . . But it

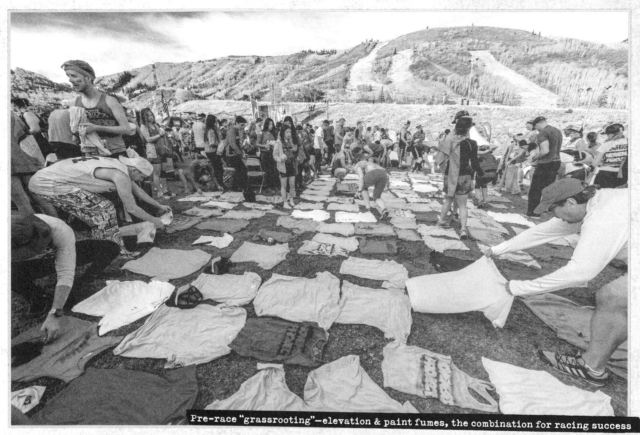

Pre-race "grassrooting"—elevation & paint fumes, the combination for racing success

makes it much more special. The last time we gave it out, the dude posted a hundred pics of himself with it, it meant so much to him."

The last item of the culture session was tagging. Graham walked around a green T-shirt that was laid out on the driveway, along with a pair of stencils, shaking a spray paint can like a maraca. "Okay," he said. "This is something I take very seriously.

"Initially, this started just because Bojan and I wanted to see people running around the Charles River in NP shirts. But when you hear stories of strangers meeting at the bottom of the Grand Canyon wearing grassroots gear and they recognize the black paint and hug it out, take a photo, it's important we do it the same."

The leaders gathered into a semicircle, their shadows casting across the asphalt as the late afternoon sun started its westward drift.

"You're gonna find all kinds of different shit that people bring that they'll want you to paint," Graham said, placing the stencils on the fabric and nudging them into place. "We paint the chests of shirts, that's it. We go into the world with November Project chest first. Not on your back, because with a backpack on it doesn't exist. What about sides? Down the leg? Sparkles? No fuckin' way. We want it to be crystal clear. Flat, black spray paint. If you have a little tiny chest, it'll read just a little bit and that's okay. You're going to be in places around world, outside of the workouts, and you're gonna see this done the exact same way and you're going to walk up to that stranger and you're gonna hug it out. Because we all do it the same way."

Graham circled the shirt like Jackson Pollock might a canvas. And then in one fluid movement, he leaned down and swept the can three times across the chest and once down each side. In less than 10 seconds, he lifted the stencils and grassroots gear appeared. "You can get a thousand shirts out of one can if you do it right," he said. "So learn this shit."

The day began to wind down and before long, the whole mob had gathered at the bottom of the driveway, many of the guys shirtless, many of the eyes tired. There had been a lot to digest. But to bake it all in, there was one last piece: a 3-mile run back to the hotel.

Graham led the way, mercifully starting off downhill. Within a quarter mile they were met with a long snaking ascent, the thin air humbling all but the fittest runners. Finally, they reached a straightaway and everyone found a comfortable pace, keeping the long line unbroken.

As the group started rolling down a winding hill, the last-line runners took off for the front as if responding to a telepathic message. Indiana Jones was on. And so it went, all the way to the hotel, long sprints with each leader cheered and high-fived as they made their way to the front and taking their turn at the pace position. The train was hurtling hard, 26 tribes moving as one. Earlier in the day, Graham and Mandaric had told the group they were aiming to bring the tribe count to 30 by the end of 2015, and that 2016 would see an overseas push—into Iceland, Serbia, maybe even Ethiopia. At that moment, the momentum and energy of the runners carving down a Park City mountain seemed to mirror the movement itself. These Indiana Jones sprints were promising to get long as fuck indeed.

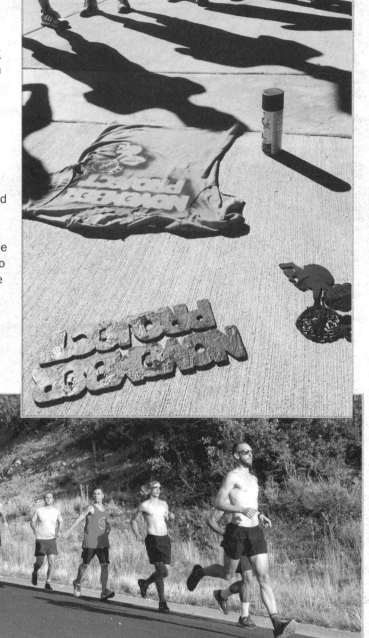

Jones'ing... Indiana Jones'ing

Saturday, September 26, 2015
7:00 a.m. Breakfast on own at hotel [complimentary]
8:00 a.m. Meet in lobby
8:10 a.m. Walk from hotel to race
10:00 a.m. Start marathon relay

Park City Mountain Resort, or simply Park City, opened in 1963 and is one of the world's premier ski destinations. Team USA trains here, and the mountain was host to several events during the 2002 Winter Olympics, including snowboarding and giant slalom. The town of Park City is also home to the Sundance Film Festival, which, each January, turns the slopes, and Main Street, into Little Hollywood. But on this sunny, late-September morning, Park City belonged to The North Face Endurance Challenge Series.

Though perhaps more accurately, it belonged to November Project. The movement that was just boozy shit-talk in a basement bar almost 4 years earlier was now taking up all kinds of space in Utah. On the grassy slopes, in the beer garden, at the picnic tables, coming out of the port-o-johns. Everywhere you looked, bright grassroots gear was stamped on shirts, trucker hats, arm sleeves, flags, across chests, across butts. On an orange turban. (Clearly, some folks hadn't received BG's tagging memo.) A neon bum rush aimed squarely at The North Face's marathon relay.

In the picnic area, music blared overhead. Beneath the bass lines and auto-tuned melodies, palms were slapping, hips were bumping, the thin air was being parted by laughs and screams and spirit fingers. The vibe was high-school-reunion-meets-Burning Man-meets-Little-Endorphin-Annie—cranked to 11. With the number of twenty-somethings initially beamed up by the Mother Ship, what with all the colleges in Boston, plenty of adventure-seeking tribe members had cycled

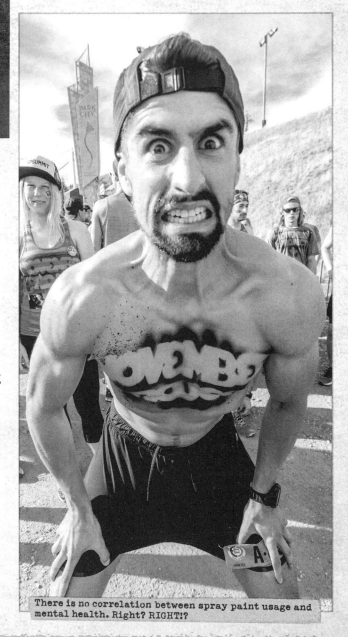

There is no correlation between spray paint usage and mental health. Right? RIGHT!?

"THE SUMMIT IS KIND OF LIKE A WEEKEND SUMMER CAMP FOR ADULTS IF A BUNCH OF AWESOME FRIENDS ARE ALL THERE FOR THE SAME REASON, TO LEARN FROM ONE ANOTHER AND SPREAD A BUNCH OF POSITIVITY AND LOVE."
—JANA GOINS, 34, EPIDEMIOLOGIST, BALTIMORE

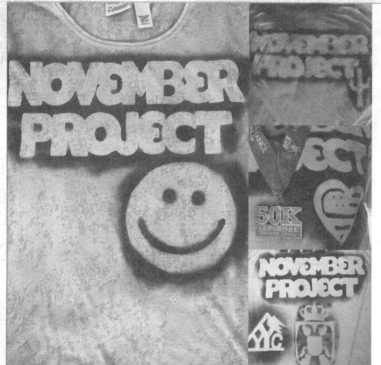

novemberproject · FOLLOW

334 likes · 1w

novemberproject What is your most rare piece of #grassrootsgear? Make 2016 the year you visit another tribe, join us at the #NPSUMMIT, or simply sign up for a race across state lines. #travel #adnventure

sinkorswag Where is the #NPSummit this year?

wooly_dang I got that primer gray Portland Pop Up stencil!

gswoodward I have a @brogan_graham tagged original. Need a 100 sections tag, a 6K & an MSP as I have done all. Goal for 2016, SFO & LA

jennyvictoriamay @mil.schip we should do the summit together one day

matt_anzur @nov_projectyyc @novemberprojectcan see you next week #verbal

novemberprojectvb @sushi_dragonfly 🏋️😍❤️ #seashore50K

Add a comment... ○○○

#NOVEMBERPROJECT

out of Beantown over the past few years, landing in other NP cities. Some had started their own tribes. Use of the #traverbal hashtag spiked. (*Note: See the glossary. Go ahead, we'll still be here when you get back.*)

But on another level, and in a real sense, this annual gathering was the inverse of a reunion. This was a coming together of friends who hadn't yet met. Strangers didn't exist here. Connections were immediate, everyone somehow familiar. Spot grassroots gear at a cafe and, boom, you had a breakfast companion. See an NPer at the same airport gate and your flight was suddenly less lonely. Get stuck in a strange city and chances were good that you'd find a place to crash and maybe even score a ride to the airport, too.

With the gun just under an hour away, most of the prerace action was taking place beyond a wooden split-rail fence that separated the picnic green and the walkway that skirted the restaurants and ski rental shops. From a distance, the sun-drenched pavement appeared to glow. Shimmering reds, pinks, yellows, oranges, blues. A Technicolor patchwork of shirts and shorts and hats lay on the ground. Many were already stenciled with civic pride: crabs (Baltimore), subway tokens with

apple leaves (NYC), spoons with cherries (Minneapolis), Fleur-de-lis (New Orleans), maple leaves (Canada), Lincoln Memorials (DC). Some shirts were covered in city tags like passport stamps. And the quilt kept growing as more fluorescent items were added, all of them thirsting for the NP Summit 3.0 stencil: a skull with a leg kicking out a crowned brain and a cloud, an original piece that Graham and newest Boston leader Chris Capozzi put together for the occasion. Meanwhile, that familiar NP tribal tune—beads rattling against hollow tin and the cat-hiss of Krylon nozzles—carried on the breeze.

Mandaric and Graham were both crouched over shirts, running their cans back and forth. The Serbian wore a dark bandanna over his mouth and an Andrew Ference T-shirt (the Oiler captain, ironically, once again had to miss the Summit because of his hockey schedule), his hands and fingers smeared with black paint. Graham was dressed in a sleeveless flannel shirt, duck hunter-style, blue knit cap, white shades, blue zinc smeared beneath his eyes and across his nose, lifeguard style. Rainbow socks. Fairly normal attire, actually. The dude was known to sport pink tutus, a giant panda head, and togas made from newspaper. In fact, Graham would only seem oddly dressed if he'd tucked a button-down into a pair of Dockers. To help handle demand, the pair was joined by taggers from San Diego, New York, San Francisco, Vancouver, and Milwaukee, plus a handful of helpers who straightened the shirts and moved the stencils.

Along one edge stood a large man with a sharp nose and a thin mustache and goatee. Every minute or so, a tribe member wrapped a pair of arms around his substantial torso and belly, and smiles and laughs would ensue. Arkansas Rich, aka Dr. Richard Eccles, a physician from Booneville, Arkansas, had become part of NP lore, having adopted the lifestyle even though he lived in a rural southern hamlet where there wasn't much hope for a tribe. In the winter of 2013, Eccles stumbled onto the NP frequency. He felt the vibe, and a few months later he sent Graham and Mandaric a note:

Also weaving through the crowd was 31-year-old Rachel White, a project manager from Minneapolis. She was wearing a purple tank, black tights, and a #NPSUMMIT hat spray-painted in California sunset colors. White had road-tripped from Minnesota with a group of tribe members. Coming here was like coming home, she later said.

"To be with so many other people at the same time who ALL feel the same way you do about this movement is just awe-inspiring. I traveled a lot last year and visited San Diego, LA, San Fran, DC, and Virginia Beach. And so many people remembered me from those trips and gave me hugs like they actually missed me and started up with conversations like we'd been friends for a while. I haven't felt this much confidence, charisma, happiness, and being comfortable in my own skin since high school."

I found you guys online (somehow) and very glad I did...

In February of this year I decided I did not want to be a fat ass anymore and set a goal to live life! Started at 398 lbs now a sleek 293 lbs down 105 lbs!! Started with just walking, then running a bit, then I found NP; stayed up most of one night reading blogs and hopefully bottling some NP love...I'm stuck in Arkansas but decided to start putting my feet on the floor at 6:30 and just, in my own way "show up."

Since then I have survived my first 5K, second one next week and ran my first 4 miles this am! I've been rocking the high school stadium bleachers each Wednesday and Plum Street (my hill) on Fridays... My deckaday is more of a go fish kids deck for now, but its everyday and getting stronger....

My goal is to come join you guys on the big steps next May for my birthday...until then my little tribe of one will stay strong and race everything!

Anyway, just wanted to say thank you for the motivation...

Thanks,
Richard

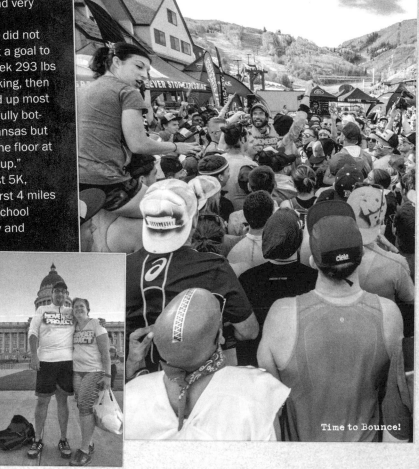

Time to Bounce!

The farther you waded into the crowd, the more colorful it grew. Two of the San Diego coleaders, Lauren Padula and Ashleigh Voychick, were dancing, pink trucker hats turned backward, each reading "Fit As F**k!" Sarah Lindstrom and Amanda Ellmaker, a pair of twenty-somethings from Madison, Wisconsin, wore cheeseheads, the orange foam wedges tagged appropriately. A tanned, spray-painted bare chest belonged to LA leader Orrin Whalen (one of a handful of tagged torsos in the crowd). There were at least three dyed Mohawks in the immediate vicinity. Nearby, an older man with a salt-and-pepper goatee was inspecting a freshly painted green shirt. Ron Buch, 50, from the DC tribe, was a federal judge for the United States Tax Court. Making the pilgrimage was a no-brainer, he would tell me.

"The members are the kind of people I want to be around. They are positive, energetic, supportive, and sometimes a little crazy, but always in a positive way. I want to be more like these people, so I surround myself with them. They make me a better person."

"ALRIGHT, ALRIGHT, ALRIGHT!!!"

There was no mistaking that cavernous voice. I'm sure the response among Boston members to the once-familiar vocal thunder was straight-up Pavlovian drool. It was 20 minutes before showtime, and Graham and Mandaric were standing in the middle of the picnic area, waving their long arms overhead, calling in the troops. It was time for the Bounce. Within moments, a crowd had gathered around them—10, 15, 20 deep. A human crop circle. Dudes were on tiptoes. Girls were sitting on shoulders. Hats were turned backward.

"Listen up!" Graham shouted. "If you're on the edges, do me a favor and take the front of your body and push it against the back of a stranger's body. Bring it in tight."

All around, internal temperatures spiked.

"OK, it's one thing to show up to a race with giant numbers and change the chemistry and the competitive nature," he continued, "but the people who are here who aren't part of November Project, let's bring them into the family. Let's give them hugs, let's encourage them on the trail. Let's make it an awesome day. Let's get a little bounce!"

Graham tomahawked his hand in the air, and he and Mandaric started jumping. Within seconds, some 800 feet were stomping and springing. A furious stampede held in place. It felt like we might bust through the grass and land in someone's basement. Then like a conductor, Graham punctuated his bounce with a long, low "AWWWW . . ." His giddy, neon orchestra synched up with its own "AWWWWW." Then he took it an octave lower before pushing it higher. The crowd responded in kind. He picked up the pace until the hundreds of voices morphed into a frequency human ears rarely hear. "AND STOP!"

Silence, but for the breeze. Graham looked around, knowing exactly how long to hold the beat, just how close to the sneeze he could go . . . "Good morning!" "GOOD MORNING!!!" "Are you good?!" "FUCK YEAH!!!" "OK, let's meet down by the starting line. Go! Go! GO!"

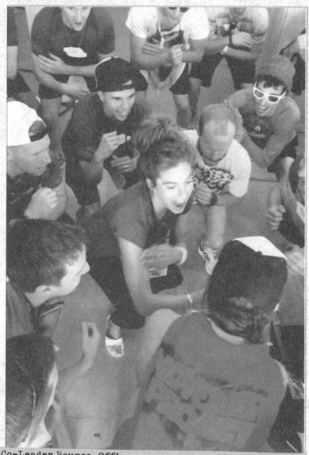
Co-Leader Bounce-Off!

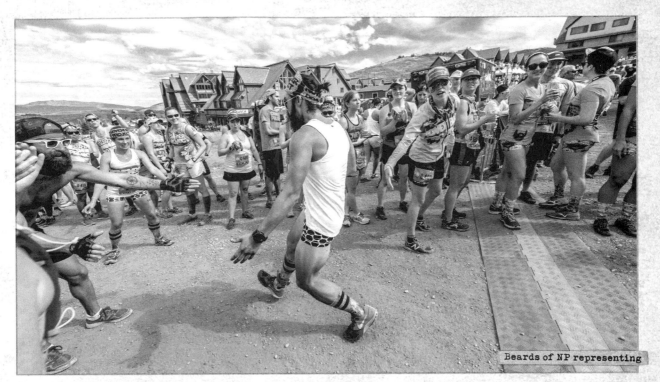

Beards of NP representing

#RaceEverything

The first two lines of racers were all coleaders, with Graham in the middle. They were gunning their engines, brimming, leaning over the timing mats, fingers on stopwatches, playfully jostling with each other. I stood a few rows back feeling nervous, nursing a leg strain. I could still feel the humiliating sting of the previous day's thin-air runs. Even though I'd run a 50-K a few weeks earlier and knocked off a full mountain marathon at altitude in Colorado a couple years before, every race felt like a reset. A nerve-fraying unknown. But that was part of the thrill. Then the horn went off and it was on. Paddy O'Leary, a coleader from San Francisco, took the lead. With every blink of the eye he edged a few yards farther ahead of the pack. Then he vanished.

After the first mile of narrow dirt switchbacks, a lot of people had down-shifted into power hiking. An Asian dude in a red NP shirt zipped by me, along with a few other young whippets. Each one greeted me with "nice work" or "you got this." I slapped them on the shoulder as they passed. Chair lift lines appeared then vanished. Around mile 2, a blond woman in a lime green tank stood at a turn and high-fived every runner who passed, some stopping for hugs. I felt good, my blood flowing strong, and I managed to power to the summit without walking. Then it was all downhill and I took flight, the twisting trails studded with rocks and spread with burnt red leaves, which I kicked through like free money.

My running partner that morning was 42-year-old Harry Mattison, a Boston software developer who'd only started running seriously a few years earlier, just before he showed up to NP. (He'd registered our team as November Project Goes Hypoxic.) Mattison completed his first marathon the previous year in 3:24. Pre-NP, his best half marathon was a 1:53. He was a smart and droll dude with the best dead-fish face this side of the Continental Divide. But his work ethic was sick, and he knocked off triple burgers (three stadium tours for 111 sections) and 50-Ks on the regs. I sprinted into the transition area, clocking in at 64 minutes. With speed and precision, Harry switched out our ankle bracelet and took off. Watching him go, in his trademark blue butterfly shorts, I thought about a blog post he wrote a few weeks earlier. In it he crystallized the NP ethos about as succinctly as any I'd ever come across:

Guest Blog: Harry Mattison of NP_BOS

🕐 31st August 2015   👤 Emily   📁 Blog   💬 0 Comments

The challenges that we all face (or invent for ourselves) bring to mind two concepts that I learned outside of November Project. Though Brogan and Bojan don't use these phrases, for me they embody the NP spirit and culture and make it so uplifting: Basking in Reflected Glory (BIRG) and We're In This Together (WITT).

I learned about Basking in Reflected Glory last year at my college reunion. In remarks to the alumni, the university president asked us to consider "How do we feel when a classmate wins a Pulitzer Prize? What is our reaction when we are part of a community whose members achieve fame and fortune?" I don't know if it is learned or innate, but haven't we all felt a flash of inadequacy when we hear news like this?

As an alternative, Basking in Reflected Glory suggests that we choose to be inspired by and share in the successes of our colleagues. When one of us in a community is honored, so is our entire community. When we #JustShowUp, we are enriching our collective lives and motivating everyone to improve. When we see #GrassrootsGear on the podium or worn in an Instagram photo of an unimaginable yoga move, BIRGing means reacting with a collective sense of accomplishment, striving to do our personal best, and lifting our spirits and aspirations.

The economist Jared Bernstein discusses "We're In This Together" in his book All Together Now: Common Sense for a Fair Economy. Everyone familiar with NP knows the power of our WITT vibe. Remembering our most #Weatherproof blizzard workouts brings a swelling feeling of camaraderie.

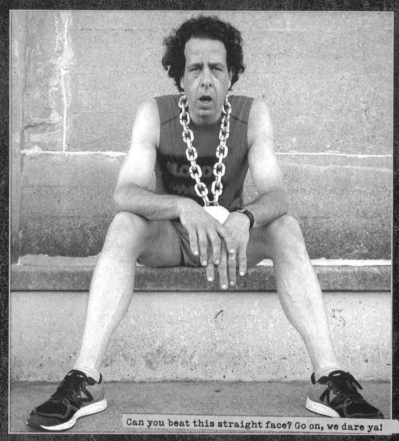

Can you beat this straight face? Go on, we dare ya!

As winter approaches and our alarm clocks ring before sunrise, it is that much easier to roll out bed because we know the tribe and their hugs will be ready and waiting for us.

Our leaders consistently emphasize how the beauty of each person builds our community and encourages everyone to strive for new levels of fitness, self-confidence, and achievement. Support at NP flows both to and from people across the entire fitness spectrum. This unconditional acceptance empowers us to embrace our individual reality and set our own goals instead of trying to measure up to a fictionalized concept of perfection.

As if on cue, Jesse Ledin stormed across the finish mats, dressed in cosmos-themed leggings, a matching ball cap turned backward, and a pair of Blues Brothers–style shades. He looked as strong as I'd ever seen him, a whisper away from reaching the 100-pound mark in his weight-loss journey. Since that sub-zero workout at MIT the previous January, Ledin had knocked off a bunch of half-marathons, the Boston Marathon, a Spartan Beast, a 100-mile bike race, a triathlon, and assorted other contests. Chicago and New York were on tap. Ledin smiled when he saw me, as gentle and kind-eyed as ever. In his hand, the worn Positivity Award he'd won the previous week at Harvard Stadium. He'd run with it the whole time.

"Sprinting towards the finish line with the PA and my grassroots gear gave me an overwhelming feeling of being free," he said. "Having the past that I did, I never felt I belonged anywhere. Most of my days were filled with gray overcast skies. Those skies only started to clear a few years ago and now the sun is permanently shining."

Meanwhile, Mattison was up and down the mountain in 58 minutes, despite having landed the day before with less than 24 hours to acclimate to the altitude. So before I knew it, I was off again. The second pass was more difficult, but I trusted my training. I trusted NP. In the battle of me versus my environment, me versus my sense of limitations, me versus me, I had a deep bench.

As I turned into my last mile, I heard steps behind me and was briefly seized by that flee-like-an-antelope feeling. It was O'Leary, moving like flood water. He patted me on the back as he passed. Jesus. He was on his final leg. I was just wrapping up number three for Team Hypoxic. A few switchbacks later, I could begin to make out the clouds of cheering from the finish. A half mile to go. The next thing I know, Whalen was upon me. "Looking strong, my man," he said, on his way to second place. Then, moments later, as I headed into the final twists before the last straightaway, I caught sight of New York coleader Paul Leak, shirtless, bearded, and focused, reeling me in. "You are a fuckin' animal, dude!" Then he flashed past, the final piece of an NP podium sweep. Sometimes, I feel a sting when I'm passed on Boston's Esplanade or around Fresh Pond, wishing I could call out, "I'm on mile 17, you know, or I'm 15 years older than you, punk." But feeling the breeze from those three turbo beasts, all four of us sporting grassroots gear, was like coal hitting the firebox. I was BIRGing hard.

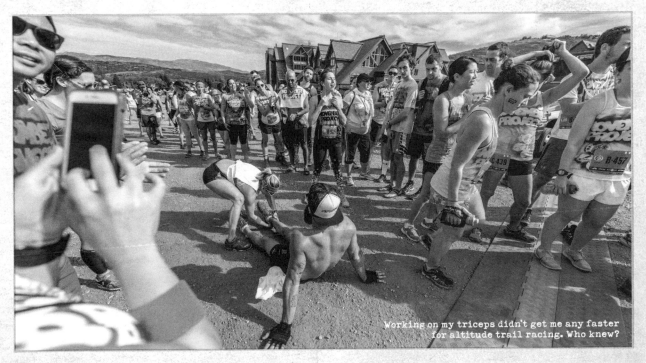

Working on my triceps didn't get me any faster for altitude trail racing. Who knew?

Meanwhile, Graham and Mandaric were leaning over the fencing at the finish line, standing about 10 feet apart, watching and clapping. Chris Heuisler, of Belmont, Mass., was taking in the scene, too. The 36-year-old sub-3:00 marathoner was also a former actor, who'd landed roles on *General Hospital* and in the reboot of *Freaky Friday* with Lindsay Lohan and Jamie Lee Curtis. Though he set aside the dream in favor of family, he was still an ardent student of human behavior. As O'Leary came barreling down the final stretch, Heuisler watched Graham hop onto the course as if to bear witness. Then, in came Whalen, followed by Leak. Respectively, they clocked a 3:08.16, a 3:10.14, and a 3:13.46. Graham stepped back to let them have their moment.

"My eyes went to Brogan," Heuisler recalled. "He just watched this group hug. And so did Bojan, who was off to the other side. Both of these giants had the exact same expressions on their face: the look of a parent who just witnessed their child do something not even they thought was possible. I got choked up because their pure joy for those leaders was palpable. And then, as if rehearsed, Brogan and Bojan made eye contact and shook their heads in disbelief. They met each other in the middle, hugged and high-fived, and then went right back at it: cheering on both finishers and relay runners who still had another leg or two ahead of them."

I later asked Graham about that moment and he said, "It was aggressive racing by our leaders. By most anyone's standards, they were extremely fast. Bojan and I weren't in the mix. We were done for the day, but seeing everyone really balls out and heartfelt, you saw this thing evolving in front of your eyes. It's not the BG and Bojan show. It's that feeling of, 'Wow, these people were not this way before coming to NP.'"

As I approached the transition area and Mattison's waiting hands, I heard a familiar female voice coming from the grassy slope on the other side. "Go, Bookman! Go! Go! Go!" There standing alone was Ann Doody, looming in red pants, tan jacket, and aquamarine grass-roots gear. The Khaleesi of November Project Nation. (Janel had arranged her trip on the sly, a surprise to BG and DG.) The two Graham brothers stood almost directly across from their mother, giant wild hands reaching for mine as I sprinted past. The spiritual geometry of the moment was perfect.

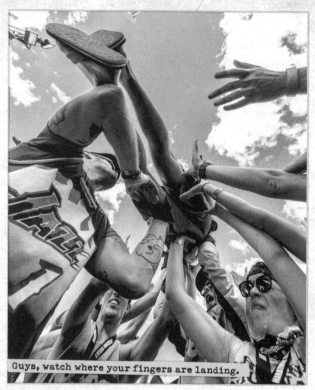

Guys, watch where your fingers are landing.

For the next hour, the cheer volume hovered at full-blast and notched up after Boston tribe member Dan West, a 30-year-old mechanical engineer, barreled down the straightaway, dust kicking up his wake. His race partner and longtime girlfriend, Sara Dyer, 30, manager of photography at Boston University, jumped onto the course and they crossed the mats hand-in-hand. And before Dyer could give her man a big squeeze, he was down on one knee, opening a ring box. Dyer squealed, put her hands over her face, then took them away to release a winged "yes" from her mouth. West was all grin. He'd tackled his two legs of the course with the ring in his fuel vest. "My heart was racing the whole time," he said. "I don't know if it was the altitude or me imagining the moment. All I know is I kept my hand on that pocket the whole time."

An hour later, the MC announced the start of the awards ceremony. First up, the Marathon Relay. Dean Karnazes stood on stage, dressed in The North Face racing gear and tinted black sunglasses, ready to hand out winner prizes. The leader teams from SF, NY, and LA were each called to the podium. The tribe had gathered in full force, cheering, screaming, laughing, fist-pumping with each announcement. Graham and Mandaric stood at the front, shredding their vocal cords. Once they were all gathered on the podium and Karnazes had shaken their hands, the chant went up: "CROWD SURF! CROWD SURF! CROWD SURF!" And one by one, O'Leary, McCloskey, Whalen, Leak, San Diego coleader Angelo Neroni, and NYC coleader John Honerkamp fell backward onto a sea of arms that began passing them all around like beach balls. Karnazes was doubled over with laughter.

After Honerkamp was finally let down to the ground, the MC began announcing the male victors for the 50-mile race. The sweaty-fluorescent-dusty-muddy-bloody crowd didn't budge. As soon as the first name was called, they cheered just as wildly for the day's top endurance athletes, none of them from November Project (*note: yet*). "CROWD SURF! CROWD SURF! CROWD SURF!" They looked confused, unsure. Then the 50-M winner, Lars Kjerengtoen (7:33.14) looked at the others and gave a "what the hell" look and jumped onto the bed of writhing hands. The others followed suit. And so it went for the female 50-M winners, then the 50-K male and female winners, then the marathon winners. Lastly, Graham and Mandaric, hoarse to the point of a whisper, pointed at Karnazes. "CROWD SURF! CROWD SURF! CROWD SURF!" He jumped in like it was a familiar mountain lake, and ultra-running's most famous body was off his feet, flying beneath the sun, the mighty Wasatch bearing witness from above.

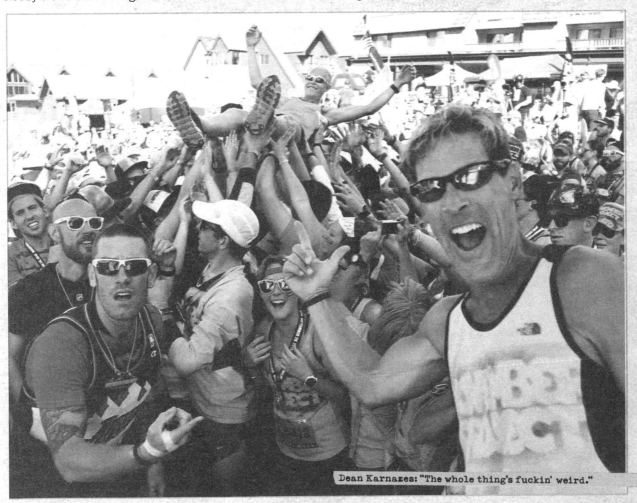

Dean Karnazes: "The whole thing's fuckin' weird."

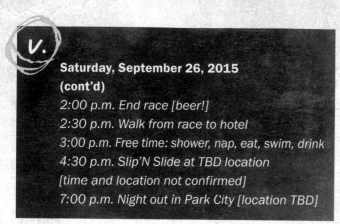

V.

Saturday, September 26, 2015 (cont'd)

2:00 p.m. End race [beer!]
2:30 p.m. Walk from race to hotel
3:00 p.m. Free time: shower, nap, eat, swim, drink
*4:30 p.m. Slip'N Slide at TBD location
[time and location not confirmed]*
7:00 p.m. Night out in Park City [location TBD]

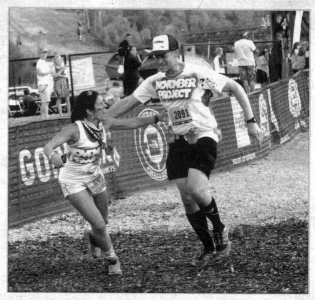

As the crowd dispersed and the NP tribe leaders made their way back to the Park City Peaks Hotel to change or hit the hot tub, there was still unfinished business taking place on the mountain. Boston tribe member Nick Flattes was at mile 19 of the marathon, one of a handful of NPers tackling the longer distances. And he was hurting, dizzy and winded from the altitude, and thirsty and burning from sun exposure. It had been a grueling 15.7-mile climb and he was halfway into the rocky 10.5-mile descent after going off course for a mile. Flattes had been on his feet since 9 a.m., almost 8 hours, and the course sweeper was now pacing him.

"I wanted redemption," he said. "In summer of 2013, I was training for the Victoria Half Marathon in British Columbia. A medial gastrocnemius tear in my right calf caused my leg to swell to twice its normal size and I had to stop my training. This also came at a low point in my life. My marriage had fallen apart and I was going through a custody battle. I put my sights on the ECS marathon to prove to myself that completing my first marathon was not a fluke and I had what it takes to finish another one."

Somehow, he pushed through the pain and loneliness and doubt, conjuring up the toughest NP workouts he'd survived last year during Boston's historic winter. Finally, he spied the last set of turns that sloped down to the finish line. Even from his vantage point, he could tell most of the runners had gone home, with mostly stragglers and volunteers milling about, the tents empty. Then with maybe yards to go, a short, tanned brown-haired woman jumped onto the course next to him. It was Maria Cesca, the first person he met at November Project during that fateful nor'easter at the stadium almost 2 years earlier.

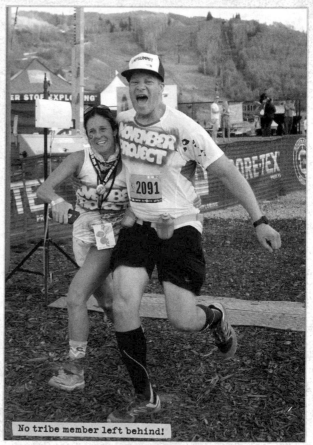

No tribe member left behind!

"I've been following Nick's journey to get physically and emotionally fit," Cesca said. "We keep in touch through Facebook, and I know how important November Project has been in his life. I also know how important it is to finish a race with people you know cheering and supporting you. I wanted Nick to have someone there to share his joy, euphoria, and sense of accomplishment."

"It was incredible that she waited for me," Flattes said. "I was shocked. It was the happiest moment of my life. All the races I had done in Vancouver, my ex-wife was never at the finish line. It was like somehow starting a new chapter in my life at that moment."

While Flattes and Cesca caught up and took some selfies, a few miles down the road, Karnazes, who was also staying at the Park City Peaks Hotel, was just getting out of the pool. He was wrapped in a towel, his golden hair slicked back. Against the white terrycloth, his tan muscles appeared carved from driftwood. The offspring of sun and rock face. Karnazes, a North Face athlete, is the face of the TNF Endurance Challenge Series, which stages eight trail races a year in the United States and Canada.

"The marathon relay used to be our smallest event and now when NP shows up, it's our biggest," Karnazes said. "November Project has brought a lot of new participants into the series. They've really adopted it. It's a good fit. You hear a lot of people saying what is this November Project? Where is it? I want to try it."

Karnazes first met Graham on the Boston Marathon course in 2013 when the ultra-runner was competing in the event. "He just jumped in beside me. I get people coming up to me all the time with ideas. Brogan reminded me of Tony Robbins on steroids, Red Bull running through his veins. I kind of held him at arm's length. But he was persistent, said, 'You gotta try it, you gotta try it. We're building something and it's more than what you think.'"

Eventually Karnazes showed up. And he was won over.

"The vibe's incredible, the positivity is incredible," he said. "I mean, look at what happened today. After they announced the marathon relay winners, they could have all walked away, but they stayed. They're so inclusive and supportive of other people. That alone says so much about the quality and character of the people involved."

From above there was a sudden series of knocks. From the second-floor windows, overlooking the indoor patio where we were talking, Graham and Whalen, on their way to the evening social on Main Street (where another NP takeover would take place), had spotted us. They began gyrating and lifting their shirts like they were in a red-light district storefront. Karnazes followed suit, waving his arms back and forth, in just his towel, laughing until they vanished, gone just as quickly as they had appeared.

"They're disrupting the fitness industry," Karnazes said, still smiling. "They're getting people out of the gym. They're getting new people into running. They're making fitness fun, which I really like. I think we're on the cusp of a new era."

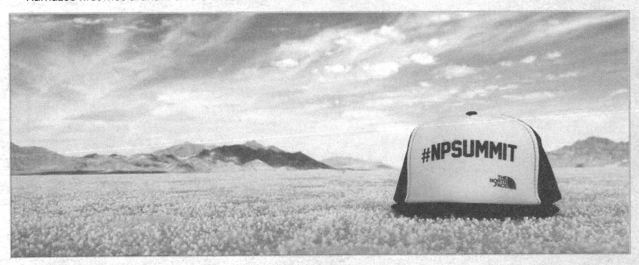

NOVEMBER PROJECT
GLOSSARY OF TERMS

BY BROGAN GRAHAM AND BOJAN MANDARIC

It's important to know the language used here at November Project if you're planning to train with, or even follow, what we're up to each week. Here is a short list of terminology we use at November Project that will help you make sense of it all. Enjoy.

#DestinationDeck: A simple hashtag term used to label our Monday workout.

We Missed You: A section of the NP website. If you glance to the top of the page you'll see the tab...go ahead, click on it. It will give you the play-by-play for those November Project members who didn't show up after dropping a "verbal" (see below for definition). Katie Deans is an example of one of our best entries.

Verbal: A verbal commitment to attend a future workout. Most commonly done via word-of-mouth, verbals can also be "dropped" online, through a text message, or on a handwritten love note. Giving a verbal is like swearing on all graves covered in holy scriptures and future loved children and grandchildren that you'll attend. Do the right thing, don't break a verbal. Ever. If someone says, "Yeah, I think I'll check out November Project this week," you can force them by saying, "Is that a verbal?" Then show them the We Missed You section. This is "hunting" or "fishing" for a verbal.

Verbal Harvest: Use this technique to gain a large number of verbals at the same time: Find a large group in person or on the World Wide Web and ask which of them are planning to come to the next morning session/workout. Pushing people to drop verbals is one thing that the NP leaders in both Boston and Madison do well.

Traverbal: Committing to attend a November Project workout in another city.

PR Pizza: Race your booty off on the last Wednesday of each month, post your personal fastest time, and you'll win a pizza-shaped trophy. It's a pizza. Kinda like BOOK IT back in the day...but less books. (Author's note: Frozen pizza has been retired. These days, you get your photo taken wearing BG's Run DMC-style gold chain, a WWE champion's belt, or with a pot-belly pig. Who knows what it will be by the time this book comes out.)

Spice: Any small change or addition to a workout that will make the work more fun, harder, more interesting, or all of the above.

November Project Worcester City Tag

217

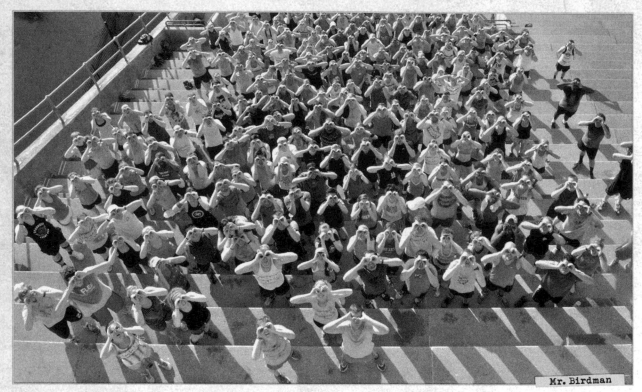

Mr. Birdman

#Dooster_Pledge: A hashtag to be placed after a photo you believe is worthy of Dooster quality, and as such the photographer ought to be made part of the team. Dooster is still just two dudes.

Stealing Wireless: The term we use for the folks who come to train with us but start at an amount of time annoyingly early or late so that "they don't have to deal with the large group." This isn't really playing fair because they're essentially soaking up the vibe and personal drive to get out of bed without doing the NP workout or making new friends the way we do. If people want less of a group, then they should train where we train on Tuesday, Thursday, and Saturday at 6:30 a.m. Boom!

Andrew Schwartz'd: In a carpooling situation, you offer someone in the group a ride in your car. Immediately, that person jumps in the back seat. That leaves the front seat empty. Does your passenger see the strangeness of this situation and get into the front seat to politely keep you, the driver, company? Or does this passenger take a ride in the back seat,

taxicab style? If the passenger doesn't move and remains in the back seat for the duration of your awkward ride as you drive to the destination...you've just been Andrew Schwartz'd.

Mr. Birdman: A group game that can be played at all times in all locations of this world. Put on the Mr. Birdman goggles—create the lenses by touching your thumb and index fingers—and make eye contact with other members. If they look into your eyes, then they must lie down on the ground for 5 seconds no matter where they're standing.

Recruiting Papers: Hand-cut circular pieces of discarded cardboard that simply read "FUCK YEAH NOVEMBER PROJECT" on them. They also have our website information and are handed out to only the nicest, fittest/fattest, and most fun people we run into here in Boston. I may hand you one at the end of your workout and tell you to bring one new person to the next workout (after you give that person the info). Recruiting Papers. Make each one count.

The "Easter Hash Hunt": The November Project spring race that makes most people in Boston a little nervous. Like everything else we do, it is held outdoors, fun as heck, and 100 percent FREE. Easter Hash Hunt is the best thing since racing shopping carts.

The Chris Marshall Rule: The Chris Marshall Rule states that every NP member who drives to the workout on Friday will park their vehicle at the bottom of the hill on Beacon Street (there are tons of metered parking spots that don't kick in until 8 a.m. on both sides of the street) or on one of the streets on the Brighton side of the hill. This will allow us to keep the passing lane on the road nice and clear and will not be obstructed by our four-wheelers lining up and down the hill.

Sebastians: Seven minutes of all-out burpees. We did this workout during the hurricane in the fall. Break 100 and you're moving pretty quick.

Bojans: When you and a partner duck, crawl, down-dog, and FLY OVER one another.

The Positivity Award: At almost every single workout you'll see the weathered oar handle from Northeastern Rowing. This award is handed to a NP member who drives the group with their positivity.

#NP_TSA: A hashtag often used when a tribe member is traveling and displaying grassroots gear while on their way to another tribe city.

#deckaday: An online check-in during the month of October of 2013. The phrase refers to the commitment to become fitter in the core by doing a deck of cards every single day throughout the month.

#deckaday tourist: The person who drops in on a good amount of the opening decks in a certain month, and then fades in and out of his or her commitment. This person is weak when it comes to sticking to a schedule but, if they play it right, this can also be pretty funny. This kind of person is usually not seen as badass at all.

Fighter Jet: A person, not a real jet, and from all we know, not a huge fighter. His real name is FJ Perfas, and he is in charge of the Sunday social/training group called Boston Brunch Runners. You'll see "Fighter Jet" at almost every single workout we host. Find and LIKE Boston Brunch Runners on Facebook. They're strong. They're fun. They're led by a Fighter Jet.

Morning Person: As in, "I'm not a morning person." The facts are simple; they don't exist. We're not morning people. No one is. Just wake up and stop talking about reasons you have to lie in bed and grow your gut. Boom.

November Project: Dude, just check out the Wikipedia page!: wikipedia.org/wiki/November_Project.

"FUCK YEAH!": This is the only answer option when anyone from your November Project tribe asks you if you're good, as in, "You good?" Without getting into how tired you are or how busy things are at work, cut through the shit and respond with "Fuck Yeah!"

Have a great day!
This week is going to be amazing.
See you Wednesday and Friday and Monday.

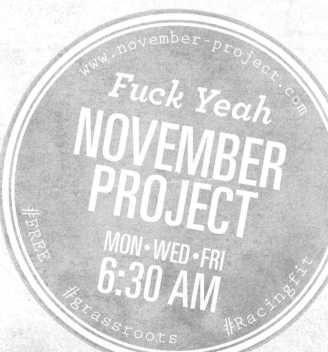

ACKNOWLEDGMENTS

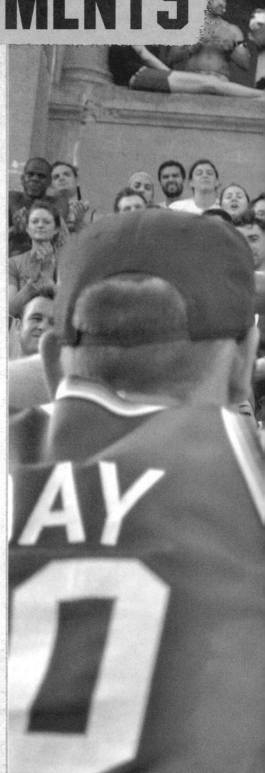

CALEB DANILOFF

There are numerous people who helped turn a bunch of hot air into the bound set of pages you're now holding in your hands. But everything starts with Brogan Graham and Bojan Mandaric. Without them—no November Project, no community, no book, no writing these acknowledgments. They are rare woodpeckers indeed, and I'm truly honored that they trusted me enough to help bang out their song. Boom shakalaka, m'dudes!

Dialing things back, I want to thank the folks at *Runner's World,* where this tale, or at least my part in it, began. To editor-in-chief David Willey who, from his first encounter, saw the magic of November Project and to senior editor Katie Neitz, who didn't flinch when I filed a piece four times the word count and dropped a cover bomb. From day one, Katie was champion.

I want to thank and applaud the talented team at Rodale Books, especially executive editor Mark Weinstein, creative director Jeff Batzli, and project editor Nancy N. Bailey, all of whom we drove crazy on a regular basis. (The hair implants are on us, guys). They helped bring this thing to life in true Fuck-Yeah fashion. Thanks, of course, to my agent Wendy Sherman, who helped guide and counsel from the get-go.

I need to thank the countless tribe members who took the time to talk with me and contributed their heartfelt thoughts, insights, and enthusiasm to the project. I owe a particularly loud shout-out to Chris "Can of Spaghetti" Cantergiani, who, at key moments, loaned a hand with the mountain of content. Also, to Tony DiPasquale, who supplied the tool that helped build that mountain. Many thanks to all the talented tribe photographers, and to Dooster and Diana Hunt, in particular.

Finally, and far from leastly, I want to thank my wife, Christine, and daughter, Shea, for their patience, understanding, and support over the last year. Living with a writer is no easy task. Living with a tribe member might be twice as hard. I love you two beyond all periods, exclamation points, and beads of sweat.

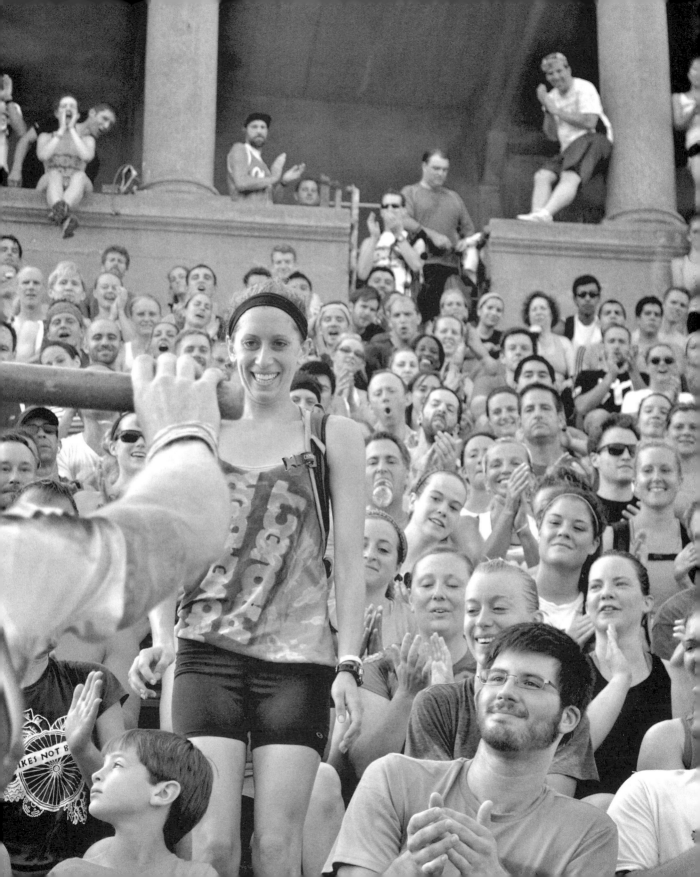

ACKNOWLEDGMENTS

BOJAN MANDARIC:

To my wife, Emilie, for making me feel like the luckiest man alive every single day. To my daughter, Marli, who inspires me to be the best version of myself. To my sister Olivera, aunts Mira and Marina, uncle Buda, cousins Sale, Andrea, Strahinja, Sonja, and the rest of the family in Serbia who love me and support me unconditionally. To my dog, Sami, who wakes me up 15 minutes before I usually would to get to the workout. To my friend and one of the most impressive humans I've ever met, Brogan Graham, who's constantly challenging me to stretch my comfort zone. To Ann Doody, my American mother. To Ethan Bookman, who got into my life as a quiet dorky journalist and stayed as a close friend who helped me put my name on the book cover.

To some of the most selfless people I have ever met: Emily Saul, Chris Payne, Chris Capozzi, Deniz Karakoyunlu, Evan Dana, Dan Graham, Pat Bauch, Jeff Morris, Ted Gurman, Ben Schwabe, Roger Huffman, Laura McCloskey (soon to be Green), Dan Clayton, Paddy O'Leary, Josh Zipin, Jennifer Ference, Nadim Chin, Tyler Sullivan, Andrew Ference, Dan Berteletti, Molly Thayer, Matthew Sellen, Ryan Wooderson (a.k.a. Timmy Ference), Danny Metcalf, Steve Christensen, Kaelan Dickinson, Lauren Padula, Ashleigh Voychick, Jess Craik, Angelo Neroni, Nick Rodricks, Sydney Van Horn, Pat O'Neal, Suzanne Allaire, Dan Layo, Bobbie Werbe, Dan German, Jason Shaw, Orrin Whalen, Stephen Selnick, Ben Otto, Tara Wall, Chris Malenab, Haley Gonzales, Stephanie Ganiban, John Honerkamp, Paul Leak, Ben Bauch, Holly Reiland, Cameron Gilly, Kate Gilly, Preston Reeder, Will Boher, Brent Cunningham, Andy Watt, Kevin Wasielewski, Brendan Scully, Rick Duha, Thomas Hall, Derek Page, Tammara Francis, Pete Nazarewycz, John DeBoer, Kris Utt, Graham Snowden, Richard Hortness, Jackie Knoll, Trevor Warren, Claire Hutchinson, Sam Hirons, Michelle Roest, Casey Winkler, Kelsey Duckett, Sam Kenary, Jim Kenary, Hank Kenary, John Kohler, Tatsiana Khvitsko, Keith Wells, Roz Hubbard, Rumon Carter, Jason Ball, Shannon Kane, Freddy Garcia, Mihajlo Jovanovic, Rakel Eva Sævarsdóttir, and all the future leaders of November Project who will continue to change fitness paradigms one member at a time without asking anything in return.

To our photographers Ryan Scura and Dylan Ladds from Dooster Film, Kelvin Ma, Samantha Goresh, Katie Hughes, Scott Yellow, Rosa Evora, Xander Miller, Diana Hunt, Alan Scherer, Matt Anzur, for always shooting gold. To the paint squad tagging millions of pieces of #GrassrootsGear. To Laura Ingalls, a.k.a. DJ Phoenix, for dropping the hottest jams that one's ear can register at 6:30 a.m. To Tony Dipasquale for being unofficial November Project CTO. To all our members, or should I say November Project Ambassadors, for loving and growing the movement. To Allie Clark for helping us incorporate. To Chris Cantergiani a.k.a. Can of Spaghetti/Filters/Book Edits/News, for sifting through thousands of pages of heartwarming content. To Mark Weinstein, Jeff Batzli, and Wendy Sherman for making this book happen. To David Willey for not laughing when we were dropping #WorldTakeover left and right. To all my coaches for teaching me how to row. To all my Husky teammates for teaching me English.

To Katie Ramage and Todd Spaletto, for believing in us, and Maeve Sloan, for dealing with our daily insanity. To Chris Heuisler for being one of our biggest fans. To everyone that I may have missed, it wasn't on purpose.

To Zdenka Mandaric for teaching me how to be a decent person—I miss you every day.

acknowledgements

☑ MEMBERS
☑ CO·LEADERS
☑ FAM.
☑ BOJ.
☑ GOLDIE
☑ HATERS?
☑ BOOKMAN

to every single person who has traded sleep for good times with us.

to every single person who has built a tribe and truly created a community.

to the Co·Leaders who host something fun and fierce, and FREE each week in any weather.

to my all·over·the·map family for always supporting my stupid ideas.

to my Co·Founder Bojan for always shooting down my stupid ideas.

to my smart/organized/amazing wife for helping "blow up" November Project.

to the people who laughed at our confidence and dreams of reaching the world.

and to Caleb "Bookman" for making this book happen. To everyone in and around this movement... thank you for all that you've done.

Brogan Graham
"BG"

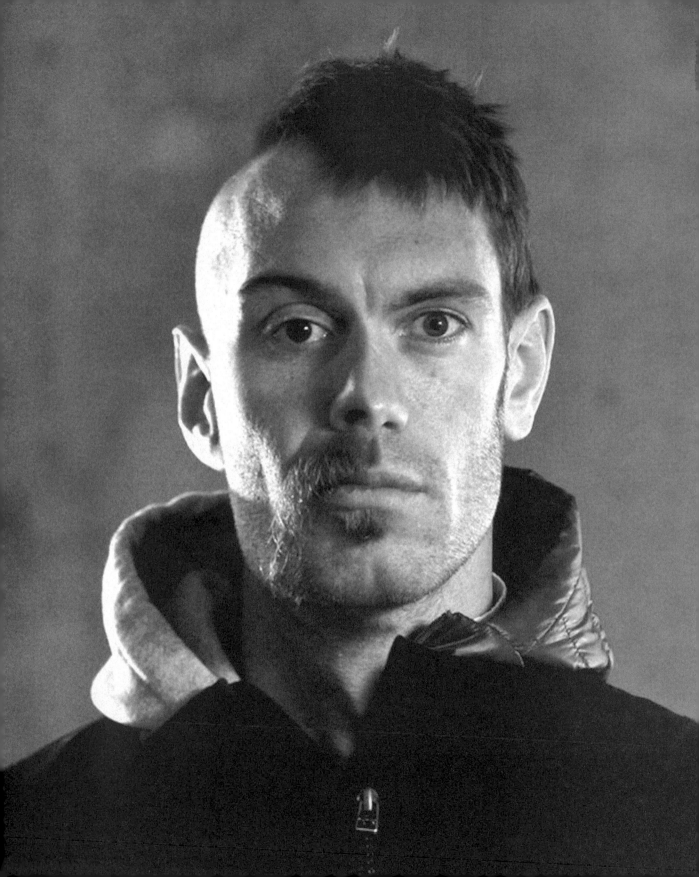

ABOUT THE AUTHORS

BOJAN

BOJAN MANDARIC grew up in Novi Sad, Serbia, and is a former rower on the Yugoslavian National Team and at Northeastern University. He has a boatload of regatta medals, speaks suspiciously fluent English, and coached rowing at Syracuse University. He is now a full-time strategist (and reluctant safety-compliance officer) at November Project. He and his wife, Emilie, have a daughter named Marli and a German shepherd named Sami. They live in Boston, Massachusetts.

BROGAN

BROGAN GRAHAM is a former rower, crew coach, world wanderer, street interviewer, pedicab driver, rap-video star, social-media strategist, tattoo canvas, and provocateur-at-large. He is now a full-time fitness fire-starter at November Project and extremely frequent flyer. He lives in San Diego, California, with his live-in yoga instructor, Goldie, whom he married in 2014.

CALEB

CALEB DANILOFF is a Boston-area freelance writer, a contributing editor at *Runner's World* magazine, and the author of *Running Ransom Road: Confronting the Past One Marathon at a Time* (Houghton Mifflin Harcourt, 2012). He is sometimes known as Ethan Bookman and no longer yells at the teens cutting across his front lawn. He lives in Cambridge, Massachusetts, with his wife, daughter, two dogs, and a cat.

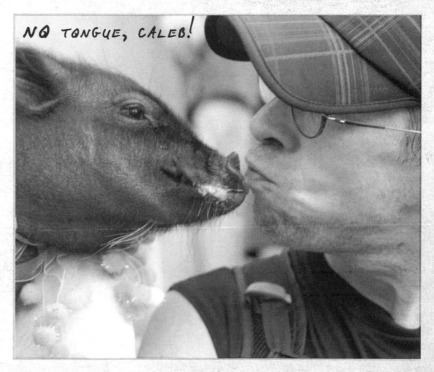

NO TONGUE, CALEB!

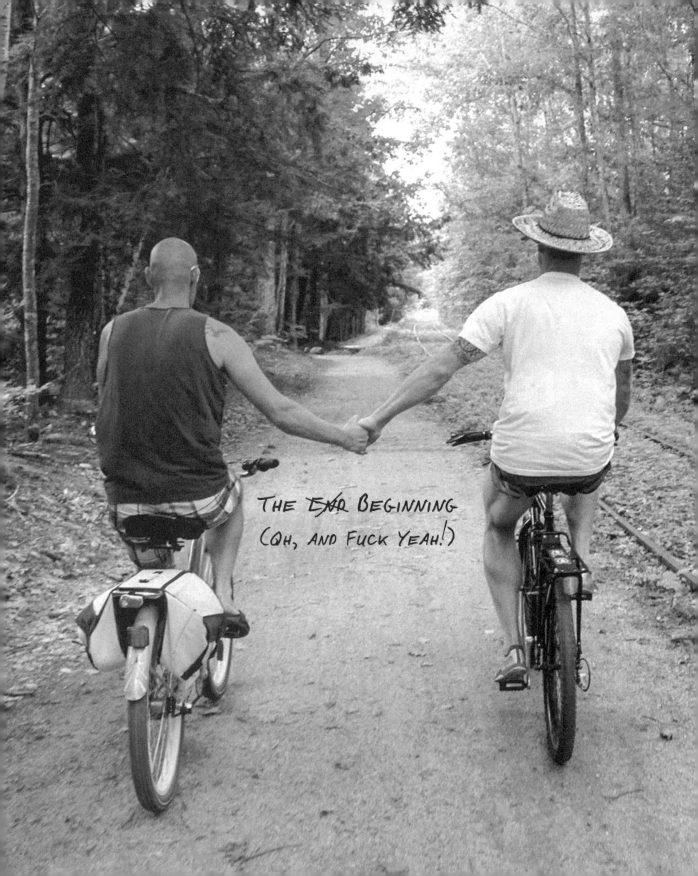

THE ~~END~~ BEGINNING
(QH, AND FUCK YEAH!)

D0691222

A TOUCH OF
FARMHOUSE CHARM

Easy DIY Projects to Add a Warm and Rustic Feel to Any Room

Liz Fourez

creator of Love Grows Wild

PAGE STREET
PUBLISHING CO.

PAGE STREET
PUBLISHING CO.

Copyright © 2016 Liz Fourez

First published in 2016 by
Page Street Publishing Co.
27 Congress Street, Suite 105
Salem, MA 01970
www.pagestreetpublishing.com

All rights reserved. No part of this book may be reproduced or used, in any form or by any means,
electronic or mechanical, without prior permission in writing from the publisher.

Distributed by Macmillan, sales in Canada by The Canadian Manda Group.

20   19   18   17   16   1   2   3   4   5

ISBN-13: 978-1-62414-292-5
ISBN-10: 1-62414-292-3

Library of Congress Control Number: 2016908618

Cover and book design by Page Street Publishing Co.
Photography by Liz Fourez and Emily Layne

Printed and bound in China

Page Street is proud to be a member of 1% for the Planet. Members donate one percent
of their sales to one or more of the over 1,500 environmental and sustainability charities
across the globe who participate in this program.

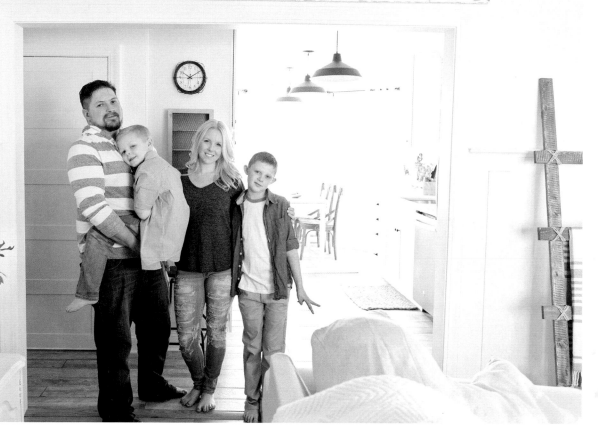

To the three amazing people I get to share this beautiful home and life with . . .

Jeremy, Alec and Wyatt

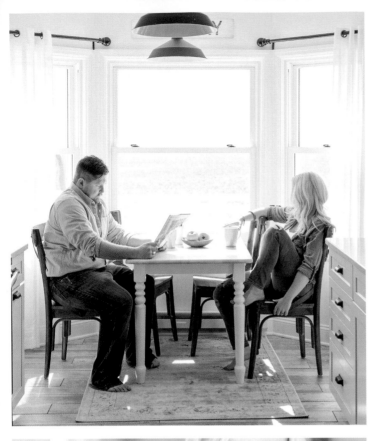

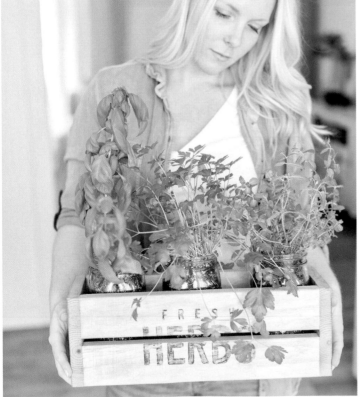

CONTENTS

INTRODUCTION

Hello, sweet friends, and welcome to our farmhouse. My husband, Jeremy, and I moved into this small Indiana home about four years ago with our two sweet boys, Alec and Wyatt, and we have been renovating room by room ever since.

Together as a family we have torn down walls, built furniture, painted every surface and restored the original charm of our 1940s farmhouse.

I think what I love most about old farmhouses is their character and the sense of history you get from them. Farmhouses were built with practical materials, and the furnishings were simple, unpretentious and collected over time. The builders used what was available to them and let nature inspire the design.

Decorating with farmhouse style today is all about blending modern amenities with elements that take you back to a simpler time. In a modern farmhouse kitchen, you might find an antique table and apron sink mixed with new white cabinetry and stainless-steel appliances.

The rooms in a modern farmhouse should feel cozy, warm, inviting and full of charm and character. Natural wood tones connect the home to the outdoors, and soft, neutral colors create a sense of calm and relaxation. Combining antiques and flea-market finds with new furniture produces a look that has evolved over time. Weathered wood, peeling paint, natural fabrics and simple, clean lines are all hallmarks of classic farmhouse style.

I've developed a huge passion for old farmhouses over the last four years and have come up with 70 easy ways you can add a touch of farmhouse charm in your own home. This book will show you everything from adding farmhouse-style details to your trim and doors to handmade, personalized décor full of vintage charm. I'll also share some simple storage solutions to organize your space and my favorite paint techniques for aging furniture.

What makes this book really special is that you will not only learn how to make all these projects, but you will also get to see how I use them to decorate our home. I'll take you on a room-by-room tour of our little farmhouse and show you how we renovated and decorated each space to turn it into the home we've always dreamed of.

My hope for this book is that you learn new skills and decorating ideas that will open up endless possibilities for your home and that you will be inspired to create a place that is warm, cozy and inviting for you and your family to enjoy. Home is all about the memories you make there together, and as I'm writing this I have flashbacks of dancing barefoot in the kitchen with my husband, giving

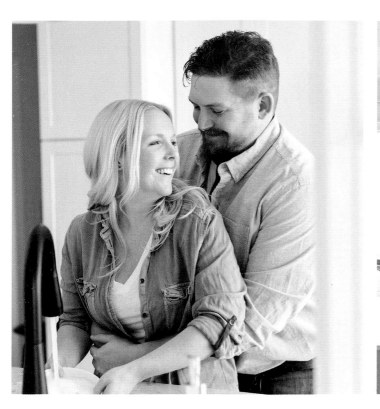
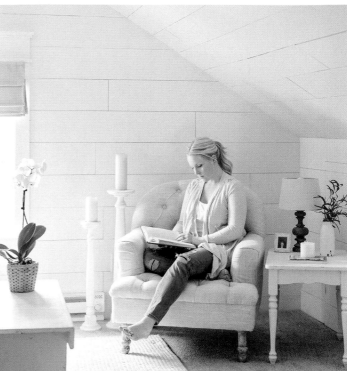

my babies bubble baths in the bathtub, having family gathered around the dining room table for holidays and snuggling together on the couch watching our favorite movies.

I'm so grateful that you picked up this book and cannot wait for you to start creating your dream home. You can keep in touch with me through my blog, lovegrowswild.com, and please share your home and project photos with me on social media!

As Dorothy would say, "There's no place like home." Let's start creating yours.

xoxo Liz

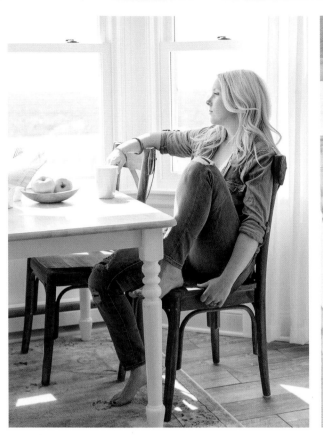
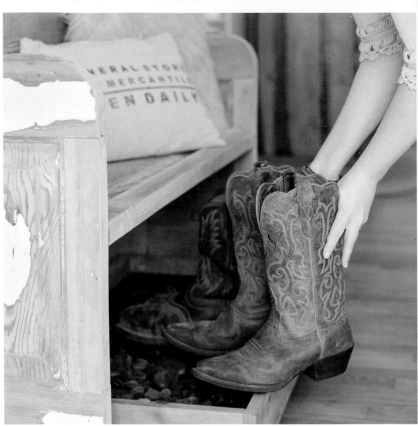
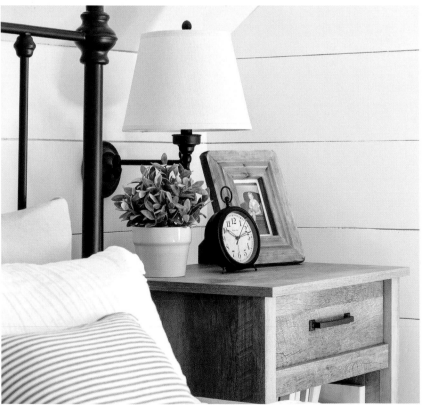
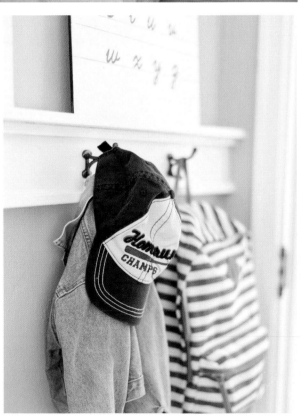

TIPS & ADVICE

Whether you are new to decorating and creating projects or a seasoned expert, there are a handful of items that will be helpful to have before getting started. Don't feel like you have to go out and buy everything all at once, but as you go through the book, add to your tool collection as your skill and comfort levels increase.

HERE'S WHAT I KEEP IN MY TOOLBOX:

- *Angled paintbrush*
- *Brad nail gun*
- *Circular saw*
- *Drill with various size bits*
- *Electronic cutting machine*
- *Hammer*
- *Jigsaw*
- *Level*
- *Metal snips*
- *Miter saw*
- *Painter's tape*
- *Paste wax*
- *Pliers*
- *Pocket-hole jig*
- *Sanding block or sandpaper*
- *Screwdriver*
- *Screws and nails in various sizes*
- *Staple gun and staples*
- *Tape measure*
- *Wall anchors*
- *White paint*
- *Wood glue*
- *Wood stain*

Most of the projects in this book are simple and don't require many tools, but some of them do call for things like a miter saw, pocket-hole jig or brad nail gun that you may not be familiar with.

HELPFUL TIPS FOR USING THESE TOOLS

- Saws—I use a few different types of saws in this book, and each one has a different purpose. A miter saw is great for cutting lumber and also allows you to cut on an angle. But the blade only cuts up to an 8- or 10-inch (20.5- or 25.5-cm) board, depending on the model you have. A circular saw is smaller and more portable than a miter saw, and I often use this one to cut big sheets of plywood that the miter saw cannot cut. When I need to make detailed cuts or rounded edges, I use a jigsaw. If you don't have access to a miter saw or circular saw, most home improvement stores will cut materials for you for a small fee. Just make sure to bring a list with you of all the cuts you need.

- Brad nail gun—This tool saves a ton of time and effort when you need to use nails on a project. You load the brad nails into the gun, and it shoots the nails into the wood for you, increasing your accuracy and speed. The nail gun I have is battery powered, but you can also purchase nail guns powered by an air compressor. If you work on home projects often, I highly recommend investing in one, but any project that calls for a brad nail gun in this book can be completed using a good old-fashioned hammer and nails as well.

- Pocket-hole jig—This tool allows you to drill holes into wood at an angle, creating a pocket for a screw. You can then connect two pieces of wood together with that screw, creating a super-strong joint and hiding the screws neatly inside the pockets. Once I started building more complex furniture projects, I decided to invest in a pocket-hole jig, and it makes woodworking go so much faster. I personally use the Kreg Jig® brand, and it comes with great instructions for learning how to use this tool. There are also many resources online you can use as well. If you do not have this tool, you can modify the projects by eliminating the pocket holes and drilling a screw straight into the wood. You will be able to see the screw heads, but you can paint over them or cover them with wood filler.

- Electronic cutting machine—This is similar to a printer that plugs into your computer, but instead of printing, it has a small blade that cuts designs into paper, vinyl, fabric and more. I use this tool most often to create stencils on adhesive vinyl that I can apply to my projects and then paint over. This tool is very versatile, especially if you do a lot of crafting, and I personally use the Silhouette CAMEO® machine. Craft stores offer a wide variety of alphabet stencils as well as other designs, and you can use those on any project that calls for a stencil in this book if you do not own a cutting machine.

Lumber sizes can be confusing if you haven't worked with them before, but this chart should help clarify. If a project calls for a 1 x 4 board, the actual size is going to be ¾ inch x 3 ½ inches (2 cm x 9 cm), but it is still called a 1 x 4. I used pine or whitewood for all the projects in this book, unless otherwise specified.

BOARD	ACTUAL SIZE
1 x 2	¾" x 1 ½" (2 cm x 3.8 cm)
1 x 3	¾" x 2 ½" (2 cm x 6.5 cm)
1 x 4	¾" x 3 ½" (2 cm x 9 cm)
1 x 6	¾" x 5 ½" (2 cm x 14 cm)
1 x 8	¾" x 7 ¼" (2 cm x 18.5 cm)
1 x 10	¾" x 9 ¼" (2 cm x 23.5 cm)
1 x 12	¾" x 11 ¼" (2 cm x 28.5 cm)

PROJECT GUIDE

Not sure which project to do first? The projects in this book have been divided into three categories: beginner, intermediate and advanced.

The beginner projects can be easily completed in a few hours or less and do not require any power tools. The intermediate projects require basic power tools and take anywhere from a few hours to one day to complete. Any of the intermediate projects that require a saw call for simple, straight cuts. The advanced projects also take up to a day to complete but use more complex power tools, and some require you to make angled cuts. These projects are also larger and may require a second set of hands to help with building.

Start with projects at the skill level you are most comfortable with and work your way up to more complex ones. Always keep safety in mind when working with power tools, and remember to have fun while creating beautiful things for your home!

BEGINNER PROJECTS

INTERMEDIATE PROJECTS

ADVANCED PROJECTS

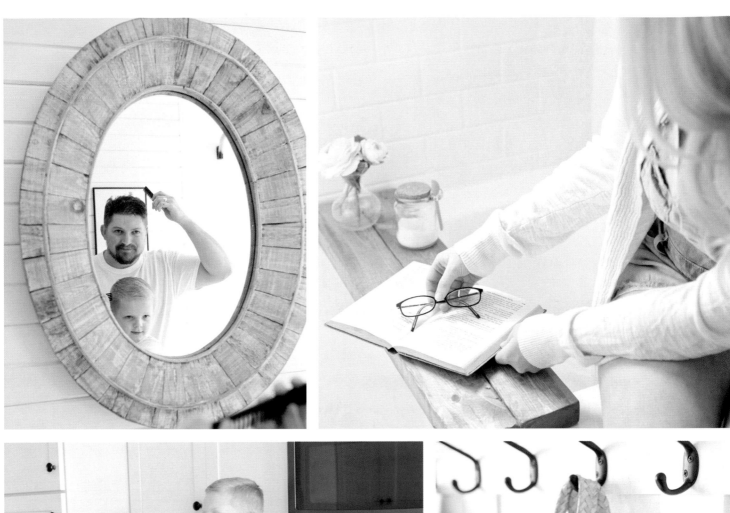

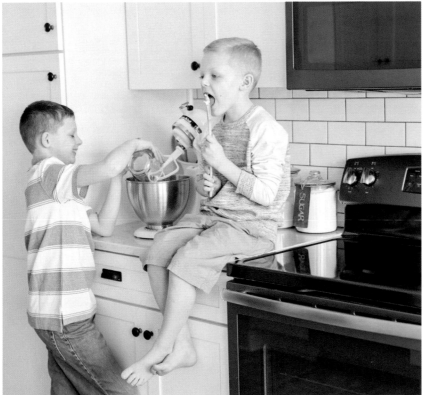

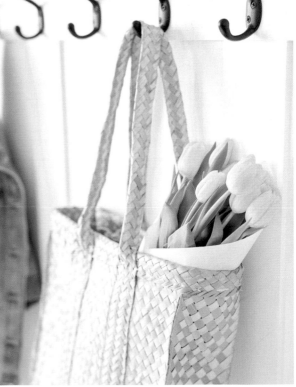

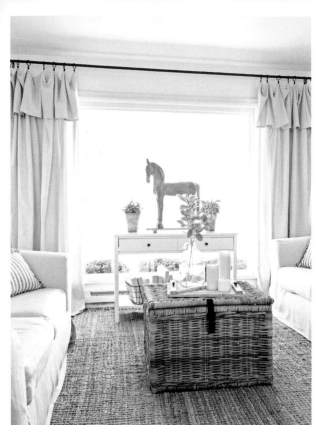
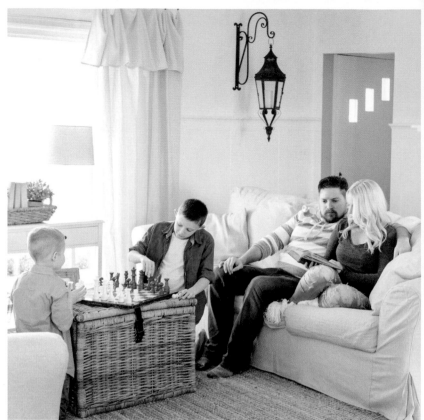
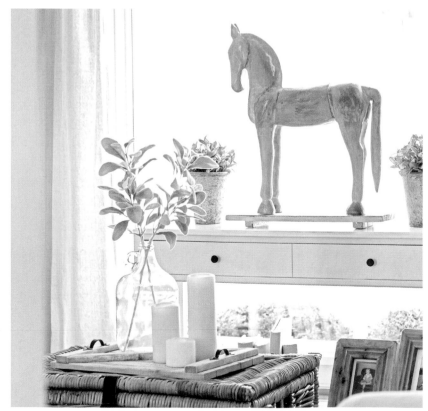
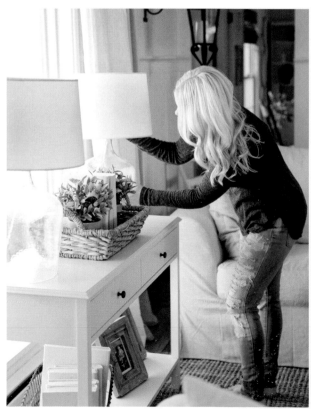

LIVING ROOM

The living room is the gathering place in your home. This is where movies are watched, parties are thrown, board games are played and afternoon naps are taken. You need enough space in which to entertain, yet you want it to feel cozy and inviting at the same time.

Our living room is open to the kitchen and dining room, so we wanted to make it all feel like one cohesive space. We painted the room a bright white and used board-and-batten trim on the walls to add extra depth and dimension. We're lucky to have several large windows that let in a lot of natural light, so we highlighted them with natural bamboo shades and curtains that I made myself from drop cloths. We also added to the character of the windows by installing farmhouse window trim above the existing trim (see the Farmhouse Window Trim project on page 40).

The rest of the room is decorated with a mix of rustic, cozy textures and light, neutral colors. I centered the entire layout of this room on our picture window and used a large jute rug as the foundation for the furniture. Our couches are slipcovered in Belgian linen that is both comfortable and durable for our family of messy boys, and a driftwood-gray wicker trunk serves as a coffee table in the center of the sofas. An antique armoire holds extra blankets and pillows, and two large iron lanterns on either side of the window add a bit of drama to the space.

In this chapter, I'll show you how to make your own inexpensive curtains (page 19), decorate with handmade pillows (page 28), add storage with a blanket ladder (page 16), personalize your room with a sign featuring your family name (page 23) and more. Get ready to curl up on the couch with a good book and enjoy your cozy new living room!

SIMPLE RUSTIC LADDER

When you're short on storage but don't want to compromise on style, sometimes you have to think outside of the box. An old wooden ladder leaning against the wall can provide storage for extra blankets in the living room, towels in a bathroom or even serve as a pot rack in a kitchen. For a decorative touch, try hanging a wreath or picture frames from the top rung.

Level of Difficulty: Intermediate

SUPPLIES

- *3 (1 x 3) boards, 8 feet (244 cm) long*
- *Miter or circular saw*
- *Tape measure*
- *Sanding block*
- *Wood glue*
- *Clamps*
- *Brad nail gun*
- *1-inch (2.5-cm) brad nails*
- *Wood stain*
- *Paintbrush*
- *Clean rags*
- *Paste wax*
- *Suede cord*

DIRECTIONS

Measure and cut two of the wood boards to 6 feet (183 cm) long using a saw. These will be the sides of the ladder. Cut the last wood board into four pieces 23 ½-inches (60-cm) long. These will be the rungs of the ladder. Sand any rough edges with a sanding block.

Lay the sides of the ladder spaced 14 inches (35.5 cm) apart from inside edge to inside edge. Place the rungs on top of the sides about 14 ½ inches (37 cm) apart from each other. Apply wood glue to each rung where it crosses over the sides of the ladder, and use clamps to hold the rungs and sides in place. Flip the ladder over and add a few brad nails where the rungs cross over the sides.

Apply stain to the entire ladder using a paintbrush. Allow the stain to penetrate for 5–15 minutes until the desired color is achieved. Then wipe the wood with a clean rag to remove any remaining stain, and allow it to dry completely, about 8 hours. To seal the wood, apply a layer of paste wax with a paintbrush and buff with a clean rag.

Wrap suede cord around each rung in an X-pattern where it crosses over the side of the ladder, then tie a knot in back to secure the suede in place.

TIP | *If you want a more rustic look for your ladder, try using furring strips for the wood boards. They are less expensive than standard boards because they often have irregularities, but the distress marks just add to the character of the wood. Just make sure to search through the pile for straight ones!*

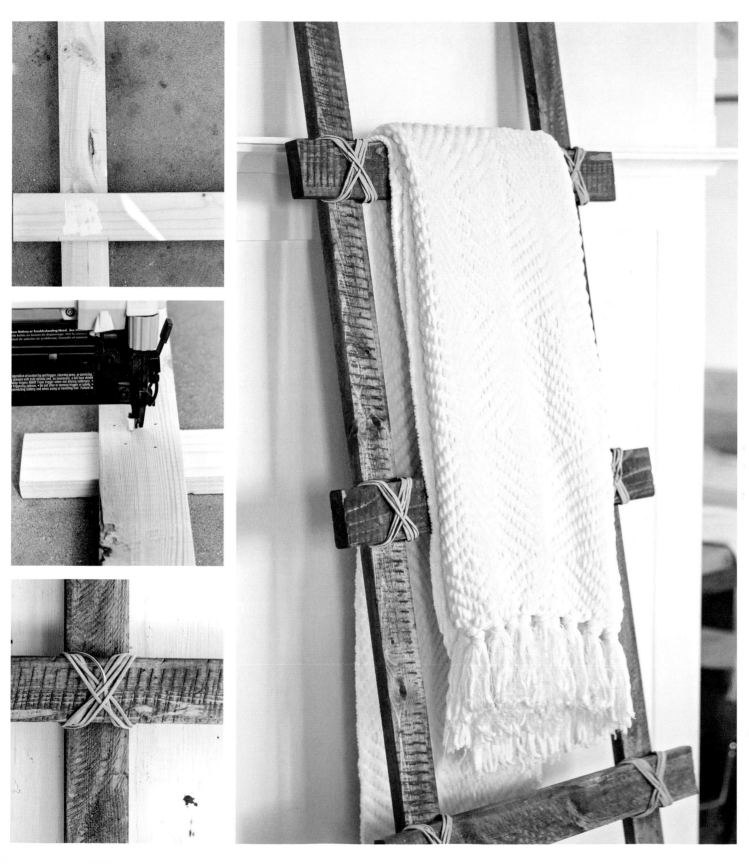

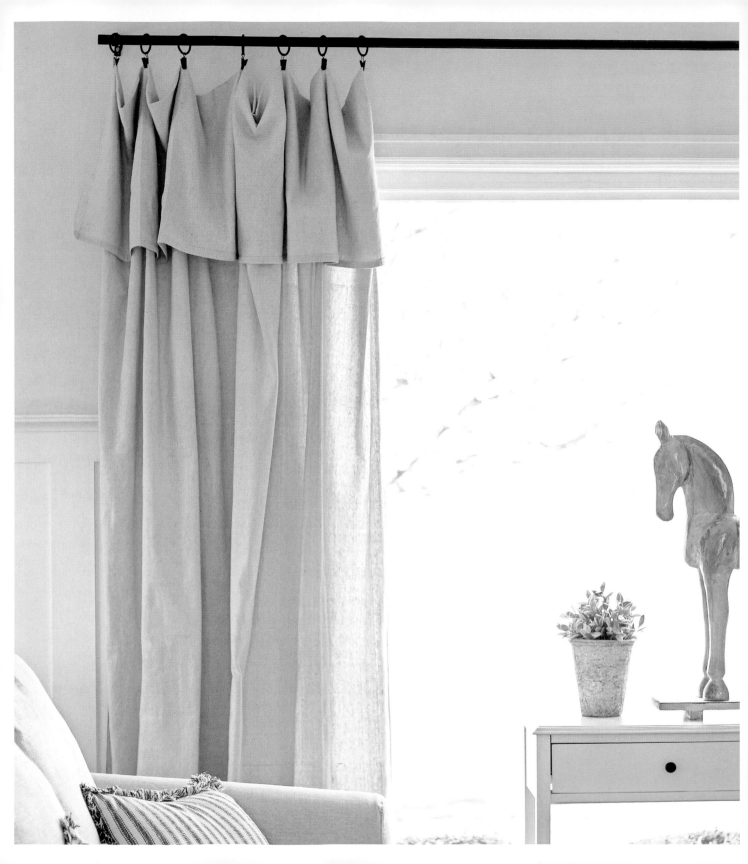

EASY DROP CLOTH CURTAINS

Finding great curtains can be expensive, especially if you have tall ceilings and need the extra length. Using a drop cloth to make your own gives you plenty of fabric to work with at a fraction of the price of store-bought curtains. The best part is how incredibly easy these are to make! Just use curtain clip rings to hang the drop cloths . . . no sewing required!

Level of Difficulty: Beginner

SUPPLIES

- *2 canvas drop cloths with hemmed edges*
- *Iron and ironing board*
- *Curtain clip rings*
- *Curtain rod with brackets*
- *Drill*

DIRECTIONS

Wash and dry the drop cloths and iron to smooth any wrinkles. Attach the clip rings evenly spaced along the top of the drop cloths.

Install the curtain rod brackets above your window using a drill. Slide the clip rings onto the curtain rod and set the rod inside the brackets.

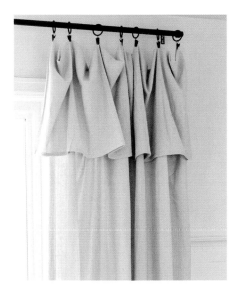

TIP | *Curtains look best when they are brushing or puddled on the floor, but if they are way too long, fold the top of the drop cloth over until they are the correct length.*

CHICKEN-WIRE CANDLEHOLDER

Centerpieces don't have to be complicated or expensive. A few candles set on a moss-covered wood plate will add instant warmth and coziness to a room. Try styling this piece on your coffee table or dining room table.

Level of Difficulty: Beginner

SUPPLIES

- *Metal snips*
- *1-inch (2.5-cm) galvanized poultry netting*
- *Pliers*
- *14-inch (35.5-cm) wood plate or charger*
- *Staple gun and staples*
- *Pillar candles in various heights*
- *Moss*

DIRECTIONS

Use metal snips to cut a piece of poultry netting about 11 inches (28 cm) high and about 30 inches (76 cm) long. Wrap the netting to form a cylinder and use pliers to wrap the loose ends of wire around each other, securing the cylinder in place.

Bend the netting on the bottom of the cylinder inward, and set the netting on the center of the wood plate. Use a staple gun to secure the bent wires to the bottom of the plate.

Set pillar candles of various heights inside the netting and cover the bottom of the plate with moss.

TIP | *Using moss around the candles adds a touch of nature and a pop of fresh color, but try using different fillers as the seasons change, such as acorns for fall or pinecones for winter.*

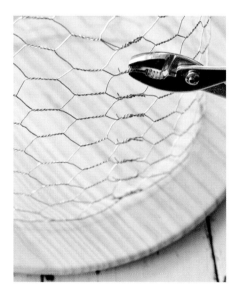
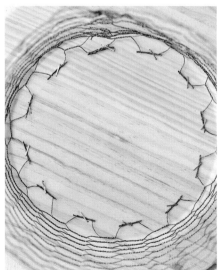

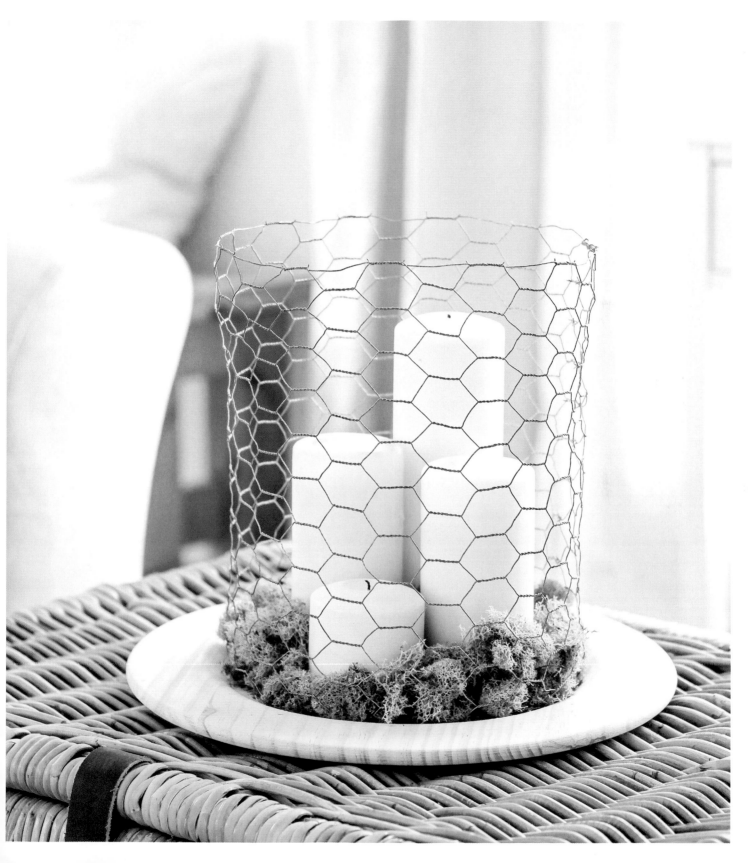

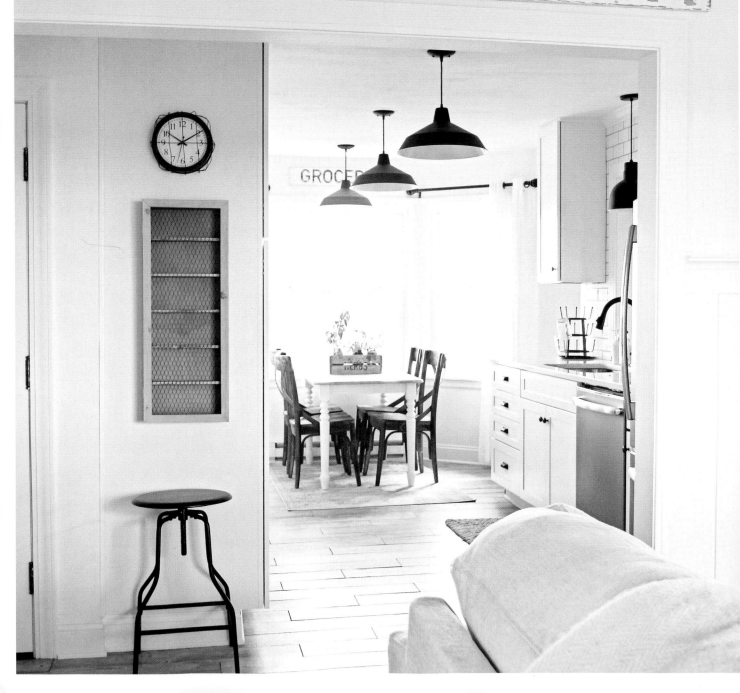

FAMILY NAME SIGN

Nothing will put a personal touch on your home more than a custom, handmade sign with your family's name on it. This tutorial will walk you through the steps of creating a painted wood sign that you can customize with any size and finish you like. Once you know how to make unique signs like these, I promise you will want to add them all over your house!

Level of Difficulty: Intermediate

SUPPLIES

- *Tape measure*
- *1 x 10 board*
- *Miter or circular saw*
- *Sanding block*
- *Clean rags*
- *Wood stain*
- *Paintbrushes*
- *White paint*
- *Alphabet stencils (including numbers)*
- *Black paint*
- *Sawtooth hanging hardware*
- *Hammer and nails*

DIRECTIONS

Measure and cut the 1 x 10 board to your desired length using a saw. (I cut mine to 8 feet [244 cm] long.) Sand the entire board with a sanding block to remove any rough edges and round the corners. Wipe off dust with a clean rag and apply stain to the wood using a paintbrush. Allow the stain to penetrate for 5–15 minutes until the desired color is achieved. Wipe the wood with a clean rag to remove any remaining stain and allow it to dry completely, about 8 hours.

Apply white paint over the stained wood and allow it to dry completely, about 4 hours. Use stencils to paint your last name and wedding date on the sign with black paint. You can also use the technique in the Vintage Label Wooden Stool project (page 125) to transfer the words using paper. Allow the paint to dry completely, about 4 hours.

If you want to add a distressed look to the sign, use the sanding block to remove layers of paint around the edges and corners, exposing the wood underneath. Add several sawtooth hangers on the back of the sign using a hammer, and hang the sign on the wall with nails.

TIP | *For a more rustic look, skip the coat of white paint and add your wording right on the wood. White letters over stained wood always look beautiful!*

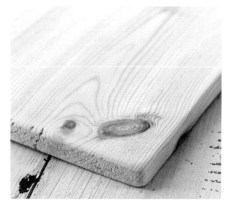

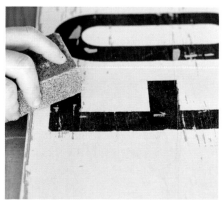

FRAMED GRAIN SACK

Old grain sacks are a staple of farmhouse décor, and this simple frame is a great way to show them off. Each grain sack is unique and has its own markings that tell a story of where it has been, which will add a ton of character to your home. Set your framed grain sack on a console table or dresser, or hang a whole collection of them on a wall.

Level of Difficulty: Advanced

SUPPLIES

- *Tape measure*
- *1 (1 x 2) board, 10 feet (305 cm) long*
- *Miter saw*
- *Cloth grain sack*
- *Drill*
- *Pocket-hole jig*
- *Wood glue*
- *1 ¼-inch (3-cm) pocket-hole screws*
- *Wood stain*
- *Paintbrush*
- *Clean rags*
- *Staple gun and staples*

DIRECTIONS

Measure and cut the 1 x 2 using a miter saw into two 34-inch (86.5-cm) pieces and two 20-inch (51-cm) pieces, mitering all the edges on a 45° angle. Measure the perimeter of your grain sack, and adjust the frame measurements if necessary before making any cuts.

Create a pocket hole in both ends of the 34-inch (86.5-cm) pieces using a drill and the pocket-hole jig. Add wood glue to the cut ends, and fit the mitered edges together to create a frame. Secure the corner joints by adding a screw to each pocket hole using a drill.

When the frame is built, apply stain to the front and sides using a paintbrush. Allow the stain to penetrate for 5–15 minutes until the desired color is achieved. Wipe the frame with a clean rag to remove any remaining stain, and allow it to dry completely, about 8 hours.

Lay the grain sack facedown on the back of the frame. Attach the sack to the frame using staples, pulling the cloth taut as you go.

TIPS | *Try searching for vintage grain sacks on websites like Etsy or eBay.*

Also, if you don't own a pocket-hole jig, you can use the method introduced in the Rustic Wooden Frame project (page 85) for creating a frame.

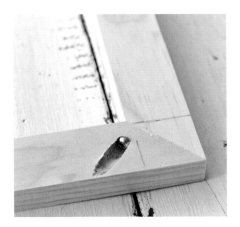 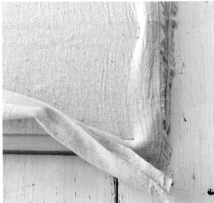

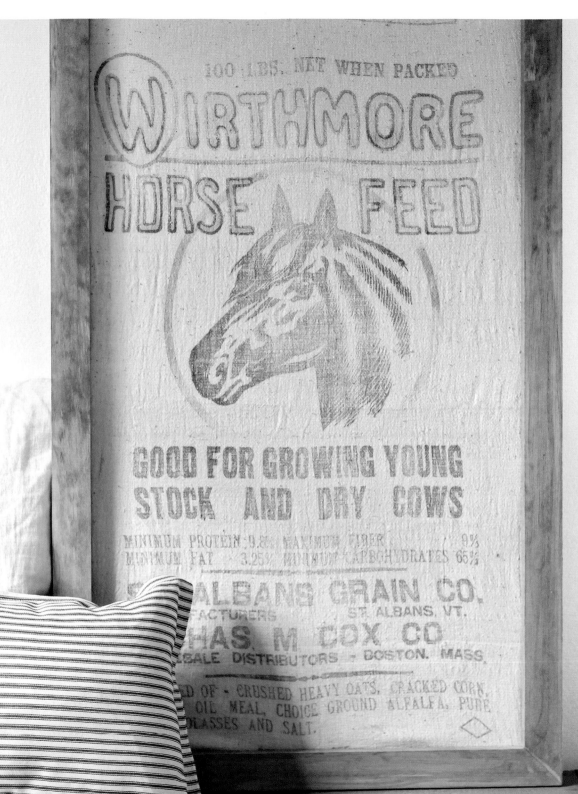

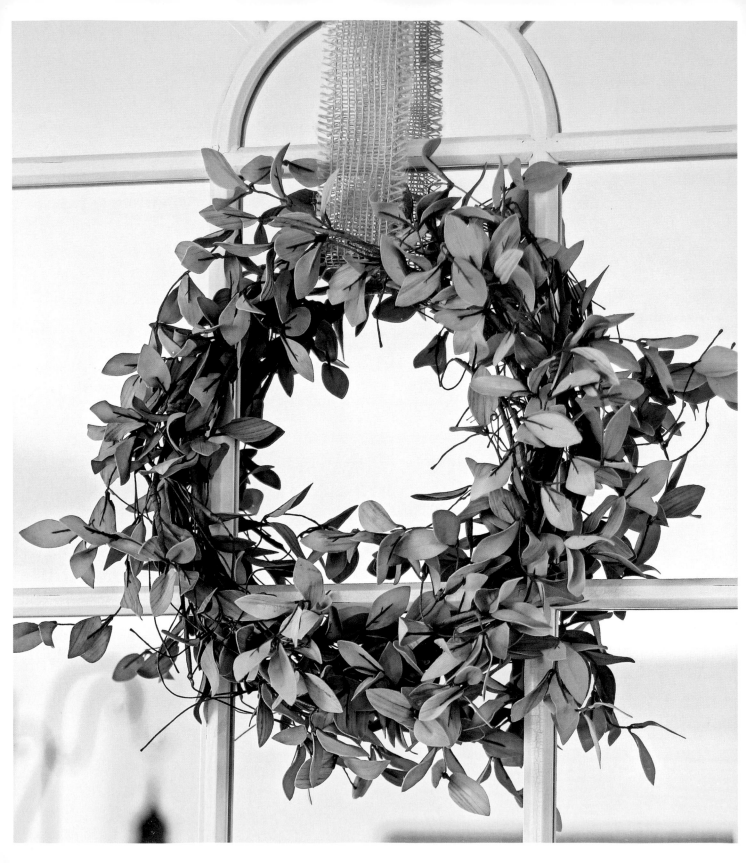

SIMPLE GREENERY WREATH

Wreaths are perfect for dressing up a front door or decorating above a mantel, and making your own is so easy and inexpensive. This tutorial will show you how to create a simple greenery wreath that looks great year round using just three supplies! You can follow this same technique to create different types of wreaths from branches, floral stems and more.

Level of Difficulty: Beginner

SUPPLIES

- *Faux greenery garland*
- *Floral wire*
- *Metal snips*

TIP | *Craft stores carry a variety of faux greenery and floral garlands, so you can make a different wreath for each season!*

DIRECTIONS

Bend the garland into a circle, overlapping as needed to get the size wreath you want.

Cut a piece of floral wire about 5 inches (13 cm) long. Wrap the wire around the overlapping garland, twisting tightly to keep the garland secure. Cut any excess wire with metal snips. Continue wrapping wire around the wreath until all loose ends are secured.

Fluff the wreath by gently bending the branches outward, making sure to conceal any exposed floral wire.

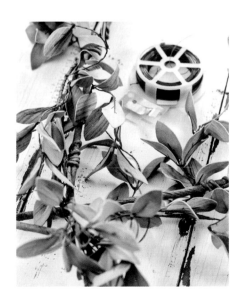
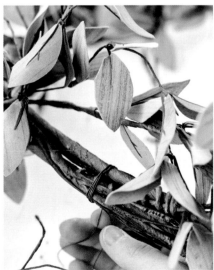
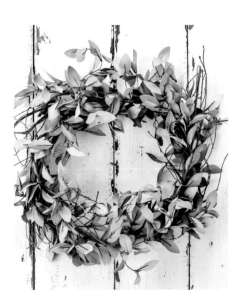

STITCHED COW PILLOW

This darling pillow will add plenty of farmhouse charm to your sofa and is really simple to make. Just cut out a cow shape from a light-colored fabric, and stitch it onto a pillow cover using dark thread. Get creative and use this technique to make a pillow with any stitched design, such as a number, letter or flower. The possibilities are endless!

Level of Difficulty: Beginner

SUPPLIES

- *Computer and printer*
- *Scissors*
- *Light-colored fabric*
- *Pencil*
- *Plain pillow cover*
- *Sewing pins*
- *Sewing needle*
- *Black thread*
- *Pillow form*

DIRECTIONS

Find a cow image online, choosing a simple silhouette that will be easy to sew. Print the image onto paper and cut out the design using scissors. Set the cow on your fabric and trace the outline with a pencil. Use scissors to cut out the cow shape on your fabric.

Place the cow centered on the front of your pillow cover and pin the fabric to hold it in place as you sew. Thread a needle with black thread and hand stitch around the outline of the cow. When finished, tie a knot in the thread on the inside of the pillow cover and insert a pillow form.

TIP | *I used a tone-on-tone look for my pillow to allow the stitching to really stand out, but play around with contrasting colors to match your décor.*

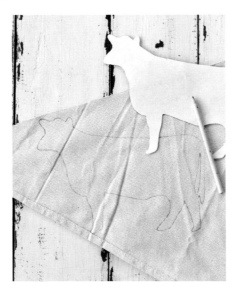
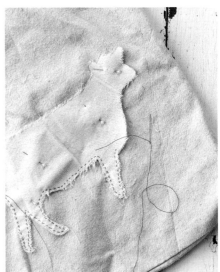

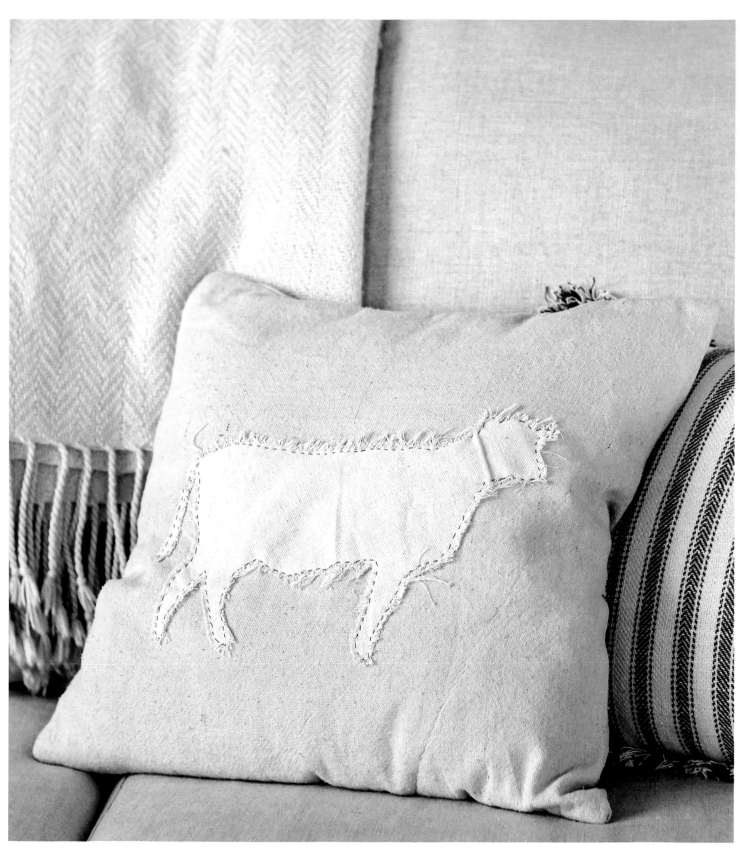

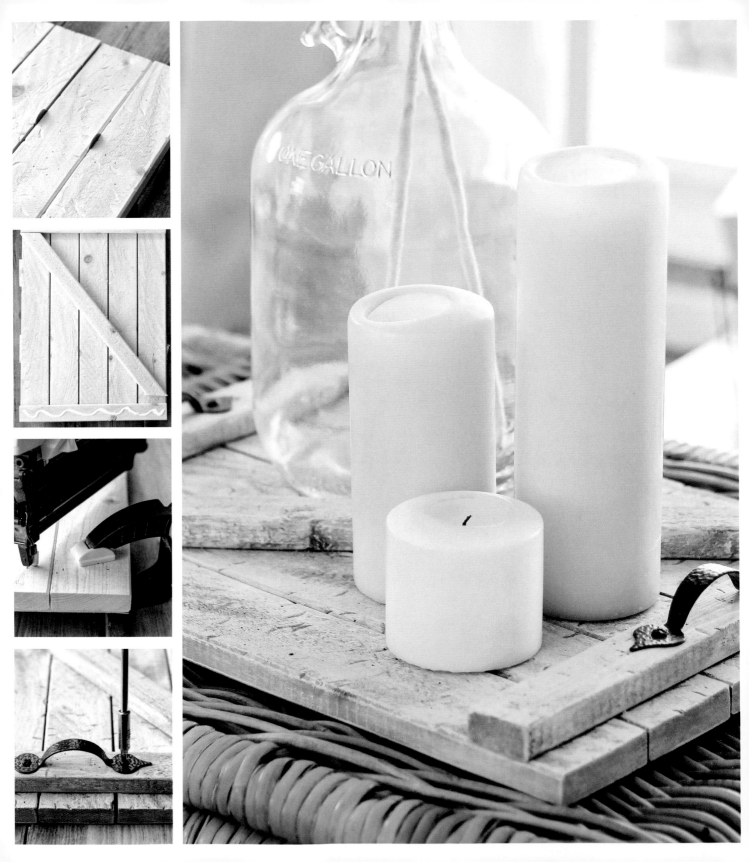

RUSTIC DECORATIVE TRAY

Trays are a great accessory to have around the home, with endless uses and decorating possibilities. On a coffee table or dining table, a tray can act as a base for a simple centerpiece. You can also use trays to corral items you keep out on the counter in a kitchen or bathroom to make the space look more organized and less cluttered. This rustic tray is made to look like the wood came right off an old barn door and even has handles that resemble what you would see on a barn.

Level of Difficulty: Advanced

SUPPLIES

- *Tape measure*
- *1 (1 x 3) board, 8 feet (244 cm) long*
- *1 (1 x 2) board, 6 feet (183 cm) long*
- *Miter saw*
- *Hammer*
- *Screwdriver*
- *Quarters, to use as spacers*
- *Wood glue*
- *Brad nail gun*
- *1-inch (2.5-cm) brad nails*
- *Paint*
- *Paintbrush*
- *Two cabinet handles*

DIRECTIONS

Measure and cut five 18-inch (45.5-cm) pieces from the 1 x 3. Cut two 12 ½-inch (32-cm) pieces from the 1 x 2. To make the new wood look old and used, hit the boards with a hammer and screwdriver to create random marks all over.

Lay the five 1 x 3 pieces next to each other, placing a quarter in between each board to act as a spacer. Place the 1 x 2 pieces across the 1 x 3 boards about 1 inch (2.5 cm) in from each end. Add wood glue to each 1 x 2, and attach them to the bottom boards using brad nails.

Measure and cut another piece of 1 x 2 to fit diagonally between the 12 ½-inch (32-cm) 1 x 2s. (It's best to wait until the other 1 x 2s are already attached to get an exact measurement.) For the diagonal piece, you'll need to use a miter saw to cut the ends at an angle. Add wood glue to the diagonal 1 x 2 and use brad nails to attach it across the tray.

When assembled, paint the tray. Allow the paint to dry completely, about 4 hours. Attach a handle centered on both ends of the tray using a screwdriver and the screws included with the handle.

TIPS | *Clamps may be helpful to hold boards together as you nail everything in place.*

For a weathered wood finish, use a sanding block to remove some of the paint, exposing the wood underneath.

When choosing your cabinet handles, look for ones with a dark or distressed finish, rather than a shiny metal finish.

WINDOWPANE MIRROR

Mirrors are great for making a space feel bigger and bouncing light throughout the room, but they certainly don't have to be basic or boring. Give your mirror the look of an old window just by adding a few simple trim pieces!

Level of Difficulty: Intermediate

SUPPLIES

- *Tape measure*
- *Rectangular framed mirror*
- *¾-inch (2-cm) wooden screen molding*
- *Miter or circular saw*
- *Paint or wood stain*
- *Paintbrush*
- *Clear superglue*
- *Two wood rosettes*

DIRECTIONS

Measure the length of your mirror (not including the frame), and cut a piece of screen molding to that length using a saw. Set the piece in the center of the mirror and measure the distance between the edge of the molding and the edge of the mirror. This will be the length of your crosspieces. Cut four pieces of screen molding to that length.

Paint or stain the pieces of molding to match your mirror frame, and allow them to dry completely. (If you would like to change the color of your mirror frame, paint both the molding and frame with your desired color.) Position the molding pieces evenly spaced on top of the mirror, and use small dabs of superglue to secure them to the mirror.

Paint or stain the rosettes, and allow them to dry completely. Add a rosette on top of the molding where the horizontal and vertical pieces intersect, using superglue to secure them to the wood.

TIP | *Look for screen molding in the trim section at your hardware or home improvement store. The wood rosettes should be located with other unfinished wood items.*

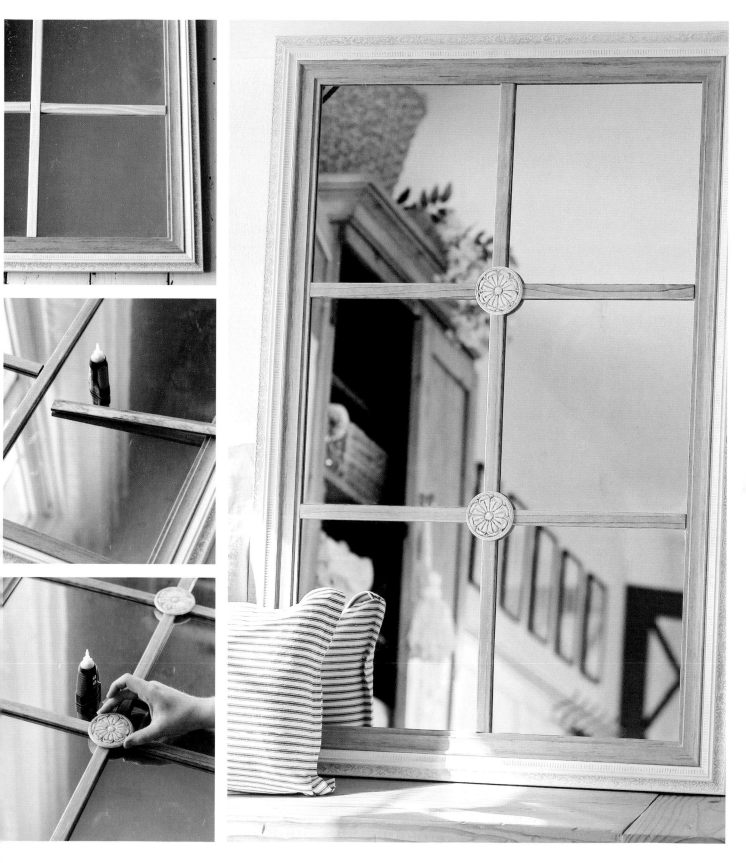

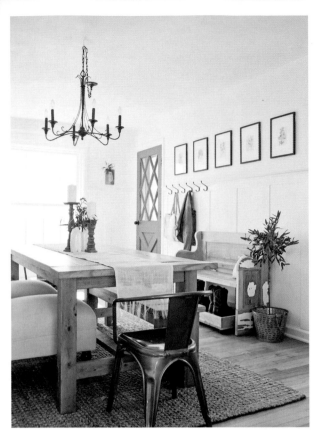
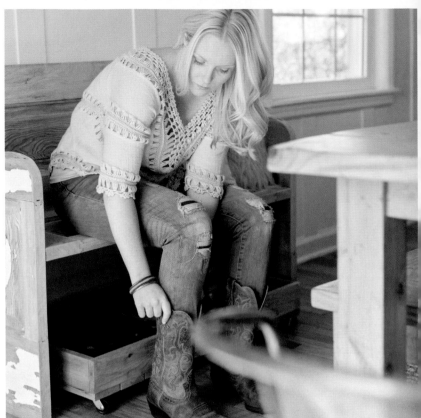
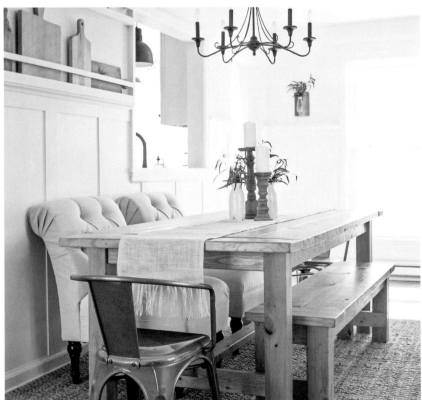
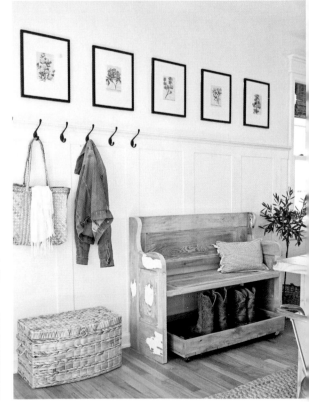

DINING ROOM & ENTRYWAY

Your dining room is the place where memories are made. Small, casual family dinners are enjoyed here as well as large holiday gatherings, both with long conversations over wine and plenty of laughter. This room should feel welcoming and intimate, with plenty of space to entertain guests and serve delicious, home-cooked meals.

Our dining room is unique in that it also serves as our entryway. This room had to fulfill a lot of purposes in a small space, so I had to get creative with the layout and furniture choices. We carried the white walls and board-and-batten trim from our living room into the dining room and painted our front door a deep charcoal gray to allow the detailed glass and wood panels to stand out.

As a family, we built a large farmhouse table that seats eight to ten people. We hung a dramatic iron chandelier overhead that makes a big impact against the white walls. We used two tufted slipper chairs on one side of the table to add some softness and elegance and built a bench for the other side that slides underneath the table to save space.

Next to the front door, I added a row of large coat hooks because we don't have a coat closet here, and built a church pew–style bench from an old door to give us somewhere to sit when slipping our shoes on and off.

In this chapter, I'll show you how to make your dining room feel more relaxed and inviting with framed book-page art (page 36), rustic hanging vases (page 39) and a fringed burlap table runner (page 43). To help organize your entryway, I'll share ideas for a wooden boot tray (page 48) and custom monogrammed doormat (page 52). You'll also learn how to create the farmhouse window trim we used on all the windows in our house (page 40). Start planning your next dinner party because you're going to be very excited to entertain in this space!

PRINTED BOOK-PAGE ART

Old books are great for decorating with, but this project showcases them in a really special way. Images are printed directly on the old book pages and framed as unique artwork that couldn't be simpler to make. Be sure to find books that you don't mind losing some pages out of!

Level of Difficulty: Beginner

SUPPLIES

- *Old book*
- *Computer and printer*
- *Picture frame*

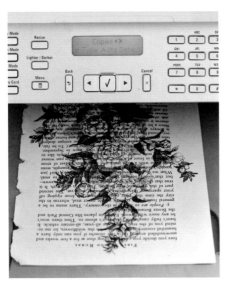

DIRECTIONS

Carefully tear a page from an old book and load the paper into your printer. Find an image you would like to use by searching online for free images such as vintage flowers or farm animals. Print the design directly onto your book page. You may need to adjust the settings on your printer for the size of paper and margins. If you would like your image to be printed in black and white, make sure to select that setting.

Mount the book page in a picture frame and hang it on the wall, or display the frame on a table or bookcase.

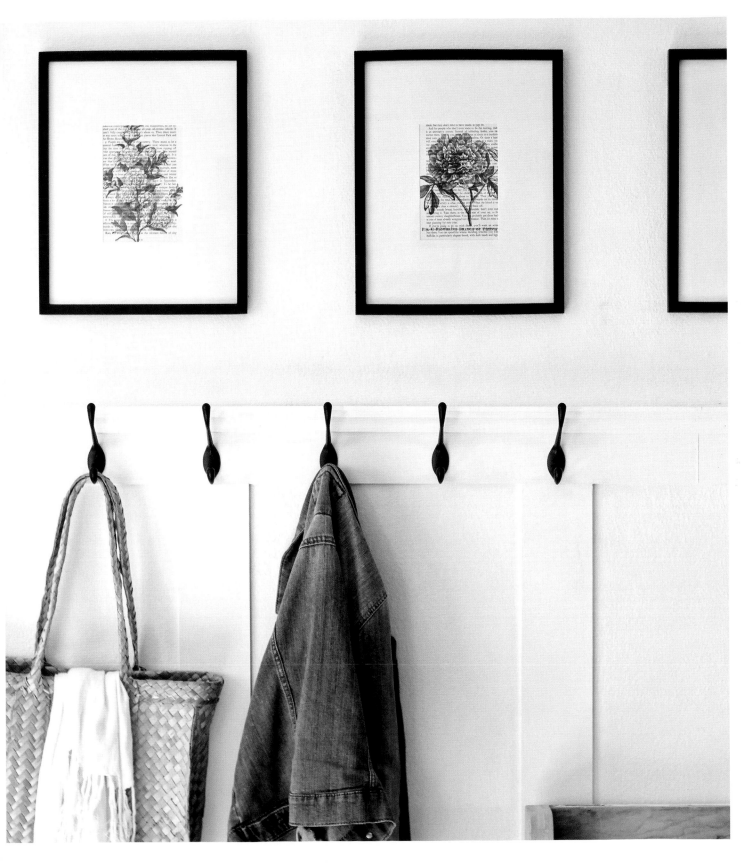

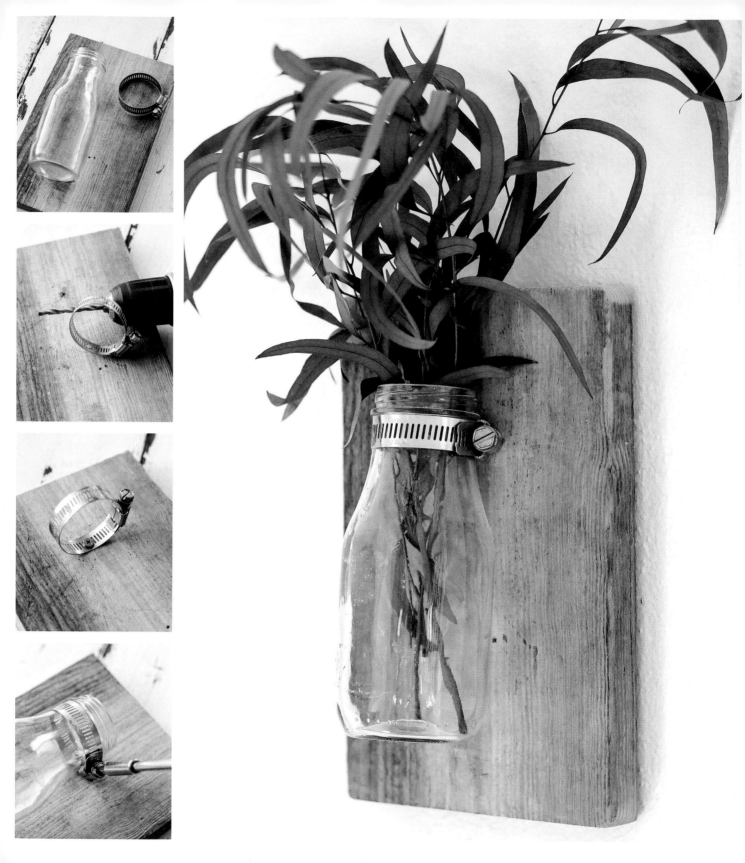

RUSTIC HANGING VASE

Flowers look beautiful in a vase sitting on a table, so why not add that same beauty to your walls? This rustic hanging vase is perfect for displaying fresh blooms and adding a bit of warmth and life to your space. The colorful flowers and lush greenery will draw your eye upward on the wall, making your space feel bigger as well. When you don't have any fresh flowers on hand, use a few stems of faux greenery or flowers for a look that will last all year long.

Level of Difficulty: Intermediate

SUPPLIES

- *1 x 6 board*
- *Miter or circular saw*
- *Tape measure*
- *Wood stain*
- *Paintbrush*
- *Clean rags*
- *Small hose clamp*
- *Drill and masonry bit*
- *½-inch (13-mm) screw*
- *Screwdriver*
- *Glass bottle*
- *Sawtooth hanging hardware*
- *Hammer and nails*
- *Fresh or faux flowers/greenery*

DIRECTIONS

Measure and cut a piece from the 1 x 6 about 9 inches (23 cm) long using a saw. Apply stain to the wood using a paintbrush. Allow the stain to penetrate for 5–15 minutes until the desired color is achieved. Wipe the wood with a clean rag to remove any remaining stain, and allow it to dry completely, about 8 hours.

Drill a small hole in the hose clamp using a masonry bit just big enough for the ½-inch (13-mm) screw to fit through. Determine where you would like the top of your bottle to be on the board, and attach the hose clamp there using a screwdriver and ½-inch (13-mm) screw. Loosen the hose clamp with a screwdriver, and slide the bottle through the clamp until the lip is resting on the top of the clamp. Tighten the hose clamp until the bottle is secure. Add a sawtooth hanger on the back of the board using a hammer, and hang it on the wall with nails. Place faux or fresh flowers in the vase.

TIP | *You can find hose clamps of all sizes at your hardware or home improvement store. I recommend taking your glass bottle when going to the store to purchase the clamp so you can get an exact fit.*

FARMHOUSE WINDOW TRIM

One way to give your home an instant upgrade is by adding this farmhouse trim detail to your windows. The bones of your home are just as important as the decorative elements, and you'll be amazed how much character just a few simple boards can add to your windows. In keeping with traditional farmhouse style, this trim is simple and substantial and won't break the bank. You can also use this trim detail over your doorways or on the Coat and Backpack Storage Rack (page 152).

Level of Difficulty: Advanced

SUPPLIES

- 1 x 4 board
- 2 (1 x 2) boards
- 1 x 3 board
- Miter or circular saw
- Tape measure
- Wood glue
- Brad nail gun
- 1 ¼-inch (3-cm) brad nails
- Caulk
- Paint
- Paintbrush

DIRECTIONS

Measure the width of the top of your window trim. Add 1 inch (2.5 cm) to that measurement and cut a 1 x 4 to that length using a saw. Add 2 inches (5 cm) to your window width and cut two 1 x 2s to that length. Add 3 inches (7.5 cm) to your window width and cut a 1 x 3 to that length.

Attach a 1 x 2 to the side of the 1 x 4 using wood glue and 1 ¼-inch (3-cm) brad nails. Attach the other 1 x 2 to the opposite side of the 1 x 4. Set the 1 x 3 on top of the last 1 x 2 and attach them together with wood glue and brad nails. Each piece should be centered.

Set the finished trim piece on top of the existing window trim and attach it to the wall using brad nails through the 1 x 4.

Caulk any seams between the boards, wall and original window trim. Paint the boards to match your existing trim, and allow the paint to dry completely, about 4 hours.

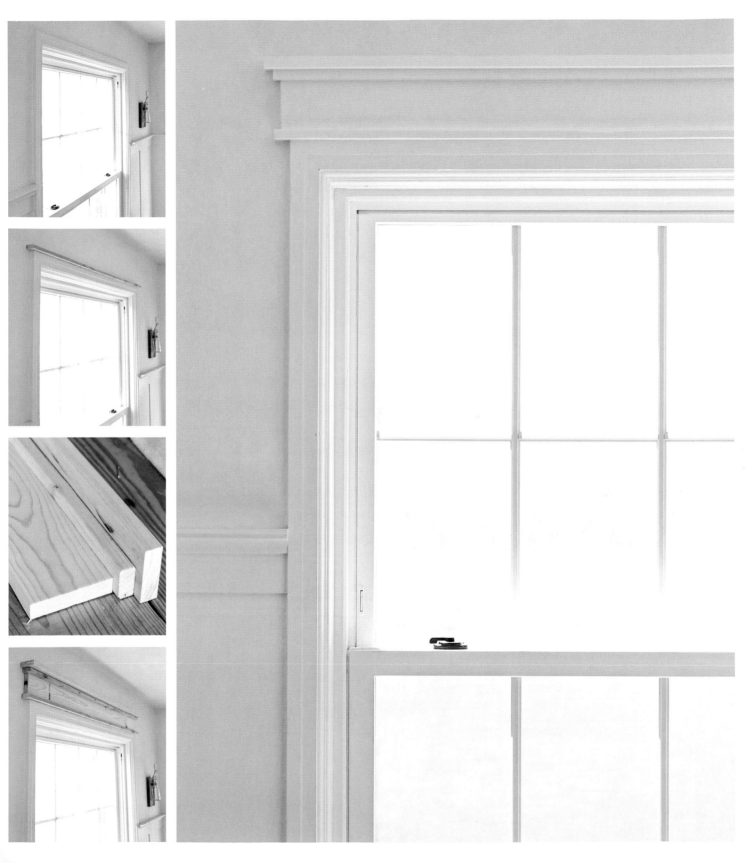

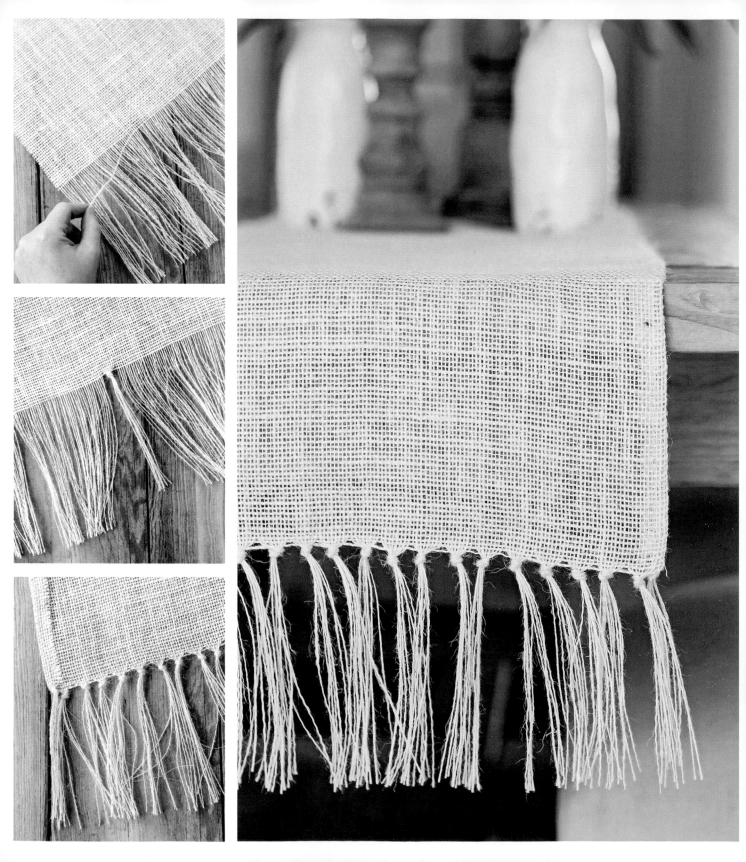

FRINGED BURLAP TABLE RUNNER

Burlap is a staple of farmhouse décor, and this gorgeous table runner with fringed edges will add both texture and softness to your dining room table. Just pull strands of burlap loose at both ends and tie a group of strands together to create long, beautiful fringed edges. They really add a special touch to this basic table runner! The runner looks great by itself or with a centerpiece added, such as the Chicken-Wire Candleholder (page 20) or the Simple, Natural Centerpiece (page 67).

Level of Difficulty: Beginner

SUPPLIES

- *Tape measure*
- *Several yards of burlap fabric*
- *Scissors*
- *Iron and ironing board*
- *Sewing machine and thread*

DIRECTIONS

Measure the length of your table and add 24 inches (61 cm). This will give you a 12-inch (30.5-cm) overhang at both ends of your table runner. Cut a piece of burlap to that length and 15 inches (38 cm) wide using scissors.

Fold the long edges of the runner under ½ inch (13 mm), and press with an iron to hold in place. Pull strands from the short edges until you have about 5 inches (13 cm) of fringe on both ends. Starting in the middle, gather eight loose strands and tie them together in a knot right at the edge of the burlap. Continue tying knots until you run out of loose strands.

When both ends of the runner have been knotted, sew along the long folded edges to hold the fold in place and prevent the runner from unraveling.

TIP | *Use hem tape and an iron in place of the sewing machine, if necessary. Just follow the instructions on the hem tape package!*

PLATE RACK

Plate racks are often found in old farmhouses to display plates and serving platters, and this tutorial will show you how to add one in your own home. This simple display that also doubles as storage is perfect for awkward walls that are hard to decorate, and you can customize your plate rack to fit a wall of any size. Add a few vintage cutting boards to your plate rack using the Vintage Cutting Board tutorial on page 47!

Level of Difficulty: Advanced

SUPPLIES

- *1 x 2 board*
- *Miter or circular saw*
- *Tape measure*
- *Brad nail gun*
- *2-inch (5-cm) brad nails*
- *Level*
- *Paint*
- *Paintbrush*
- *1 ¾-inch (4.5-cm) lattice strip*
- *1-inch (2.5-cm) lattice strip*
- *Caulk*

DIRECTIONS

Measure the space for your plate rack on a wall and using a saw, cut four 1 x 2 pieces to create a frame. Nail the frame into the wall and/or ceiling using 2-inch (5-cm) brad nails.

Measure the distance between the inside edge of the left and right 1 x 2s, and cut another piece of 1 x 2 to create a shelf. Place the shelf piece centered vertically inside the frame, and make sure the shelf is level before securing it to the wall with brad nails. Paint the plate rack frame and shelf, and allow all pieces to dry completely, about 4 hours.

Measure the outside edge of your plate rack frame and cut two pieces of 1-inch (2.5-cm) lattice strip to that length. Cut two pieces of 1 ¾-inch (4.5-cm) lattice strip to that same length. Use brad nails to attach the 1 ¾-inch (4.5-cm) lattice over the middle and bottom 1 x 2s. The lattice should be sitting flush with the bottom of the 1 x 2. Attach the 1-inch (2.5-cm) lattice above the other lattice using brad nails, leaving about a 2-inch (5-cm) gap in between.

Caulk any seams between the boards and the wall. Finish painting the lattice strips on the plate rack. When dry, display your favorite plates on the shelves.

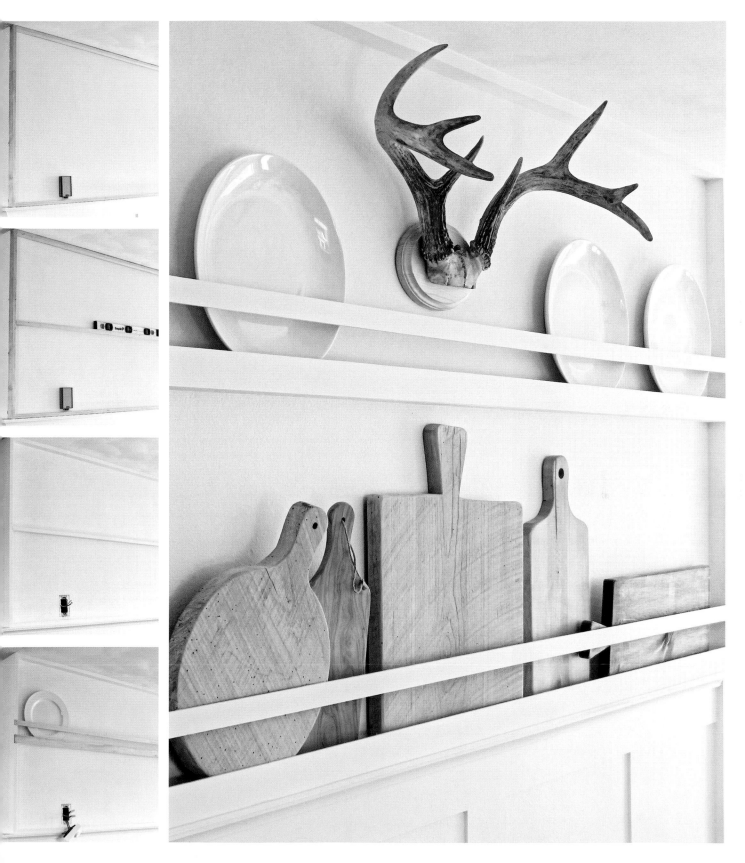

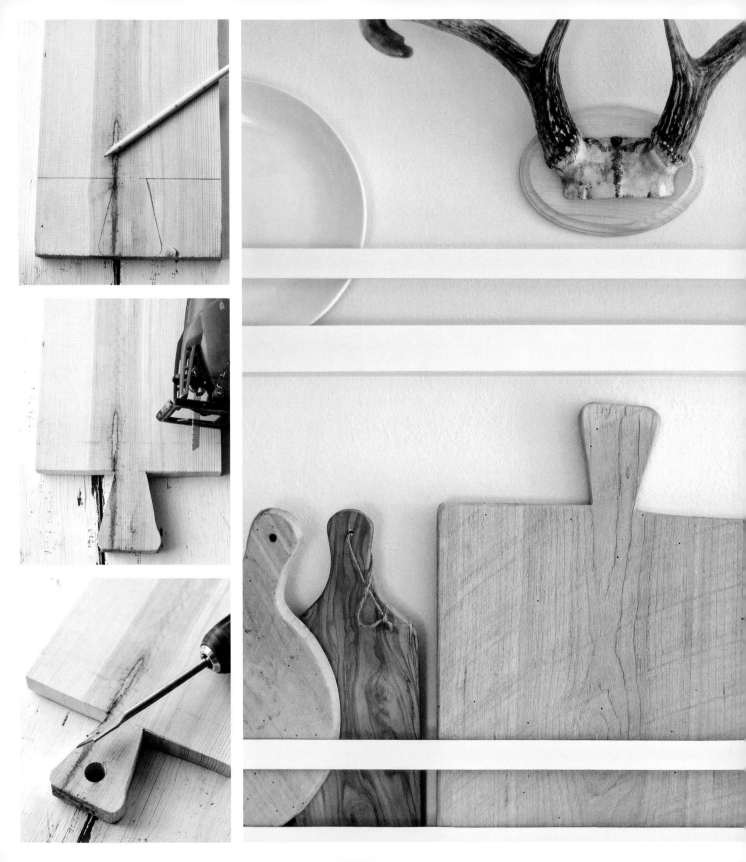

VINTAGE CUTTING BOARD

Antique cutting boards are often found in farmhouse decorating for the warmth and vintage charm they add to a space. Finding authentic antique boards will cost you a pretty penny, but luckily they are really simple to replicate. Play around with different shapes and sizes to build a collection of boards you can display on the Plate Rack shown on page 45.

Level of Difficulty: Intermediate

SUPPLIES

- *Tape measure*
- *1 x 8 board*
- *Miter or circular saw*
- *Pencil*
- *Jigsaw*
- *Drill (optional)*
- *½-inch (13-mm) paddle bit (optional)*
- *Sanding block*
- *Clean rags*
- *Wood stain*
- *Paintbrush*
- *Paste wax*

DIRECTIONS

Measure and cut a piece of 1 x 8 to 15 inches (38 cm) long using a saw. Use a pencil to draw a handle shape on one end of the board, then cut along the handle outline using a jigsaw. Optional: use a paddle bit to drill a hole in the center of the handle.

Sand the entire board using a sanding block, focusing on the corners and edges to round them. Wipe off dust with a clean rag, and apply stain to the board using a paintbrush. Allow the stain to penetrate for 5–15 minutes until the desired color is achieved. Wipe the wood with a clean rag to remove any remaining stain, and allow it to dry completely, about 8 hours. To seal the wood, apply a layer of paste wax with a paintbrush and buff with a clean rag.

TIP | *Vintage cutting boards are perfect for decorating, but if you want to use your board for food, use a food-safe finish like mineral oil, walnut oil or beeswax instead of wood stain.*

WOODEN BOOT TRAY ON CASTERS

Wet, muddy boots and shoes need a place to dry off, and this wooden boot tray is the perfect place. Caster wheels are added to the bottom of the box so you can easily slide the tray under a bench (like the Simple Wooden Bench on page 82) and out of the way. Your clean floors are going to thank you for this one.

Level of Difficulty: Intermediate

SUPPLIES

- *Tape measure*
- *3 (1 x 4) boards, 10 feet (305 cm) long*
- *Miter or circular saw*
- *Wood glue*
- *Hammer*
- *1 ½-inch (3.8-cm) nails*
- *Sanding block*
- *Clean rags*
- *Wood stain*
- *Paintbrush*
- *Paste wax*
- *Four small caster wheels*
- *½-inch (13-mm) screws*
- *Screwdriver*
- *Rubber boot tray liner (approximately 17 x 35 inches [43 x 89 cm])*

DIRECTIONS

Measure and cut two pieces of 1 x 4 to 36 ¾ inches (93.5 cm) in length and two pieces to 17 ½ inches (44.5 cm) in length using a saw. Create a box with the two short pieces sitting inside the ends of the two long pieces. Apply wood glue to the cut ends of the short pieces, and secure the box with nails.

Cut ten pieces of 1 x 4 to 19 inches (48.5 cm) in length for the bottom of your boot tray. Line the boards up across the bottom of the box you built, and attach them using wood glue and nails.

Sand the entire boot tray with a sanding block, and wipe off dust with a clean rag. Apply stain to the tray using a paintbrush. Allow the stain to penetrate for 5–15 minutes until the desired color is achieved. Wipe the wood with a clean rag to remove any remaining stain, and allow it to dry completely, about 8 hours. To seal the wood, apply a layer of paste wax with a paintbrush and buff with a clean rag.

Attach a caster wheel to each corner on the bottom of the tray using ½-inch (13-mm) screws and a screwdriver. Insert a rubber liner into the boot tray.

> TIP | *Boot trays come in all different sizes, so if you're unable to find a rubber liner in the suggested size, simply adjust the measurements to create a custom fit for yours.*

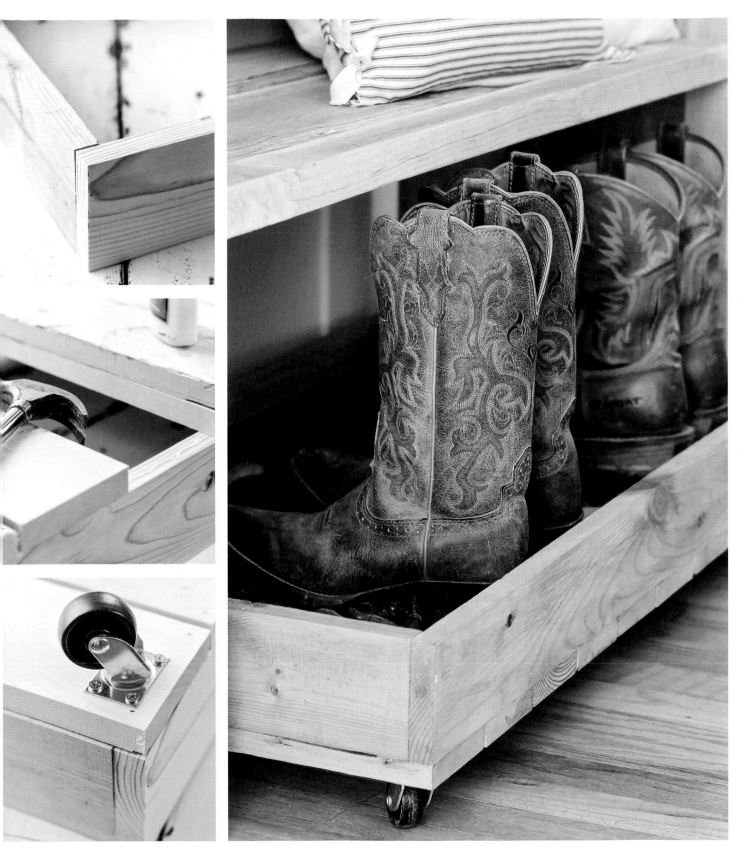

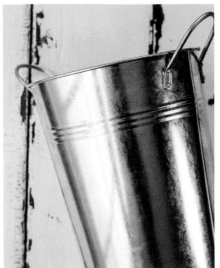

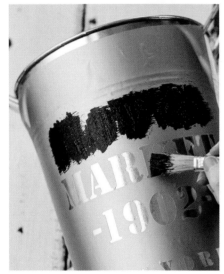

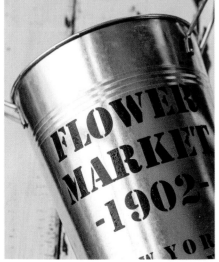

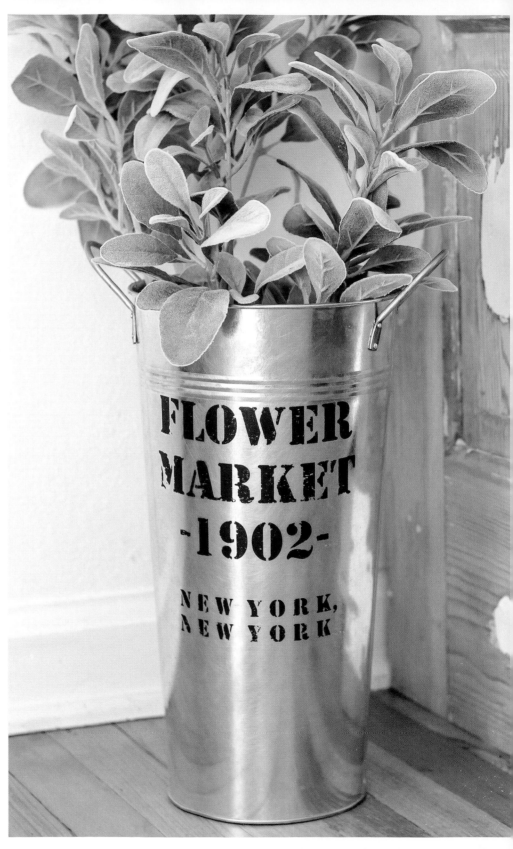

GALVANIZED METAL FLOWER BUCKET

Metal buckets are great for storing items all over the house and are also a beautiful contrast to the wood tones and neutral colors often found in farmhouse décor. This plain bucket is customized with stenciled lettering that gives the piece plenty of character with minimal time and effort. Use this flower bucket to hold umbrellas by the front door, hand towels in a bathroom or the obvious—a big, beautiful fresh bouquet of flowers.

Level of Difficulty: Beginner

SUPPLIES

- *Alphabet stencils*
- *Galvanized metal bucket*
- *Tape*
- *Black paint*
- *Paintbrush*
- *Sandpaper*

DIRECTIONS

Add stencils to one side of the bucket to spell FLOWER MARKET - 1902, NEW YORK, NEW YORK (or other wording, as desired). Place individual stencils side-by-side, using tape to hold them in place on the bucket, or paint each letter one at a time, waiting for the previous letter to dry before starting the next, if the stencils are all on one sheet. Apply black paint over the stencil, dabbing gently to avoid pushing paint underneath the stencil. After all the letters are painted, remove the stencil and allow the paint to dry completely.

Lightly sand over the painted letters to give the bucket an aged appearance.

TIP | *Metal buckets can be found at craft stores as well as farm-supply stores. To make brand new galvanized metal look old, try the aging technique in the Aged Galvanized Metal Bin project (page 140).*

MONOGRAMMED DOORMAT

Welcome guests inside your home with a fun monogrammed doormat sitting just inside your front door. The painted design will add a personalized touch to your entryway and give guests a pretty place to slip their shoes off. This doormat is best used indoors, but it can also be placed outside on a covered porch.

Level of Difficulty: Beginner

SUPPLIES

- *Painter's tape*
- *Coir or sisal doormat*
- *Black enamel paint (made for exterior use)*
- *Paintbrush*
- *Computer and printer*
- *Scissors*
- *Permanent marker*

DIRECTIONS

Use painter's tape to create a border around the edge of your doormat. Apply paint in the taped area using a paintbrush, then remove the tape.

Print a large monogram from your computer, and cut the monogram out with scissors. Place the monogram in the center of your mat and trace around the edges with a permanent marker. Fill in the outline with paint, and allow the rug to dry for 48 hours before using.

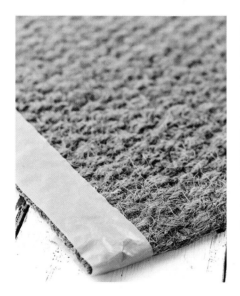 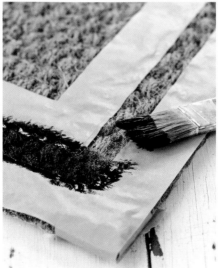 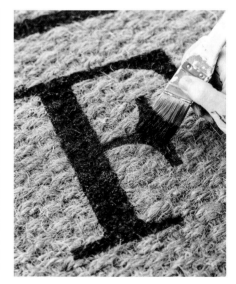

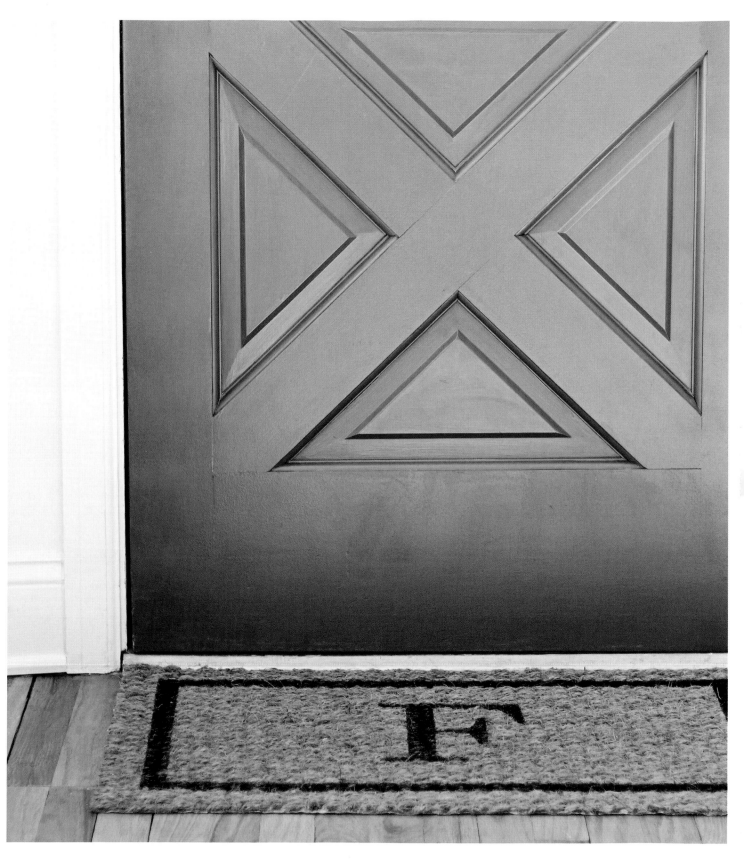

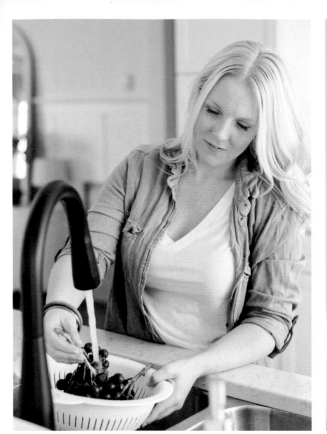

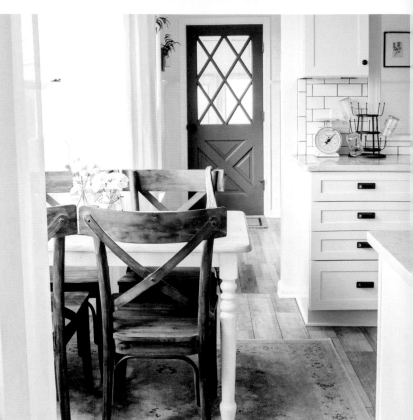

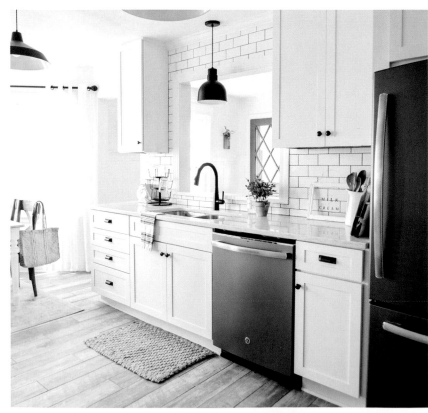

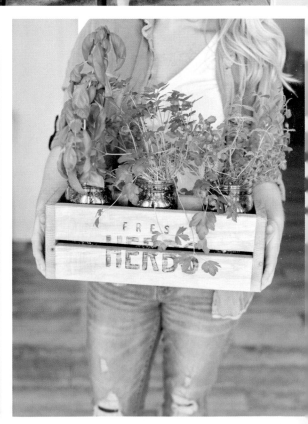

KITCHEN

If your family is like mine, you consider the kitchen the heart of your home. It's where you start your morning with that first cup of coffee and end your evenings preparing dinner together and sharing stories of how the day went. Kitchens are mostly about function and less about fashion, but there are many ways you can sneak some farmhouse style into your space.

The kitchen was the last room we renovated because we wanted to make sure we knew exactly what we wanted before spending any money. We replaced everything in the old, outdated kitchen from the cabinets and countertops to the flooring and appliances. We also opened up the wall between the kitchen and living room and tore out an old chimney that took up precious cabinet space.

We kept the space light and bright with white walls, white Shaker-style cabinets and light quartz countertops that have the look of marble. For our flooring, we chose porcelain tile that looks like old planks of barn wood, which helped to warm up the space and give it a more rustic feel. Then we added barn-style pendant lights, a matte-black sink faucet and dark cabinet hardware to contrast all the white.

One side of our kitchen has big, beautiful bay windows that ended up being the perfect place to create a breakfast nook. I added a small farmhouse table and chairs and hung long, sheer curtains to frame the space. This has become one of my favorite spots in the house to sit and look out the window at our farm, and we probably use this table for meals more often than we do our dining room table.

Connected to the kitchen is a small wash sink and closet right off our back door. When our house was first built, this space was intended for the farmers to use when they came in from the field. They would slip off their muddy boots here and wash up at the sink so they didn't track dirt all through the house. I kept this space as it was originally intended and bumped up the farmhouse charm with an old stool, soap pump and towel holder that I made from an antique grater.

In this chapter, you'll learn how to give your kitchen a farmhouse feel with projects like aged terra cotta pots (page 63), wooden cake stands (page 64), an herb planter box (page 56) and chalkboard canister labels (page 59). I'll also share my trick for creating the perfect cracked paint finish (page 71) and how to turn a plain, flat door into a paneled one (page 72).

HERB PLANTER BOX

Enjoy the convenience of having fresh herbs growing right in your kitchen with this darling herb planter box. Building the box is an easy afternoon project that will prove to be useful time and time again. You can also use the box to hold mason jars full of silverware, fresh flowers or cooking utensils.

Level of Difficulty: Intermediate

SUPPLIES

- *Tape measure*
- *1 (1 x 6) board, 6 feet (183 cm) long*
- *1 (1 x 3) board, 6 feet (183 cm) long*
- *Miter or circular saw*
- *Wood glue*
- *Brad nail gun*
- *1 ½-inch (3.8-cm) brad nails*
- *1 (1 x 4) board, 6 feet (183 cm) long*
- *Sanding block*
- *Clean rags*
- *Wood stain*
- *Paintbrush*
- *Paste wax*
- *Herb plants*
- *3 quart-size (1 L) mason jars*

DIRECTIONS

Cut two pieces of 1 x 6 to 5 ¼ inches (13.5 cm) long using a saw. Cut four pieces of 1 x 3 to 14 inches (35.5 cm) long. Apply wood glue to the ends of two 1 x 3 pieces, and attach a 1 x 6 piece on either end so that the bottoms sit flush. Add brad nails through the 1 x 6 pieces to secure the 1 x 3s.

Cut a piece of 1 x 4 to 14 inches (35.5 cm) long and set the board in between the 1 x 3s to create a bottom for your box. Again, secure the board with wood glue and brad nails.

Attach the last two 1 x 3 boards to the 1 x 6s using wood glue and brad nails with the top of the boards sitting flush. This should leave about a ½-inch (13-mm) gap between the 1 x 3s.

Sand the entire box with a sanding block to remove any rough edges, and wipe off dust with a clean rag. Apply stain to the box using a paintbrush. Allow the stain to penetrate for 5–15 minutes until the desired color is achieved. Wipe the wood with a clean rag to remove any remaining stain, and allow it to dry completely, about 8 hours. If desired, use the technique used on the Vintage Label Wooden Stool (page 125) to add a label on the front of the box. To seal the wood, apply a layer of paste wax with a paintbrush and buff with a clean rag.

Plant herbs in mason jars and set the jars inside the box. Place the herb box next to a window to give the plants plenty of sunlight.

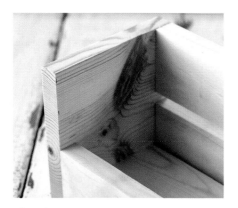

TIP | *This planter box is made to fit three quart-size (946-ml) mason jars, but you can easily adjust the measurements to accommodate differently sized planters.*

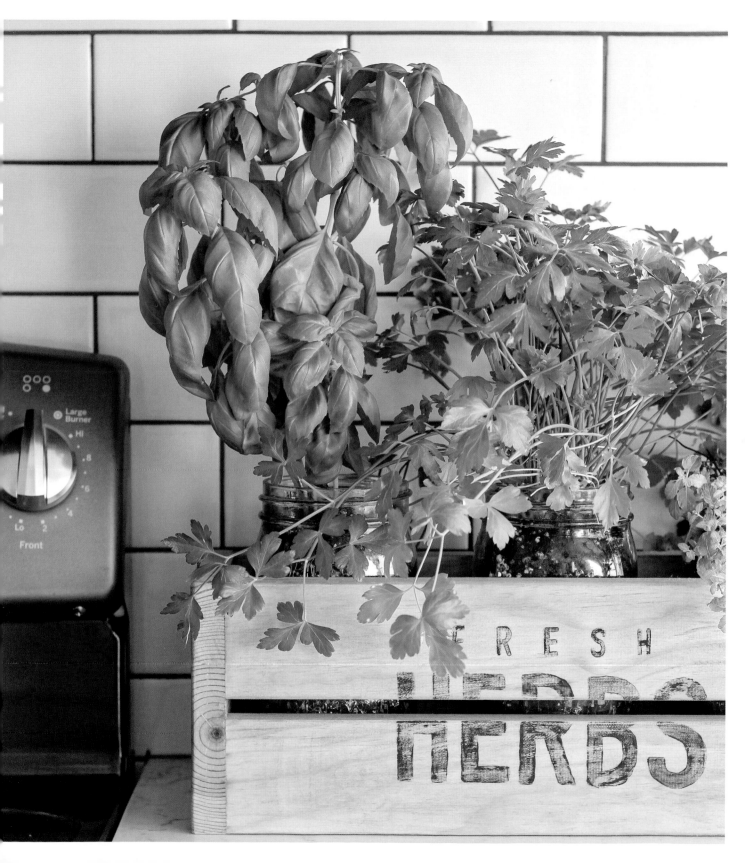

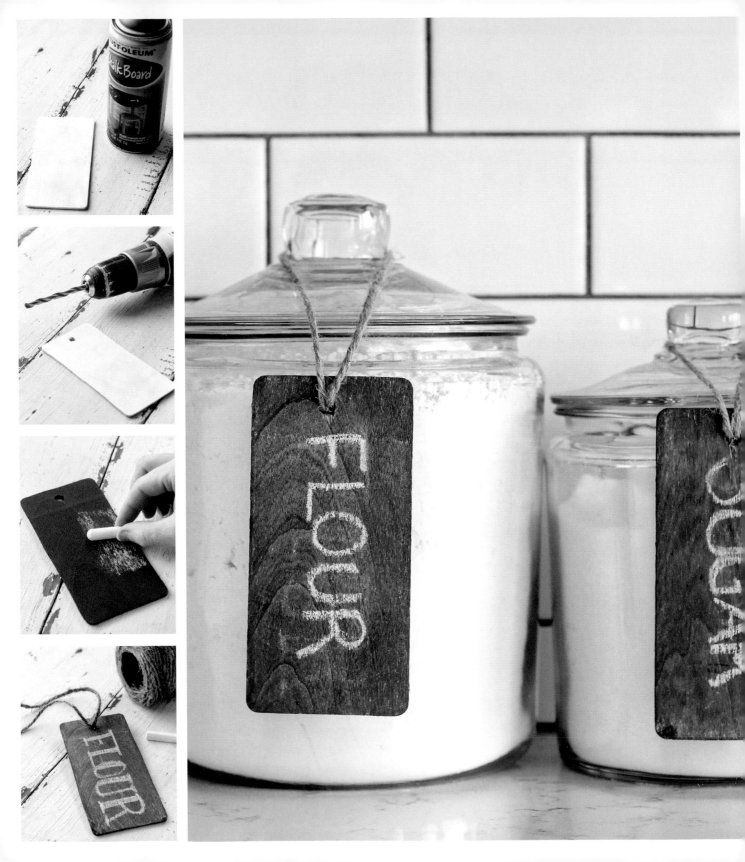

CHALKBOARD CANISTER LABEL

Farmhouse style is all about simplicity and decorating with what you already have. Glass canisters lined up on a kitchen counter are perfect for storing things like flour, coffee and pasta and make a beautiful display of the ingredients. To add an extra decorative touch, create some of these chalkboard labels using craft wood and twine to label each jar. You can erase and change the labels as often as your ingredients change!

Level of Difficulty: Beginner

SUPPLIES

- *Drill and drill bit*
- *Thin craft wood rectangle*
- *Chalkboard spray paint*
- *Chalk*
- *Dry cloth*
- *Twine*
- *Scissors*
- *Kitchen canister*

DIRECTIONS

Drill a hole centered in the top of your wood rectangle using a drill bit just big enough to make a hole you will be able to slide the twine through. Apply several light coats of chalkboard spray paint to the wood and allow the paint to dry completely, about 4 hours.

To prepare the chalkboard for use, condition the surface by rubbing the side of a piece of chalk over the entire chalkboard. When the surface is thoroughly covered in chalk, erase the board with a dry cloth.

Cut a piece of twine with scissors and slide both ends through the hole from the front of the chalkboard. Tie a knot in both ends of the twine, creating a loop to hang the chalkboard label from. Hang the label on the lid of a canister, and write the contents on the chalkboard using chalk.

TIP | *Look for thin plywood rectangles in the unfinished wood section of a craft store.*

RUFFLED STOOL SLIPCOVER

Slipcovered furniture is common in farmhouse décor for the casual, relaxed look it gives, and this simple stool slip-cover is a great way to get that look for less. The sewing is simple and straightforward, and the sweet ruffle detail with lace trim gives this project a ton of charm. For a different look, try switching out the ticking fabric for linen, gingham or even burlap!

Level of Difficulty: Intermediate

SUPPLIES

- *Tape measure*
- *Stool*
- *Ticking fabric*
- *Scissors*
- *Sewing pins*
- *Sewing machine*
- *Thread*
- *Lace trim*

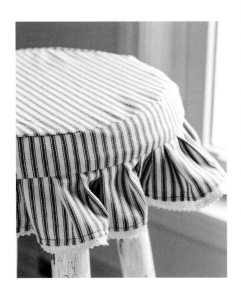

DIRECTIONS

Measure the circumference of the seat of your stool using a tape measure. Cut a piece of ticking fabric to that length and 2 ½ inches (6.5 cm) wide (or wide enough to cover the stool completely) with scissors. Wrap the fabric around the stool seat with the right side of the fabric facing the stool. Pin the fabric ends together where they meet, and sew the seam together using a sewing machine. Place the fabric back on the stool right side down.

Measure the width of the top of the stool seat and cut a circle of fabric large enough to cover the seat. Set the fabric circle face down on the seat, and pin the edges of both fabric pieces together. Sew the pinned edges with a sewing machine.

Cut a piece of fabric twice as long as the seat circumference and 3 ½ inches (9 cm) wide for the ruffle. Place the ruffle fabric right side down and fold one edge up ½ inch (13 mm). Lay the lace trim on top of the folded edge and pin the pieces together. Sew the ruffle fabric and trim together with a sewing machine.

Attach the ruffle onto the bottom of the slipcover by folding the ruffle fabric every few inches as you sew to create a pleated look. Again, both pieces should have the right sides facing down as you sew.

When you are finished sewing, turn the slipcover right side out and fit the cover over the stool seat.

TIP | *You can also sew the slipcover by hand, but it is definitely easier and much faster to use a sewing machine.*

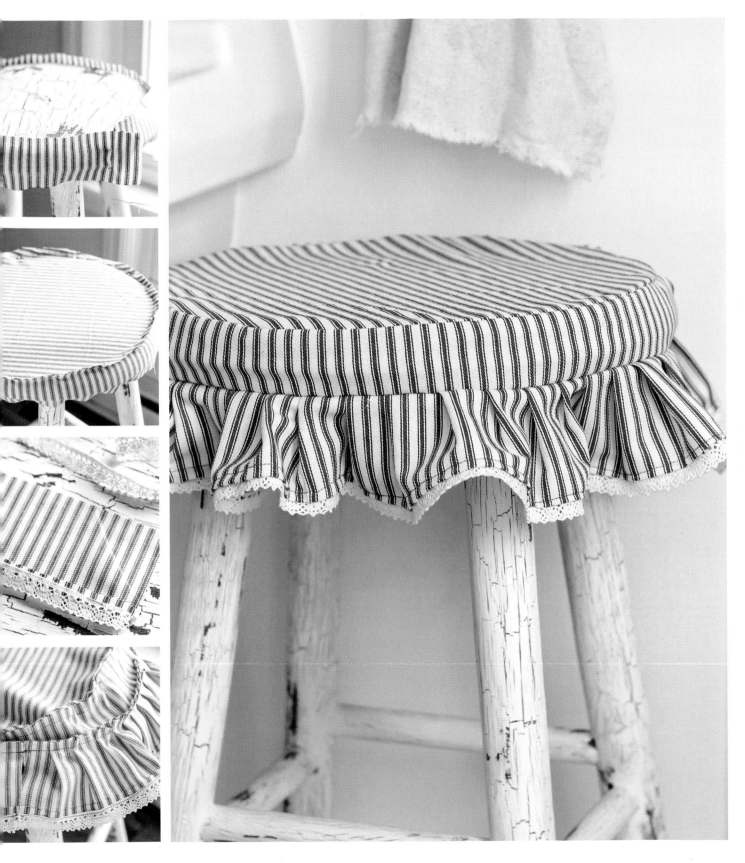

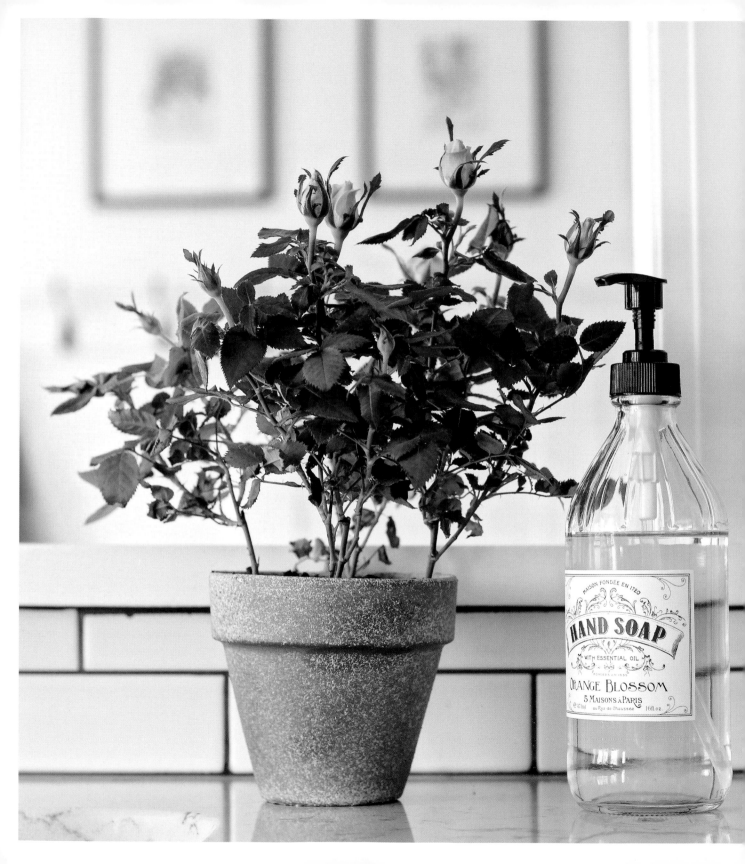

AGED TERRA COTTA POT

If you love vintage style, you'll agree that brand-new terra cotta pots do not look nearly as pretty as ones with some age on them. To give new pots an old look, use a textured spray paint to build up some texture on the pot, then antique the paint with dark wax. When you're finished, you'll have pots that look like they've been sitting in the garden for decades. You can plant flowers or herbs in the pots or even just stack them together on a shelf for a casual look.

Level of Difficulty: Beginner

SUPPLIES

- *Stone-textured spray paint*
- *Terra cotta pot, any size*
- *Paintbrush*
- *Dark paste wax*

DIRECTIONS

Shake the can of spray paint for one minute, then lightly spray the pot in short bursts. Don't worry about completely covering the pot; you want to be able to still see some of the terra cotta underneath. Do one coat for a lightly aged look or multiple coats to build up the texture. Let the pot dry completely overnight.

Lightly brush dark paste wax over the pot to blend in the spray paint and give it an aged appearance.

TIPS | *You can find the stone-textured spray paint at most hardware or home improvement stores next to the regular spray paint.*

To give the pots a moss-covered look, lightly brush a little bit of green paint over the textured parts before adding the dark wax.

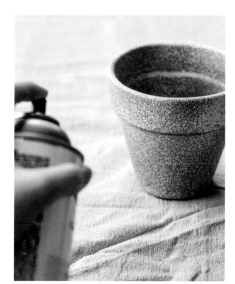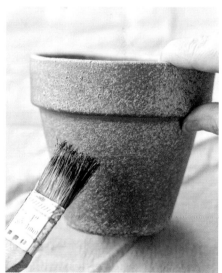

WOODEN CAKE STAND

Every kitchen needs a place to set the freshly baked cookies and cakes that come out of the oven, and this lovely little cake stand fits the bill perfectly. You can stain the wood to match the colors in your kitchen, and guests will be truly wowed when you serve them a treat from this handmade, rustic piece.

Level of Difficulty: Intermediate

SUPPLIES

- 12-inch (30.5-cm) wooden round panel
- Tape measure
- Drill and drill bit
- 4-inch (10-cm) bun-foot table leg
- 4-inch (10-cm) wooden disc
- 5-inch (13-cm) wooden disc
- 2 ½-inch (6.5-cm) screw
- Screwdriver
- Wood stain
- Paintbrush
- Clean rags
- Paste wax

DIRECTIONS

Find the center of the 12-inch (30.5-cm) wooden round with a tape measure and drill a hole about halfway through the wood. Use a drill bit slightly smaller than the screw on the top of the bun-foot table leg. Screw the bun foot into the bottom of the wooden round until it fits tightly.

Drill a hole all the way through the center of the 4-inch (10-cm) and 5-inch (13-cm) wooden discs and partially into the bottom of the bun foot. Use a drill bit the same size as your 2 ½-inch (6.5-cm) screw. Insert the screw through the 5-inch (13-cm) disc, then through the 4-inch (10-cm) disc using a screwdriver. Insert the end of the screw into the bottom of the bun foot and tighten with a screwdriver until all the pieces are secure.

Apply stain to the entire cake stand using a paintbrush. Allow the stain to penetrate for 5–15 minutes until the desired color is achieved. Wipe the wood with a clean rag to remove any remaining stain and allow it to dry completely, about 8 hours. To seal the wood, apply a layer of paste wax with a paintbrush and buff with a clean rag.

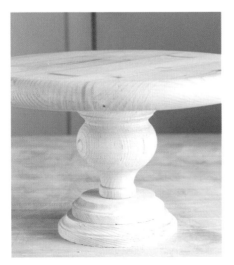

TIPS | *The large wooden round and bun foot can be found in hardware and home improvement stores, and the smaller wood discs are available in craft stores.*

For food safety, use a piece of parchment paper when setting food on the cake stand.

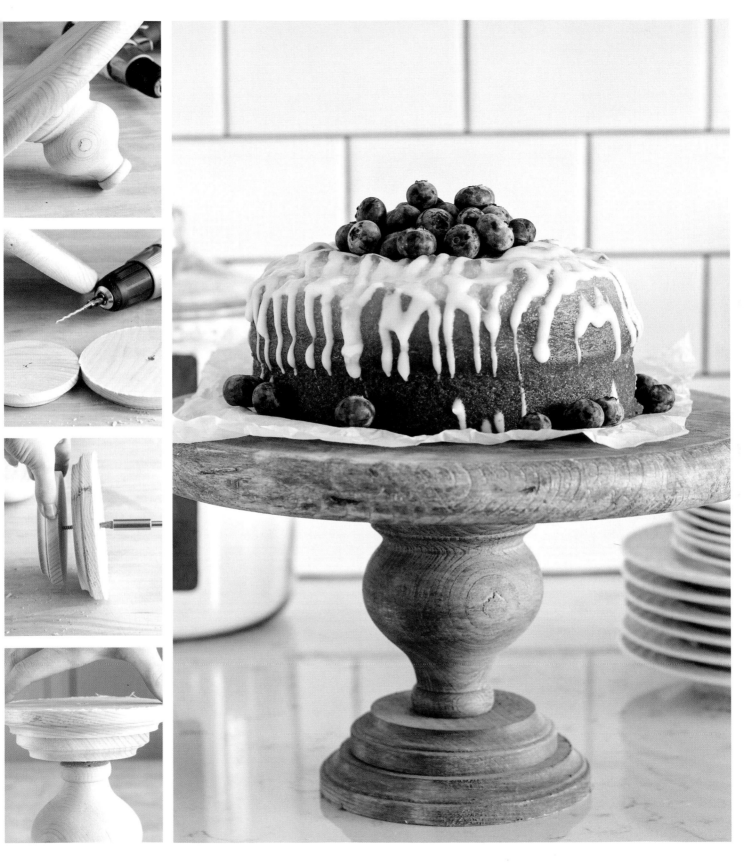

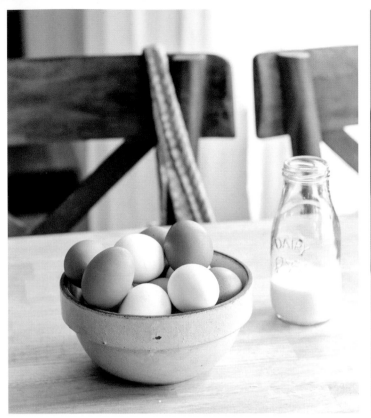
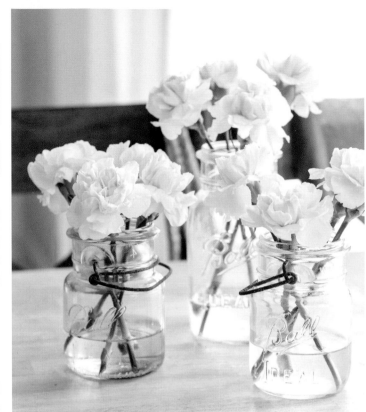
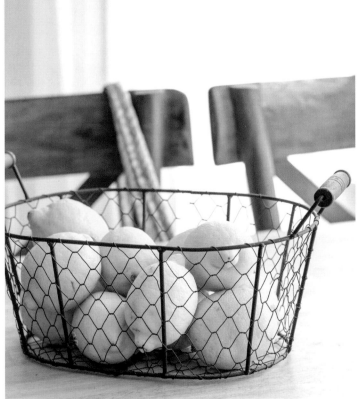
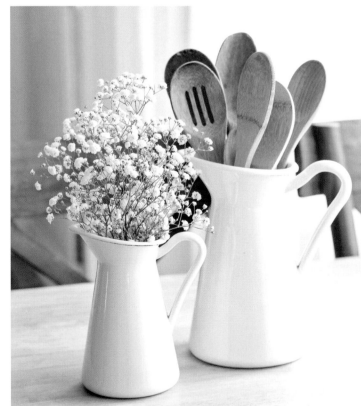

SIMPLE, NATURAL CENTERPIECE

The heart of farmhouse style comes from the simple and organic beauty found in nature. When you need a quick centerpiece, look around your home and use what you have available to you. Eggs set in a wooden bowl, wildflowers in a ceramic pitcher, lemons in a basket or fresh garden clippings in a mason jar—these ideas don't cost a lot of money or require a lot of work. Let your creativity flow and remember that simple is always beautiful! I've included a few examples to get you started.

Level of Difficulty: Beginner

CONTAINER IDEAS

- *Wood bowl*
- *Wire basket*
- *Mason jar*
- *Pitcher*
- *Wine bottle*
- *Lantern*
- *Pottery*
- *Teacup*

FILLER IDEAS

- *Eggs*
- *Fruit or vegetables*
- *Flowers or greenery*
- *Pinecones*
- *Tree-branch clippings*
- *Pebbles*
- *Moss*
- *Seashells*
- *Candles*

FARM-FRESH EGGS IN A BOWL

Fill a bowl with farm-fresh eggs, using a mix of white and brown eggs to add interest. A simple white bowl will give the centerpiece a more modern look, while a wood or pottery bowl will give it a more rustic feel. Rotate new farm-fresh eggs in the bowl every few days so they don't spoil before you are able to cook them.

FRESH-FRUIT BASKET

Use a wire basket to hold lemons, apples, oranges or bananas. They make a beautiful, colorful display as well as a great snack!

SIMPLE FLORAL JARS

Gather a collection of old mason jars and fill them halfway with water. Purchase a bouquet of fresh flowers from the store or clip some from your garden. Trim the stems on an angle to fit inside the mason jars, and add two or three flowers to each jar. Using just a few stems in each jar gives the display a casual look and also stretches the bouquet further.

BABY'S BREATH BOUQUET

Set a bunch of baby's breath (also called gypsophila) in a white pitcher. Baby's breath is very inexpensive and looks even more beautiful as it dries out over time.

MAKE YOUR OWN CENTERPIECE

Select a container large enough to fit your filler. Fill the container with all one item for a simple, soothing look or layer the container with a variety of items to create a unique, multidimensional display. Remember to change the water frequently for fresh flowers or greenery.

FRAMED GLASS SIGN

Give an old picture frame new life with this simple tutorial for creating a gorgeous framed glass sign. If you can trace over some letters with a marker, this project will be a piece of cake for you! Dig through your closet to find an old frame you're not using anymore, or shop the thrift store to find a wide variety of inexpensive ones.

Level of Difficulty: Beginner

SUPPLIES

- *Picture frame with a removable back*
- *Paint (optional)*
- *Paintbrush (optional)*
- *Computer and printer*
- *Fine-tip permanent marker*
- *Picture-hanging wire*
- *Metal snips*
- *Staple gun and staples*
- *Hammer and nail*

DIRECTIONS

Remove the back and glass from the picture frame. If desired, paint the frame and allow it to dry completely.

Use a computer to print the wording or image you would like for your sign. Place the printed paper underneath the glass, and use a fine-tip permanent marker to trace over the design onto the glass. Allow the ink to dry for several hours before touching.

Cut a piece of picture-hanging wire several inches longer than your frame using metal snips and tie a knot at each end. Staple the wire to the back of the frame near the top corners. Add the glass back into the frame (discard the backing), and hang the sign on the wall with a nail.

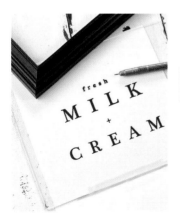
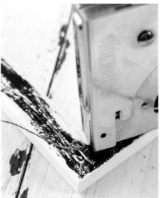
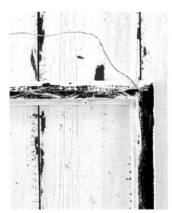
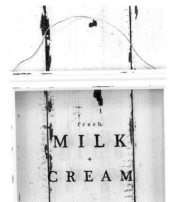

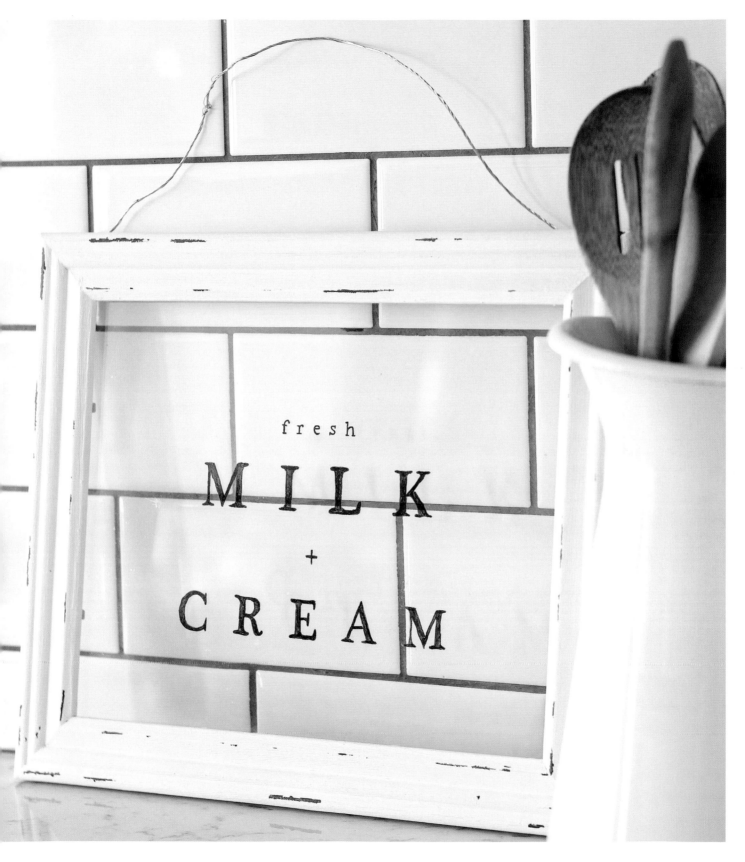

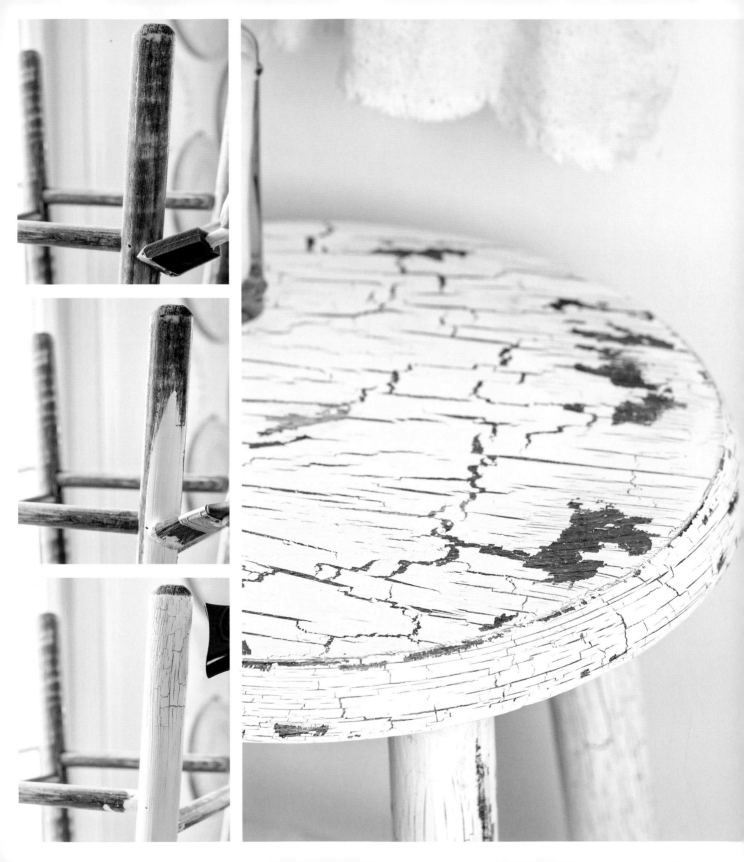

CRACKED PAINT FINISH

If you like the look of old peeling paint on furniture, you are going to love this technique! To get this cracked paint finish, apply a thin layer of glue before adding your paint, and then sit back and watch the magic happen as it dries. This finish looks beautiful when painted over wood and can be used on furniture, picture frames or handmade signs like the Family Name Sign (page 23) or Wooden Arrow Sign (page 147)! Keep in mind that smaller pieces of décor and furniture (like the stool shown here) work best for this technique, as you have to work in small sections at a time.

Level of Difficulty: Beginner

SUPPLIES

• *White school glue*
• *Wooden stool*
• *Paintbrushes*
• *Paint*
• *Hair dryer*
• *Sanding block (optional)*

DIRECTIONS

Working in small sections, no more than one square foot at a time, apply a thin layer of glue on the stool using a paintbrush. Immediately apply a thick layer of paint over the glue before it starts to dry. Use the highest heat setting on a hair dryer to quickly dry the paint. As the glue begins to dry, you will see the paint crack and separate. Make sure to use a thick enough paint layer to completely cover the wood underneath. Adding a second layer of paint will cover the cracked finish you've created.

If desired, use a sanding block to lightly remove some of the finish along the corners and edges for an authentic aged look. Make sure the paint finish is completely dry before sanding.

TIP | *Don't worry about applying the glue and paint perfectly. Having some areas with cracks and some without will make the piece look more natural.*

PANELED DOOR

One of the hallmarks of an old farmhouse is having doors with character. Even if the doors in your house are nothing special, you can easily add detail to a flat, plain door by using strips of plywood to create the look of a paneled door. This is one project that will definitely give you a big bang for your decorating buck!

Level of Difficulty: Advanced

SUPPLIES

- *Plain, flat interior door*
- *Tape measure*
- *¼-inch (6-mm) plywood*
- *Circular saw*
- *Sanding block*
- *Wood glue*
- *Brad nail gun*
- *1-inch (2.5-cm) brad nails*
- *Spackling paste*
- *Putty knife*
- *Clean rag*
- *Paint*
- *Paintbrush and/or paint roller*
- *Drill and drill bit*

DIRECTIONS

Remove the door from its hinges and set it on a flat surface. Remove the door handle and all of the hinges. Cut the plywood into 4-inch (10-cm) wide strips using a circular saw. Sand the edges of the plywood to remove any rough edges.

Measure the length of the door, and cut two strips of plywood to that length. Lay a strip on both long sides of the door and secure with wood glue and brad nails.

Measure the distance between the two plywood pieces on the door, and cut six more strips to that length. Use a tape measure to space them evenly across the door and use wood glue and brad nails to secure them in place.

Apply spackling paste to all the seams and nail holes using a putty knife, and allow the spackle to dry completely. When dry, sand over the spackle to give the door a smooth, seamless finish. Wipe off dust with a clean rag, and paint the door and trim in your desired color.

When the door is dry, drill a hole through the trim where the door handle goes, and reinstall the handle and hinges. Hang the door inside the doorframe and make sure it closes well.

TIP | *Ask your home improvement store if they will cut the plywood into strips for you. Most will do it for a small fee!*

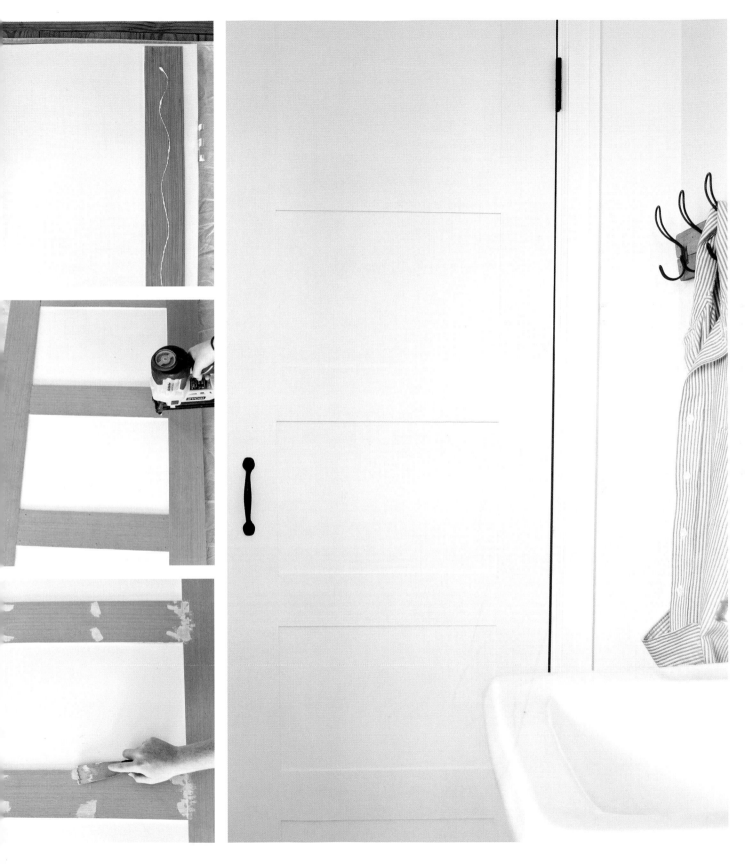

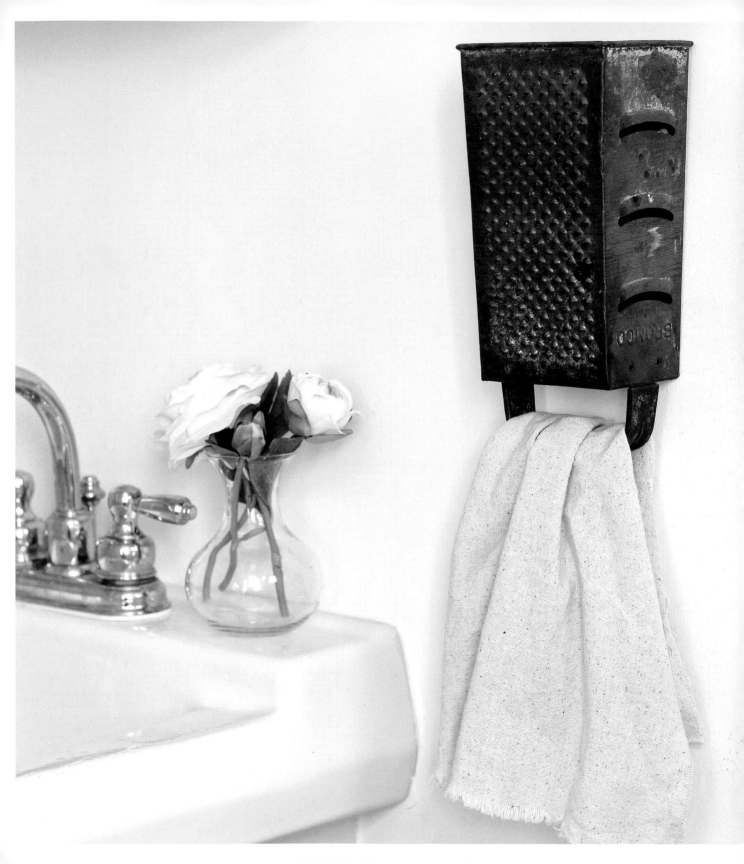

ANTIQUE GRATER TOWEL HOLDER

Farmhouse style is all about repurposing vintage pieces in new ways, and this sweet, little antique grater towel holder does just that. Instead of a traditional towel bar by your kitchen or bathroom sink, try using an unexpected item like this grater to really turn up the farmhouse charm. It takes just a few minutes to install and can be hung either on the wall or on the side of a cabinet.

Level of Difficulty: Beginner

SUPPLIES

- *Antique box grater*
- *Pencil*
- *Hammer and nails*
- *Hand towel*

DIRECTIONS

Hold a box grater upside down on the wall where you would like your towel to hang. Mark on the wall through two of the grater holes using a pencil, then hammer two nails into the wall over your pencil marks. Hang the grater on the nails and slide a towel through the handle of the grater.

TIP | *For an extra decorative touch, slide a thin vase inside the grater to hold fresh flowers.*

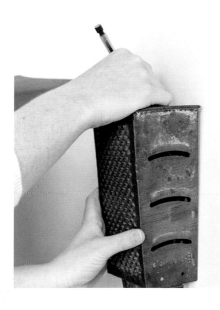 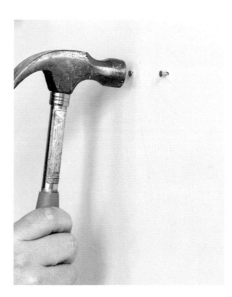 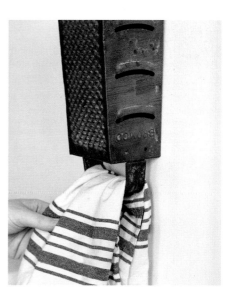

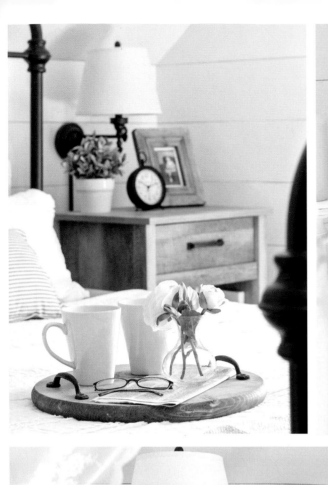
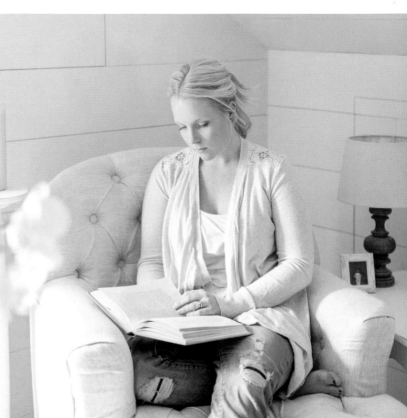
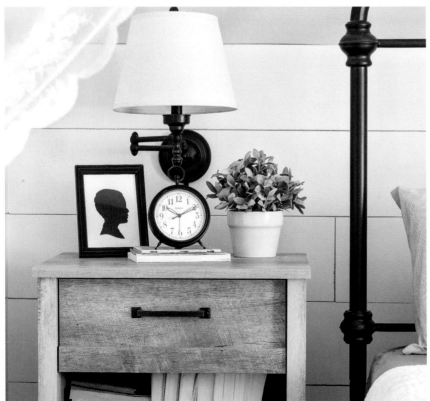
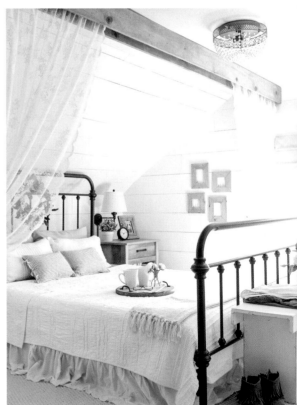

MASTER BEDROOM

Your bedroom is the first thing you see each morning, so make this a space you are excited to wake up to. It should feel like a relaxing retreat where you can curl up with a good book or sip the morning's first cup of coffee with your sweetheart.

Our master bedroom was an unfinished attic when we first moved into the farmhouse. To give this newly constructed space the same charm and character as the rest of our 1940s home, we decided to add wide wood planks on all the walls. The room instantly felt more cozy and rustic, but rather than leaving the planks natural, we painted them white to keep the space open and airy. We created a special nook for our bed by installing a faux wood beam overhead and soft lace curtains on either side. A simple iron bed frame paired with fresh, white bedding and a variety of handmade décor completes our cozy farmhouse bedroom.

In this chapter, I'll share some easy decorating ideas to give your room a warm, inviting feel with a touch of vintage charm. You'll find candleholders to add ambiance (page 78), custom artwork for a personal touch (page 86) and organizing ideas that are as functional as they are beautiful. Go ahead and turn off that alarm clock. . . . You won't want to leave your bed for a while.

TABLE LEG CANDLEHOLDER

Large antique candleholders can be very expensive, but you can make your own with this quick tutorial. Grab an old table leg or buy one new from the hardware store and add a few wooden discs to create a sturdy base. Any size or shape will work, but the more curves and details it has, the better! Stain the wood for a natural look or paint it to match your space. These also look great in a dining room and add a beautiful rustic elegance.

Level of Difficulty: Intermediate

SUPPLIES

- *Drill and drill bit*
- *Two large and two small wooden discs, about 4–6 inches (10–15 cm) wide*
- *Table leg*
- *Screws*
- *Paint*
- *Paintbrush*
- *Pillar candle*

DIRECTIONS

Drill a hole the size of your screws in the center of each wooden disc and the table leg. Line up the holes and add a screw using the drill. Attach the wooden discs to both ends of the table leg.

Paint the candleholder, and allow it to dry completely, about 4 hours.

Place the finished candleholder on a flat, even surface and set a pillar candle on top.

ALTERNATIVE | *Use a spindle in place of the table leg and wood glue instead of screws to attach the pieces.*

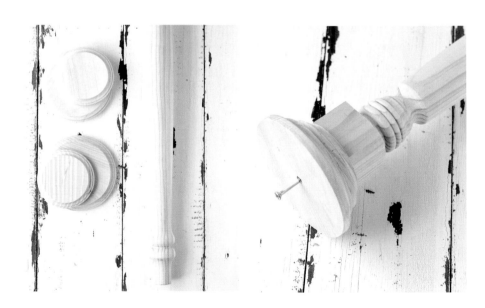

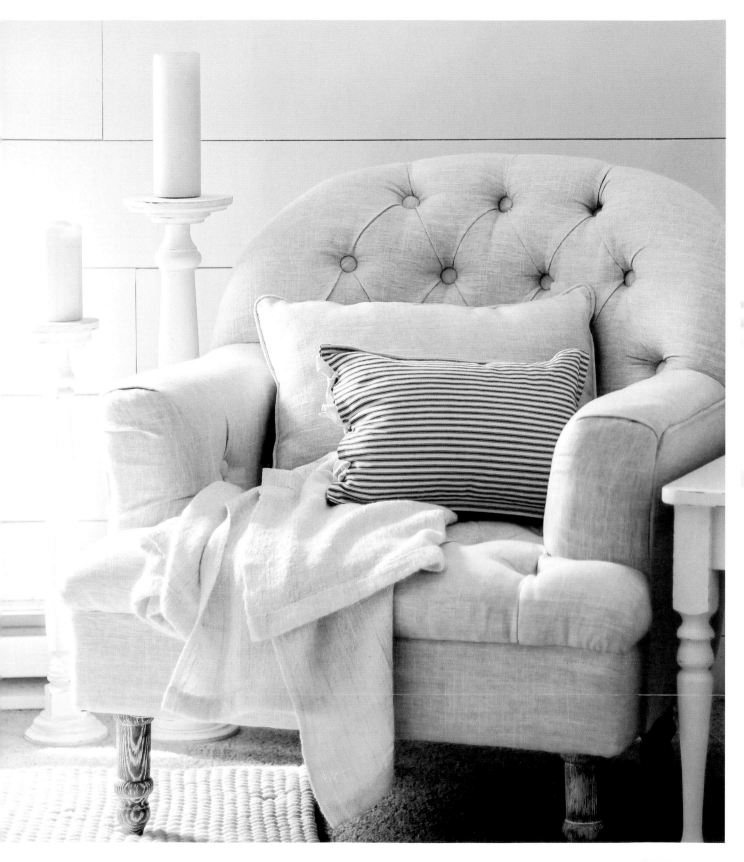

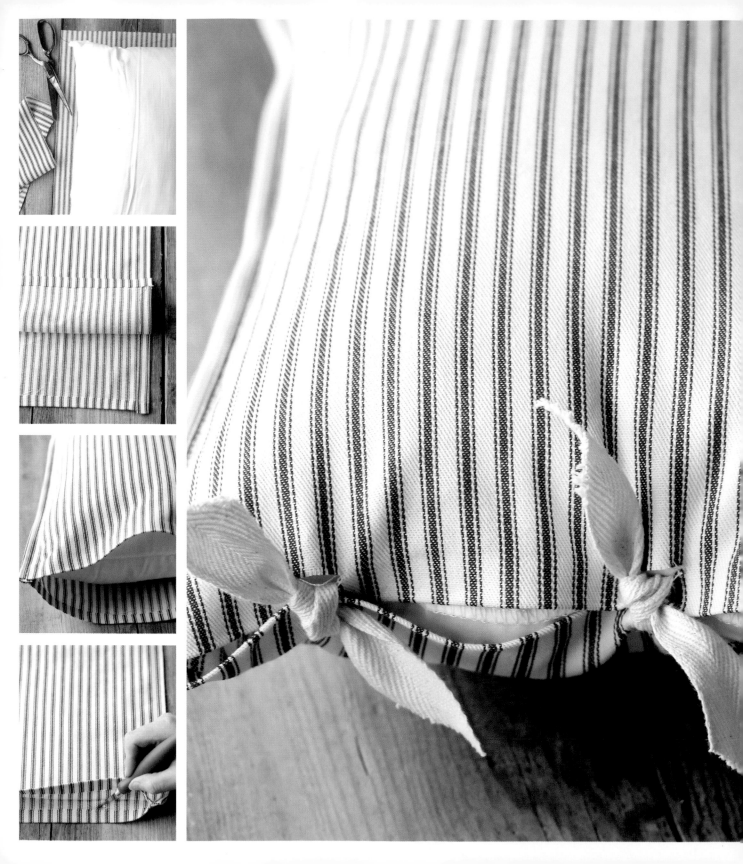

TIED PILLOW COVER

This sweet little pillow cover with ties on the side will bring an instant touch of vintage charm to your bed or sofa. Use fabrics like linen, toile, burlap, muslin, grain sacks and anything with ticking stripes to give it an authentic farmhouse feel!

Level of Difficulty: Intermediate

SUPPLIES

- *Iron and ironing board*
- *Fabric*
- *Tape measure*
- *Pillow form*
- *Scissors*
- *Sewing machine*
- *Thread*
- *Utility knife*
- *Ribbon*

DIRECTIONS

Wash, dry and iron your fabric. Measure the length and width of your pillow form and add 1 inch (2.5 cm) to each measurement. Cut two pieces of fabric to those measurements.

Sew a ½-inch (13-mm) hem on all four edges on both pieces of fabric. Place the hemmed fabric pieces together right-side out and sew them together along three sides, leaving one side open. Stuff the pillow form in the open end of the pillow cover.

Make three small, evenly spaced slits right below the hem on the open end of the pillow cover using a utility knife. Cut three pieces of ribbon about 5 inches (13 cm) long, and slide one ribbon through each slit. Tie a double knot in each ribbon to hold the pillow inside the case. Trim the edges of the ribbon, if necessary.

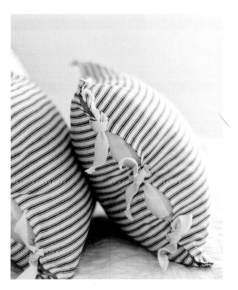

ALTERNATIVE | *Even if you don't have access to a sewing machine, you can still easily make these pillow covers! All you need is a roll of hem tape and an iron. Just follow the instructions on the hem tape package any time sewing is called for in the instructions above.*

SIMPLE WOODEN BENCH

Benches are great for extra seating and storage, and this primitive bench is full of farmhouse charm. If you are new to furniture building, this is a great place to start! You can paint the wood to match your décor and distress the finish as much or as little as you like. Or, you could stain your bench. That is the beauty of making your own furniture! Set the bench at the end of your bed or in an entryway to create a sweet, little resting place for tired feet. You can use a hammer and nails to attach the bench pieces if you don't have a brad nail gun, but be sure to use wood glue to hold all the joints in place.

Level of Difficulty: Advanced

SUPPLIES

- *Tape measure*
- *1 (1 x 12) board, 8 feet (244 cm) long*
- *Miter or circular saw*
- *Jigsaw*
- *Pencil*
- *Wood glue*
- *Drill*
- *Pocket-hole jig*
- *1 ¼-inch (3-cm) pocket-hole screws*
- *1 (1 x 4) board, 10 feet (305 cm) long*
- *Brad nail gun*
- *1 ½-inch (3.8-cm) brad nails*
- *Sanding block*
- *Clean rags*
- *Paint*
- *Paintbrush*
- *Paste wax*

DIRECTIONS

Measure and cut a piece of 1 x 12 to 38 inches (96.5 cm) long using a saw for the bench seat. Cut two pieces of 1 x 12 to 18 inches (45.5 cm) long for the bench legs. Cut a triangle out of the bottom of both bench leg pieces using a jigsaw. To create the triangle, mark 3 inches (7.5 cm) in from either side along the bottom of the board with a pencil. Then make a mark in the center of the board about 6 inches (15 cm) up from the bottom. Draw lines to connect the marks and use them as guides to cut out the triangle.

Measure 5 inches (13 cm) in from the ends of the bench seat, and attach the bench legs to the seat using wood glue, pocket holes and 1 ¼-inch (3-cm) pocket-hole screws.

Cut two pieces of 1 x 4 to 38 inches (96.5 cm) long for the sides of the bench. Lay the bench on its side and place the 1 x 4 flush with the top of the bench. Attach the 1 x 4 to the legs and seat using wood glue and brad nails. Repeat on the other side with the remaining 1 x 4.

Cut two pieces of 1 x 4 to 11 ¼ inches (28.5 cm) long to use as a support piece underneath the bench. Turn the bench upside down and place the 1 x 4s just inside the bench legs. Use wood glue and brad nails to secure the 1 x 4s to the bench.

Sand the entire bench with a sanding block to remove any rough edges, and wipe off dust with a clean rag. Paint the bench and allow it to dry completely, about 4 hours. To seal the wood, apply a layer of paste wax with a paintbrush and buff with a clean rag.

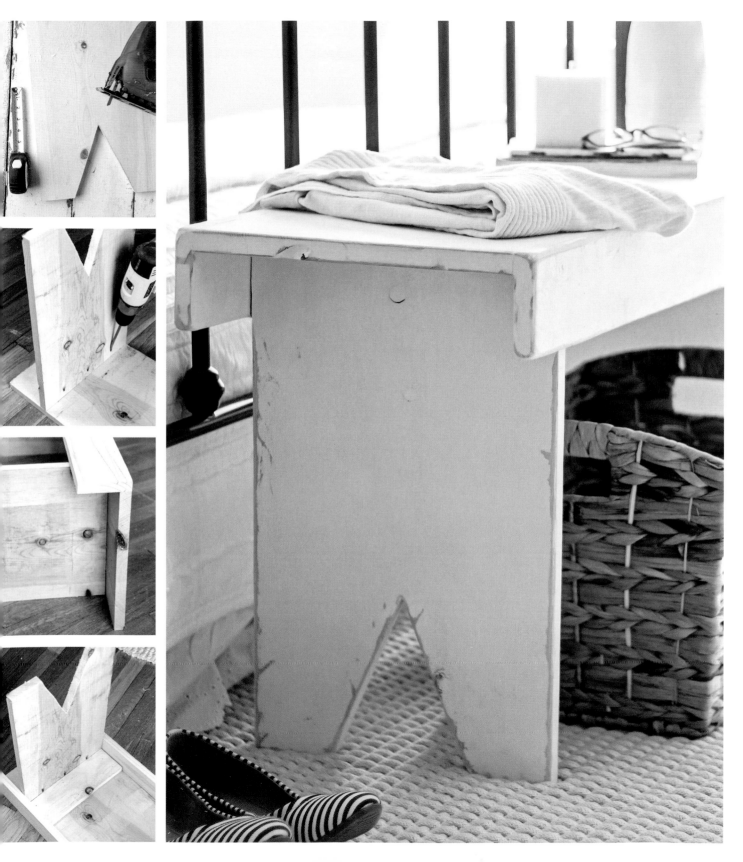

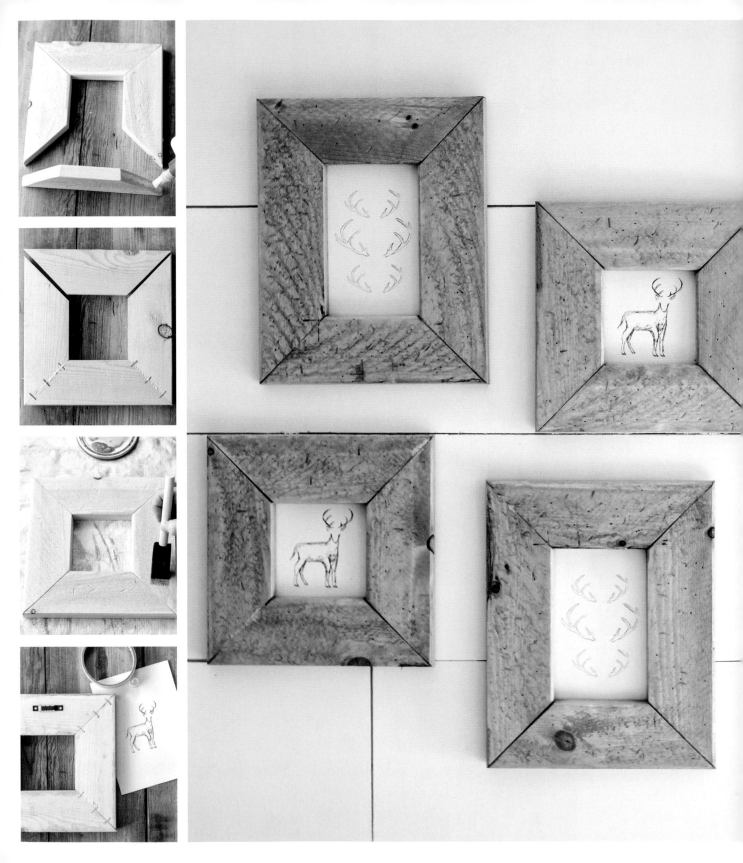

RUSTIC WOODEN FRAME

These wooden frames are perfect for when you want something a little more rustic than a standard picture frame, and you can stain them to look like you pulled the wood right out of an old barn. You can make these frames in any size to hold your favorite photos or artwork. Try making one large frame as a statement piece or a collection of smaller frames to use in a gallery wall.

Level of Difficulty: Intermediate

SUPPLIES

- *Miter saw*
- *1 x 3 board*
- *Tape measure*
- *Sanding block*
- *Clean rags*
- *Wood glue*
- *Staple gun and staples*
- *Wood stain*
- *Paintbrush*
- *Hammer and nails*
- *Sawtooth picture hanger with nails*
- *Masking tape*

DIRECTIONS

Using a miter saw, cut the 1 x 3 into four pieces with the edges mitered on a 45° angle. Sand any rough edges on the boards, then wipe them with a clean rag to remove sawdust.

Fit the mitered edges of the boards together to create a frame with the front side facing down. Apply wood glue to the mitered edges of the boards and press the seams together firmly. Add a few staples down the seams to hold the frame in place. Flip the frame over and place a heavy object on top to keep the seams tight while the glue dries, about 1 hour.

When the glue is dry, apply stain to the front and sides of the frame using a paintbrush. Allow the stain to penetrate for 5–15 minutes until the desired color is achieved. Wipe the frame with a clean rag to remove any remaining stain, and allow the wood to dry completely, about 8 hours.

Use a hammer to attach a sawtooth hanger to the back of the frame with nails. To fill your frame, simply tape a photo or piece of art to the back and hang it on the wall with a nail.

> TIPS | *The stain will not soak into the wood where there is glue, so if some gets on the outside of the frame, try to wipe it up immediately.*
>
> *To make the new wood look older and more rustic, use a hammer, screwdriver or other tools to beat up the boards a bit before assembling the frame. The marks left by the tools will give the wood lots of character!*

FRAMED SILHOUETTE

These classic framed silhouettes give a nod to the past and remind us of a time before camera phones and the digital era. You can easily replicate these silhouettes at home and have unique portraits of your family that bring a vintage touch to any space. Add a silhouette to your nightstand or mantel, or for a bigger impact, create an entire gallery wall of silhouettes.

Level of Difficulty: Beginner

SUPPLIES

- *Camera*
- *Computer and printer*
- *White printer paper*
- *Pencil*
- *Black scrapbook paper*
- *Tape*
- *Scissors*
- *Utility knife*
- *White scrapbook paper*
- *Double-sided adhesive*
- *Photo frame*

DIRECTIONS

Take a photo of someone standing against a light wall or window at a 90° angle from you, focusing on the head and shoulders. Upload the photo to your computer and print onto white printer paper.

Hold the photo against a window with the back facing you and trace around the outline of the head and shoulders with a pencil. Add details like eyelashes, hair curls, bows, collars or buttons if desired.

Set the silhouette on top of a piece of black scrapbook paper and tape at the top and bottom to hold in place. Carefully cut out the silhouette with scissors. To cut out the small details, use a utility knife.

Cut a piece of white scrapbook paper to fit inside the photo frame. Attach the black silhouette to the center of the white paper using double-sided adhesive, and place the paper inside the photo frame.

TIP | *You may need to resize your photo a bit to fit inside your frame. To do this, paste the photo into a word processor document on the computer, then click and drag the corner of the photo to change the size.*

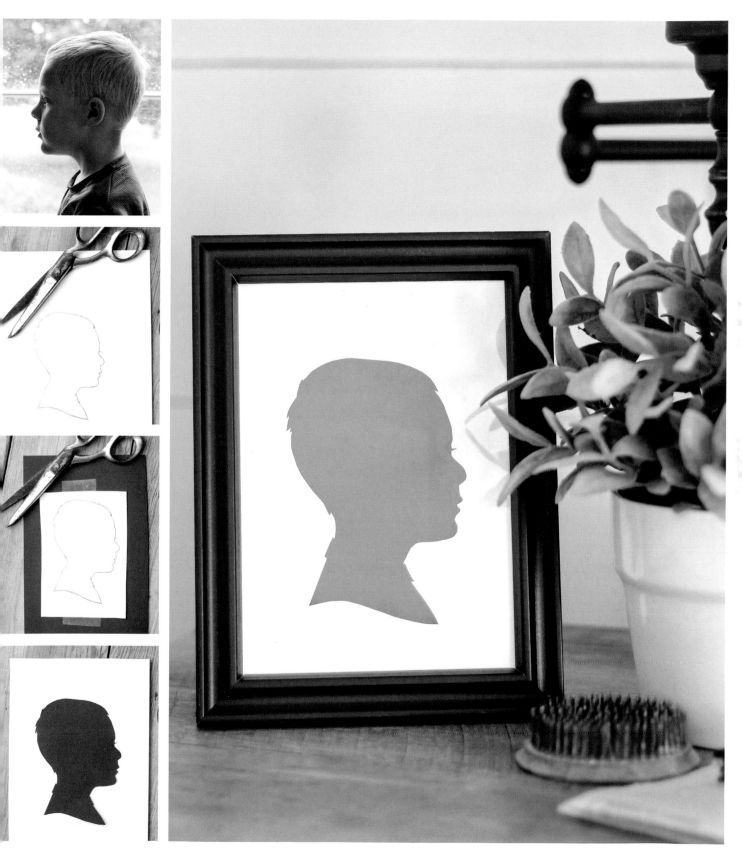

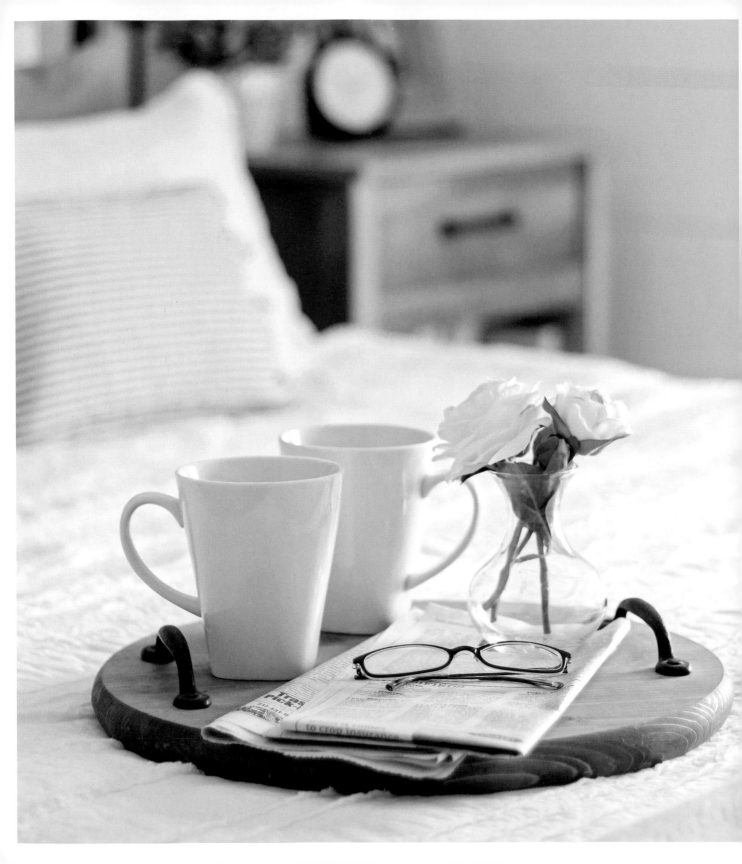

ROUND WOODEN SERVING TRAY

This simple round tray is a quick and easy project that will serve you for many years to come. Made with a basic wooden panel from the store (no cutting required!) and kitchen drawer pulls, this tray is perfect for when you are entertaining guests or serving breakfast in bed to your sweetheart.

Level of Difficulty: Intermediate

SUPPLIES

- *Wood stain*
- *15 x 1-inch (38 x 2.5-cm) round wooden panel*
- *Paintbrush*
- *Clean rags*
- *Paste wax*
- *Drill and drill bit*
- *Two drawer pulls*
- *4 (1 ¼-inch [3-cm]) machine screws*
- *Screwdriver*

DIRECTIONS

Apply stain to all sides of the round wooden panel using a paintbrush. Allow the stain to penetrate for 5–15 minutes until the desired color is achieved. Wipe the wood with a clean rag to remove any remaining stain, and allow it to dry completely, about 8 hours.

To seal the wood, apply a layer of paste wax with a paintbrush and buff with a clean rag.

Drill a hole the size of your screws through the wood where each drawer pull will go. Position the drawer pull over the holes, and insert the screws through the bottom of the wooden panel using a screwdriver.

TIP | Your drawer pulls will most likely come with screws already in the package, but they won't be long enough to go all the way through the wood. Check the thickness of your wood and the screw size you'll need while you're at the store.

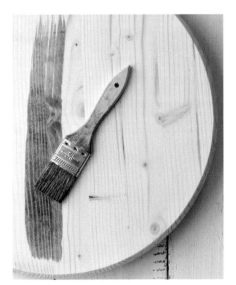
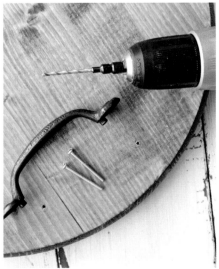

PAINTED STEP STOOL WITH EASY DISTRESSING

Furniture with a distressed, timeworn finish is common in farmhouse décor, and this trick is the fastest way I've found to get that look with paint. Instead of sanding away layers and layers of dry paint, this technique uses petroleum jelly as a barrier that prevents paint from adhering to the furniture. The paint wipes right off, saving loads of time and elbow grease!

Level of Difficulty: Beginner

SUPPLIES

- *Petroleum jelly (such as Vaseline)*
- *Wooden step stool*
- *Cotton swabs*
- *Paint*
- *Paintbrushes*
- *Sanding block*
- *Clean rags*
- *Dark wax*

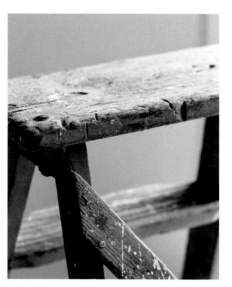

DIRECTIONS

Apply a thin layer of petroleum jelly to the edges and corners of the stool using a cotton swab. The paint will not adhere anywhere you apply the jelly, so use it only in places the paint would naturally wear off over time, such as the edges, corners, steps, near metal hardware and any place you would like some distressing.

Paint the stool using a paintbrush, and allow the stool to dry completely, about 4 hours. When dry, use a sanding block on the areas where petroleum jelly was applied. Those spots will still have a "wet" look to them and will be slightly darker than the dry paint, so you'll know exactly where to sand. The paint should come off easily, exposing the bare wood underneath.

When the entire stool has been distressed, wipe it down with a clean rag to remove dust. Then, seal the stool by applying a layer of paste wax with a paintbrush and buff with a clean rag.

TIP | *Try using flat-sheen paint to give your project a timeworn look. Matte finishes are much more common in farmhouse style than high-gloss finishes.*

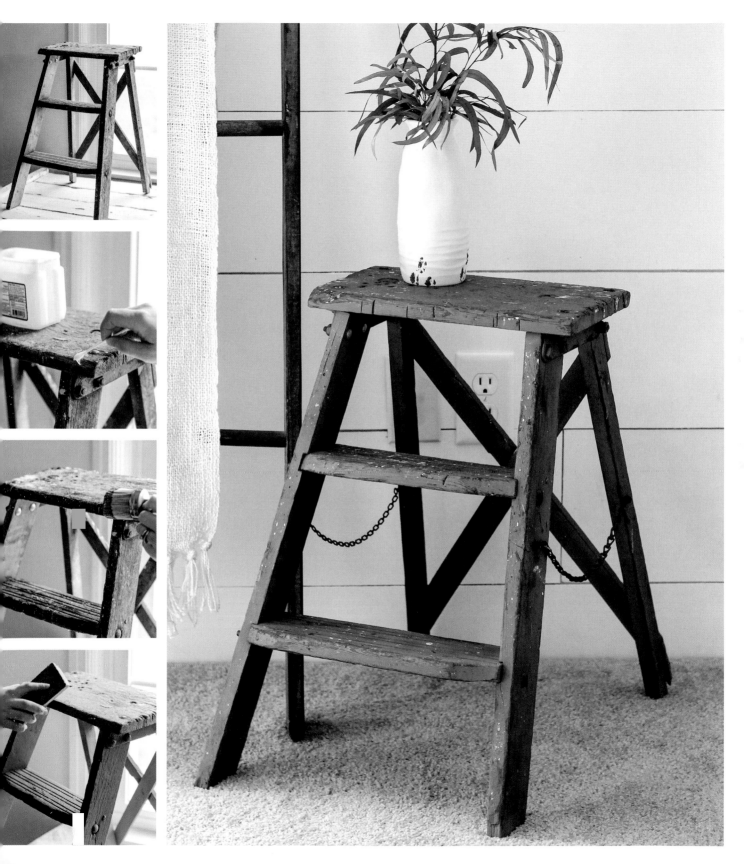

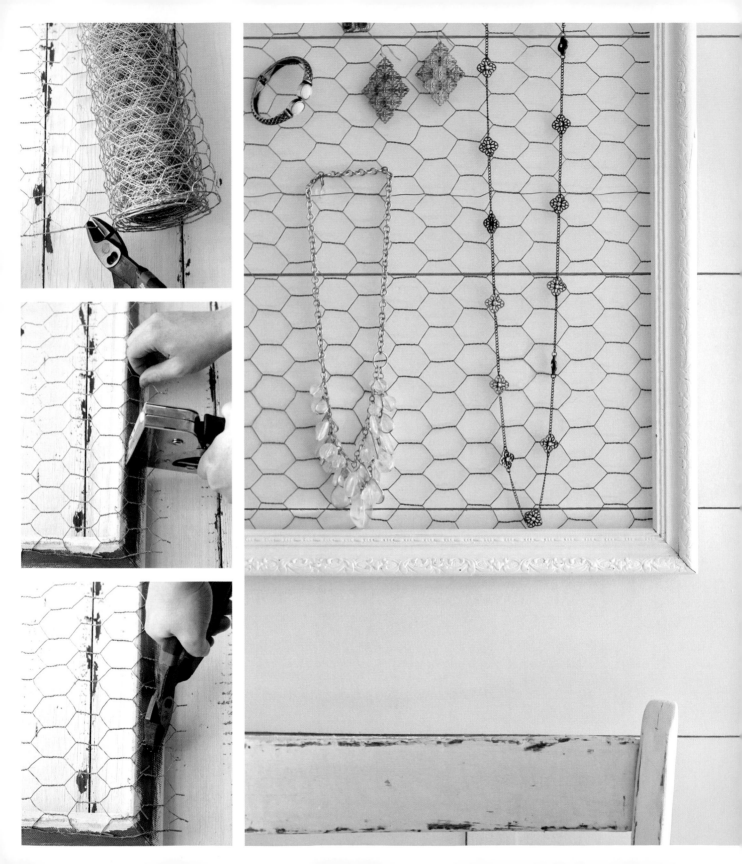

CHICKEN-WIRE JEWELRY DISPLAY

This framed jewelry display allows you to easily organize your favorite earrings and necklaces without them being hidden away in a jewelry box. The jewelry hangs on the chicken-wire, which adds the perfect touch of farmhouse charm. You can add the framed display to an empty wall or simply lean it against the wall on top of a dresser.

Level of Difficulty: Beginner

SUPPLIES

- *Large photo frame*
- *1-inch (2.5-cm) galvanized poultry netting*
- *Metal snips*
- *Spray paint*
- *Staple gun and staples*
- *Hammer and nails*
- *Sawtooth picture hanger*
- *Small s-hooks*

DIRECTIONS

Remove the glass and backing from the photo frame. Cut a piece of poultry netting using metal snips to fit behind the frame. Spray paint the netting (if desired), and allow the paint to dry completely. Place the frame right-side down and set the netting on top. Staple one side of the netting to the back of the frame, then stretch the netting tightly across the frame and staple the other side. Finish adding staples all the way around the frame to secure the netting in place.

Use a hammer to attach the sawtooth hanger to the back of the frame with nails. Hang earrings on the netting, or use small s-hooks to hang necklaces and bracelets.

TIP | *Thrift stores are great places to buy large, old photo frames. They are much less expensive than buying new and often have beautiful detailing.*

WIRE LAUNDRY HAMPER

Why use a cheap, plastic laundry basket when you can have a hamper that looks this good? Sometimes it's the small details that really make a space, and this industrial-style hamper will fit in perfectly with your décor. By adding caster wheels to the bottom, you can roll this hamper straight from the bedroom to the laundry room, and a simple pillowcase makes the perfect laundry bag.

Level of Difficulty: Advanced

SUPPLIES

- *Wood stain*
- *12 x 1-inch (30.5 x 2.5-cm) round wooden panel*
- *Paintbrush*
- *Clean rags*
- *Metal snips*
- *2 x 4-inch (5 x 10-cm) 14-gauge galvanized welded wire*
- *Pliers*
- *Staple gun and staples*
- *Four caster wheels*
- *¾-inch (2-cm) screws*
- *Screwdriver*
- *White king-size pillowcase*
- *White adhesive-back Velcro for fabric*

DIRECTIONS

Apply stain to all sides of the round wooden panel using a paintbrush. Allow the stain to penetrate for 5–15 minutes until the desired color is achieved. Wipe the wood with a clean rag to remove any remaining stain, and allow it to dry completely, about 8 hours.

Using metal snips, cut a piece of welded wire wide enough to wrap around the wooden panel with a slight overhang. Trim the length of the wire to 32 inches (81.5 cm), and tightly wrap the cut wires around the opposite edge of the wire using pliers. Trim any excess wire with the metal snips so no sharp edges stick out.

On the bottom edge of the wire cylinder, use the snips to cut off every other wire around the circle. Position the wooden panel to sit just above the bottom row of wire rectangles and bend those bottom rectangles underneath the wood. Use a staple gun to secure each wire rectangle to the panel.

Add equally spaced casters on the bottom of the wooden panel using screws and a screwdriver. Place the pillowcase inside the hamper, folding the open edge over the top wire. Add small pieces of Velcro along the top edge of the pillowcase to hold it in place on the hamper.

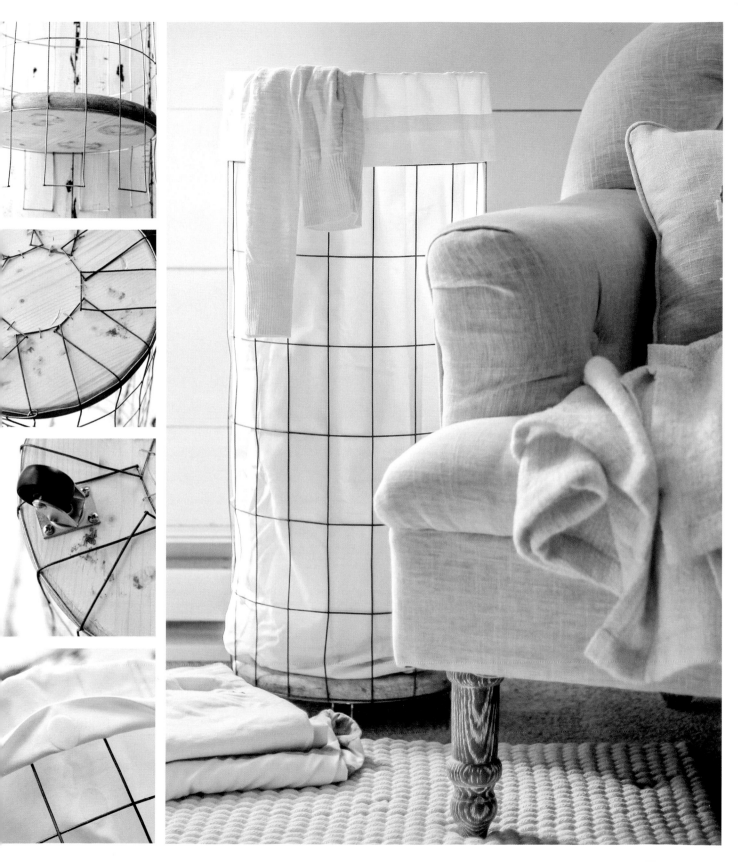

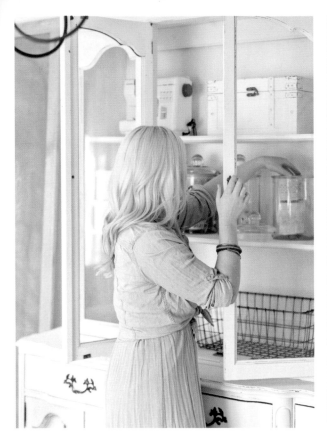
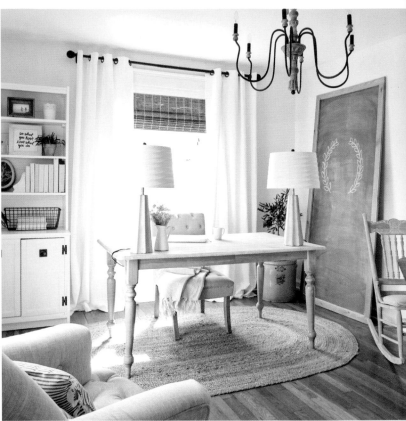
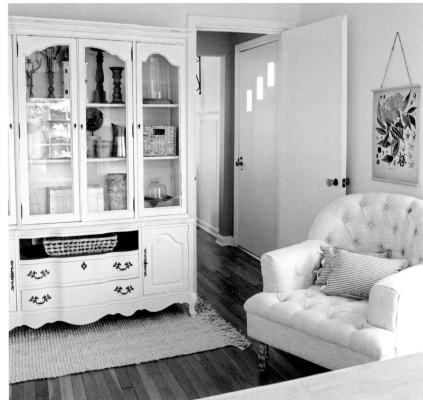
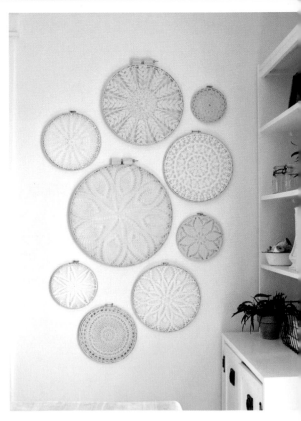

OFFICE

Your office might be the place where you work from home, catch up on homework, store your library of books or create your latest masterpiece, but, however you use it, make this a beautiful space to work in. Include plenty of storage in your design so the space feels uncluttered and tidy, and give yourself a place to organize your schedule and to-do lists. Most of all, create an office that speaks to you, motivates you and inspires you.

I work from home, which means I probably spend more hours in my office than I do my own bed, so my first task in designing the office was creating different zones for how I use this space. I needed a desk where I could run my website and business, a worktable to create my projects and tons of storage for my supplies and equipment.

I kept all the walls white for a light, bright space, but used plenty of wood tones, creamy neutrals and texture to keep the design interesting. I repurposed a large farmhouse dining table as my desk and floated it in the middle of the room to become the focal point. For storage, I moved a large china hutch that used to be in our dining room into the office and gave it a distressed white paint finish. A bookcase in the corner adds extra storage for books and décor, and an X-leg table along one wall gives me plenty of space to work on projects. For the final touch, a large, dramatic chandelier was hung in the center of the room, adding character and vintage charm.

In this chapter, I'll show you how to make a variety of vintage-inspired décor like hanging botanical prints (page 101), wooden spools (page 102) and a doily gallery wall (page 98). You'll learn how to create a large framed chalkboard (page 109) and also paint techniques for lime washing furniture (page 113) and creating a layered paint finish (page 114). Step into my office . . . we have some work to do.

DOILY GALLERY WALL

Have a blank wall in need of some artwork? Try this display of vintage crocheted doilies hung in embroidery hoops to give your walls a dose of pattern, texture and gorgeous neutral colors. Search for doilies at garage sales, thrift stores and antique stores if you don't already have some that either you have made or family members have passed down to you. Collect doilies with a variety of patterns, scale and color to add interest to your gallery wall!

Level of Difficulty: Beginner

SUPPLIES

• *Embroidery hoops*
• *Round crocheted doilies in various sizes*
• *Hammer and nails*

DIRECTIONS

Find an embroidery hoop just smaller than the size of your doily. Loosen the screw on the top of the hoop and remove the center hoop. Place the doily centered on top of the outer hoop and slide the inner hoop back inside, sandwiching the doily in between the hoops. Tighten the screw on top to secure the doily inside.

Repeat with the remaining doilies and hoops, and hang the hoops on a wall using a hammer and nails. Try hanging them together in a group with the largest hoops toward the center and the smaller hoops scattered around the outside.

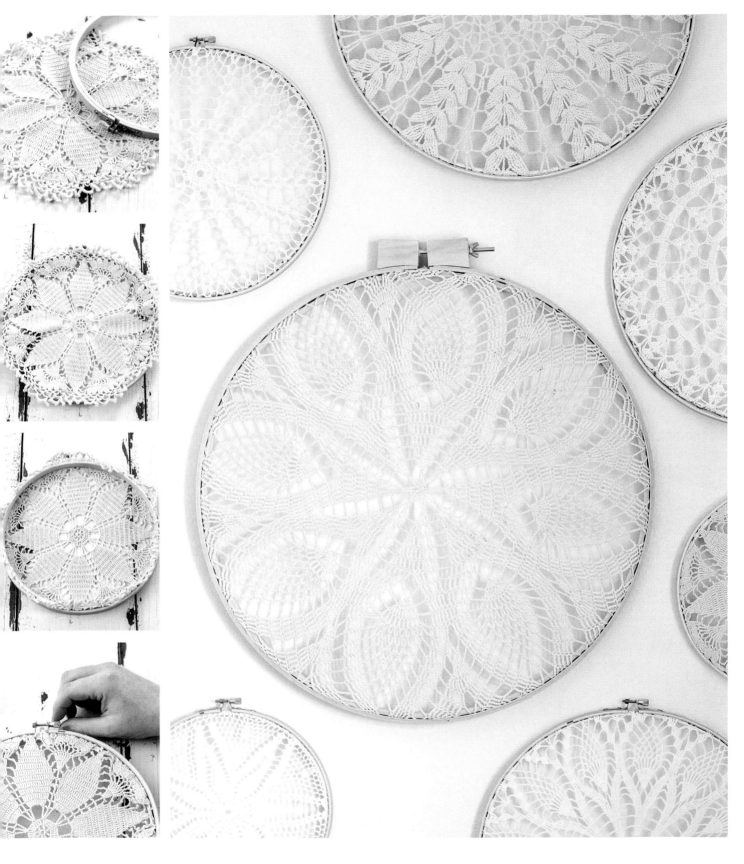

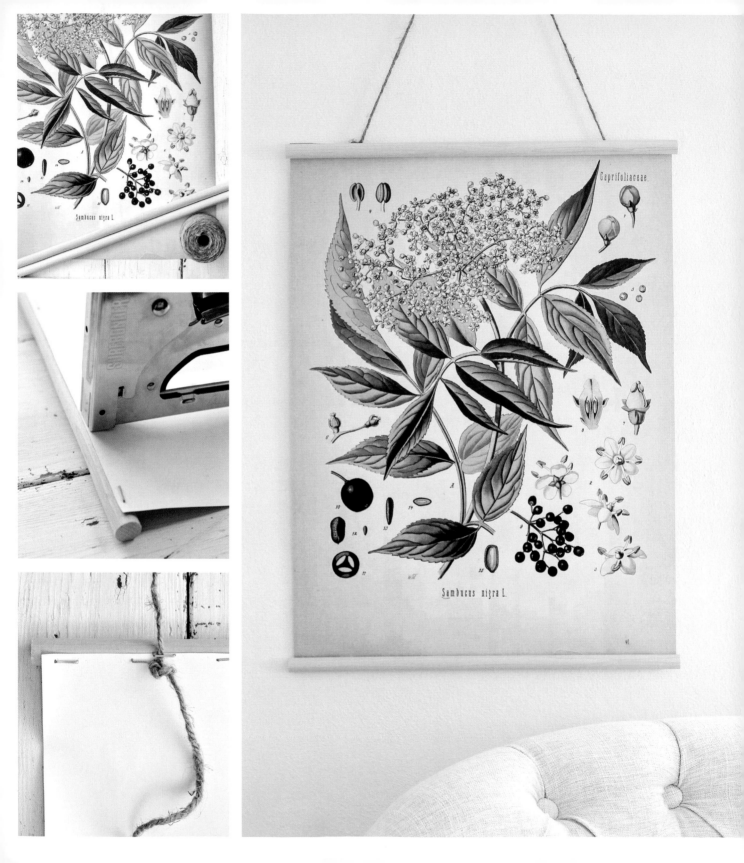

BOTANICAL WALL HANGING

Decorating with vintage botanical prints is a great way to add a touch of nature to your space without having to worry about watering any plants. And let's face it . . . they are really pretty to look at! This piece of art is easily made with an enlarged print, a few dowel rods and a piece of twine. Simple, beautiful and full of vintage charm!

Level of Difficulty: Intermediate

SUPPLIES

- *High-resolution botanical print, enlarged to desired size (mine is 16 x 20 inches [40.5 x 51 cm])*
- *Tape measure*
- *¾-inch (2-cm) dowel rod*
- *Miter or circular saw*
- *Staple gun and staples*
- *Jute twine*
- *Scissors*
- *Hammer and nail*

DIRECTIONS

Measure the width of your botanical print using a tape measure. Measure and cut two pieces from the dowel rod ½ inch (13 mm) longer than the width of the print using a saw.

Staple the top of the print to one of the dowel rods from the backside of the paper. Then staple the other dowel rod to the bottom of the print.

Cut a piece of jute twine about 30 inches (76 cm) long, and tie a double knot on each end of the twine. Staple one end of the twine behind the top dowel rod about 3 inches (7.5 cm) in from one end of the dowel. Place the staple just above the knot to hold it in place. Repeat the same steps to attach the twine to the other side of the top dowel rod. Hang the botanical print on the wall using a hammer and nail.

TIPS | *You can find a wide variety of vintage botanical prints online that are free to use. When you find one you like, download it to your computer, enlarge it to the desired size and print it at a local printing shop. Be sure that the image you choose has a high resolution so that the print doesn't appear pixelated.*

Instead of using a staple gun, you could also use a hot-glue gun to attach the dowel rods and twine.

VINTAGE WOODEN SPOOL

Small accessories are like the icing on a cake when decorating. They fill the space and add character and personality, especially when using items like this darling vintage wooden spool. You can easily make several of them with a few pieces of wood found at a craft store, and adding a faded stamp on the end gives them an authentic look. Stack a few together on a shelf or add them to a bowl set on a table.

Level of Difficulty: Intermediate

SUPPLIES

- *Tape measure*
- *1 ¼-inch (3-cm) dowel rod*
- *Miter or circular saw*
- *Drill*
- *2 (2-inch x ³⁄₁₆-inch [5-cm x 5-mm]) wood discs*
- *½-inch (13-mm) paddle bit*
- *Rubber stamp*
- *Black ink pad*
- *Wood glue*

DIRECTIONS

Measure and cut a 3-inch (7.5-cm) piece from the dowel rod using a saw. Drill a hole in the center of both wood discs using a ½-inch (13-mm) paddle bit.

Lightly stamp a design on one side of the wood discs with black ink. Attach a disc to both ends of the dowel rod using wood glue. Place something heavy on the spool while the glue dries.

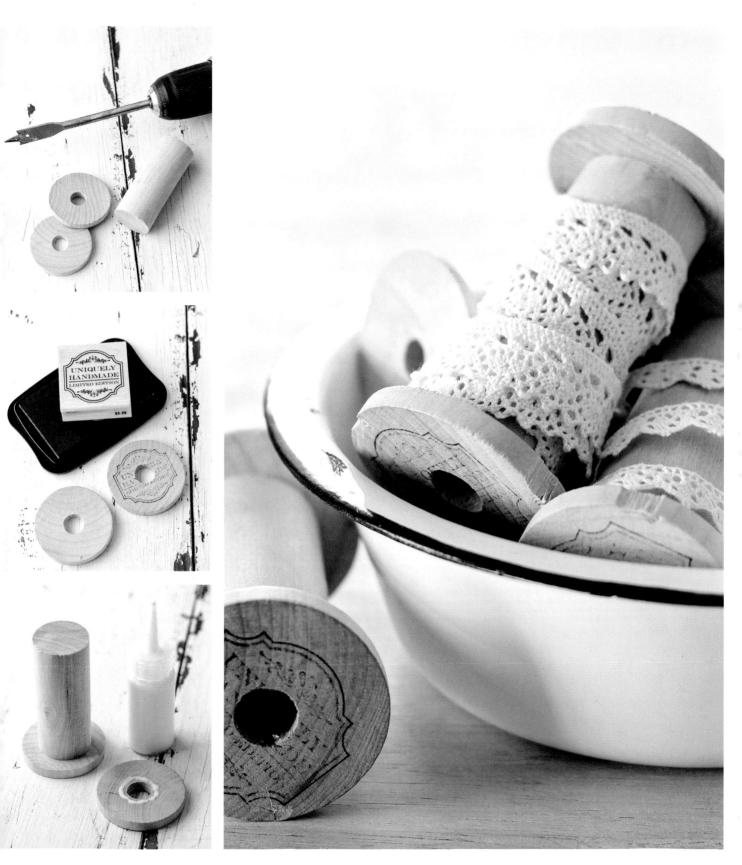

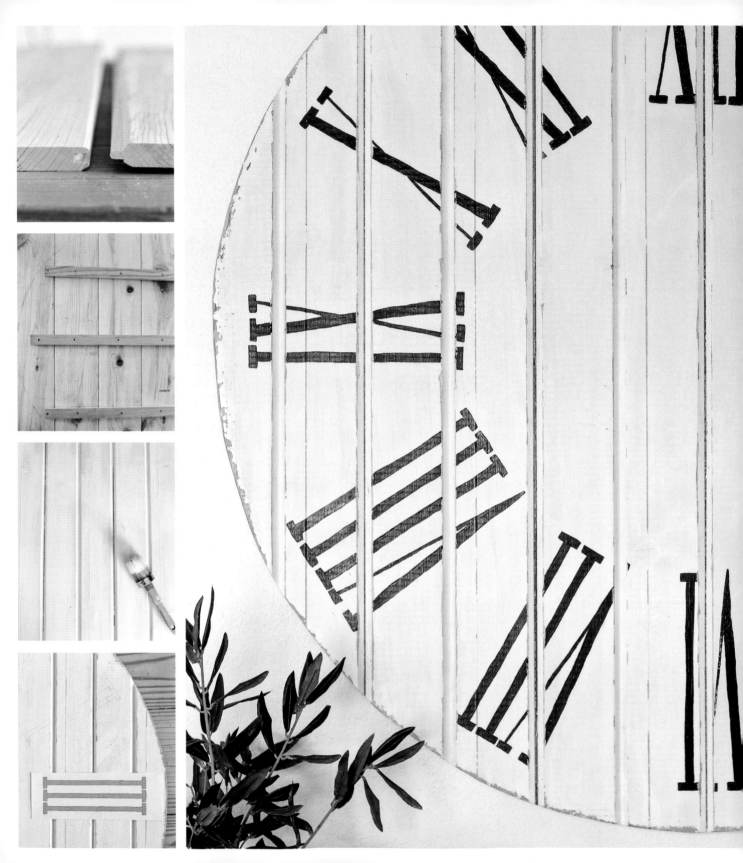

LARGE ROMAN-NUMERAL CLOCK

Large-scale clocks are a great way to fill a blank wall, but they can be pretty pricey if you have to buy one. This oversized clock gets its character from the tongue-and-groove boards and Roman numerals it is made with. This piece looks beautiful with or without clock hands, but if you want to turn it into a functioning clock, you can purchase a kit at a home improvement store. Be sure to buy one large enough to fit the tongue-and-groove boards.

Level of Difficulty: Advanced

SUPPLIES

- *Tape measure*
- *2 (1 x 8) tongue-and-groove boards, 10 feet (305 cm) long*
- *Miter or circular saw*
- *Wood glue*
- *1 (1 x 3) board, 8 feet (244 cm) long*
- *Drill and drill bit*
- *1 ¼-inch (3-cm) screws*
- *Pencil*
- *Jigsaw*
- *White paint*
- *Paintbrush*
- *Computer and printer*
- *Ballpoint pen*
- *Black paint*
- *Sanding block*
- *Two D-ring hangers with screws*
- *Screwdriver*
- *Optional: clock movement kit*

DIRECTIONS

Measure and cut six tongue-and-groove boards to 40 inches (101.5 cm) long using a saw. Apply wood glue in each groove and fit the boards together. Allow the glue to dry for about an hour before moving on to the next step.

Cut two pieces of 1 x 3 to 30 inches (76 cm) long and one piece of 1 x 3 to 34 inches (86.5 cm) long. Attach the 1 x 3s to the back of the tongue-and-groove boards using a drill and 1 ¼-inch (3-cm) screws. The longest 1 x 3 should be in the center and shorter pieces should be spaced 9 inches (23 cm) away on either side. Make sure you have one screw going into each tongue-and-groove board on each piece of 1 x 3.

Draw a 39-inch (99-cm) circle on the back of the tongue-and-groove boards and cut along your pencil line with a jigsaw. The 1 x 3s should all fit inside the circle.

Paint the front of your clock white, and allow it to dry completely, about 4 hours. Use the technique described in the Vintage Label Wooden Stool project (page 125) to print Roman numerals I–XII from your computer, and transfer them onto the clock. Paint the transferred numbers with black paint and allow the paint to dry completely, about 4 hours. If desired, use a sanding block to distress the paint along the edges.

To hang the clock on the wall, screw two D-ring hangers on the back of the clock using a screwdriver.

TIP | *The tongue-and-groove boards give the clock great character, but you can also use 1 x 8 boards instead.*

LINEN-COVERED BOOK

Books are great decorative accessories, whether they are lined up on a bookshelf or stacked on a table. To give the colorful covers a cohesive look, use this technique for wrapping them in a beautiful linen fabric. For an elegant, polished look, face the covered edge of the book out, or if you want to see a little contrast, face the pages of the book out. Either way, this simple trick will add a sense of calm and peacefulness to your space. If you don't want glue getting on your favorite books, pick up a stack of old ones from the thrift store!

Level of Difficulty: Beginner

SUPPLIES

- *Linen fabric*
- *Hardcover book*
- *Scissors*
- *Spray adhesive*
- *Hot-glue gun*
- *Rubber alphabet stamps*
- *Black ink pad*

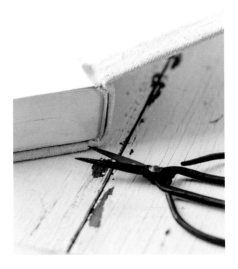

DIRECTIONS

Cut a piece of fabric to cover the outside of the book, leaving about 2 inches (5 cm) of overhang on all the edges. Spray the front and back cover of the book with spray adhesive and wrap the fabric around the book, making sure to smooth out any wrinkles.

Cut two slits in the fabric on each side of the book spine on the top and bottom of the book. Open the front cover of the book and apply hot glue along the top and bottom edges. Fold the fabric over the cover and hold for a few seconds while the glue sets.

Cut the corners of the fabric on the side of the book to make it easier to fold. Apply hot glue along the side of the book and fold the fabric over the cover. Flip the book over to the back cover and repeat the process to secure the fabric on the cover.

Trim the piece of fabric where you made the slits just long enough to tuck into the book spine. Use a small drop of hot glue to secure the fabric inside the spine.

Use rubber alphabet stamps pressed in black ink to add the book title along the spine of the book.

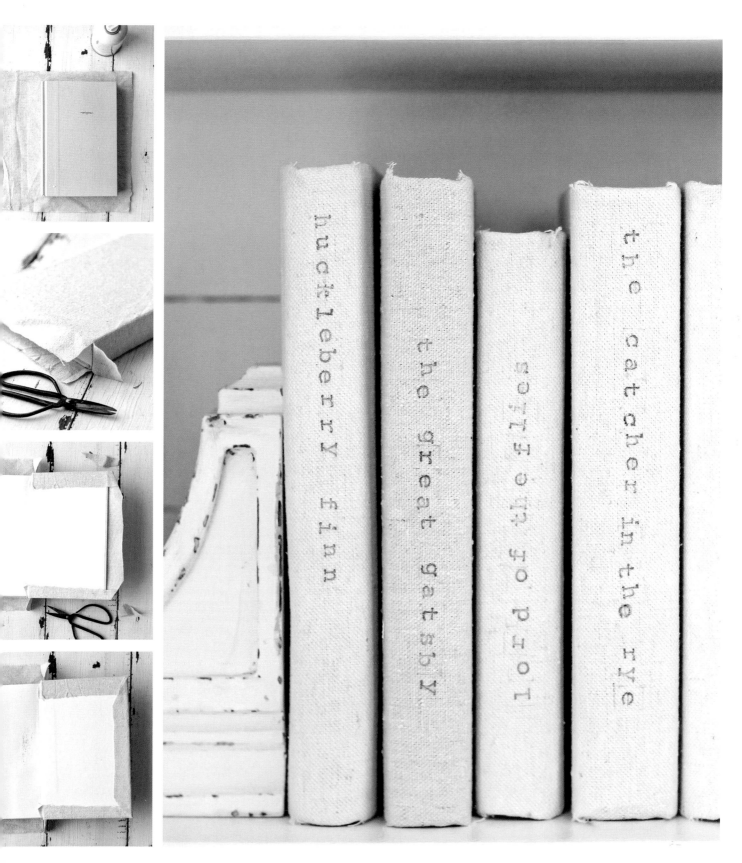

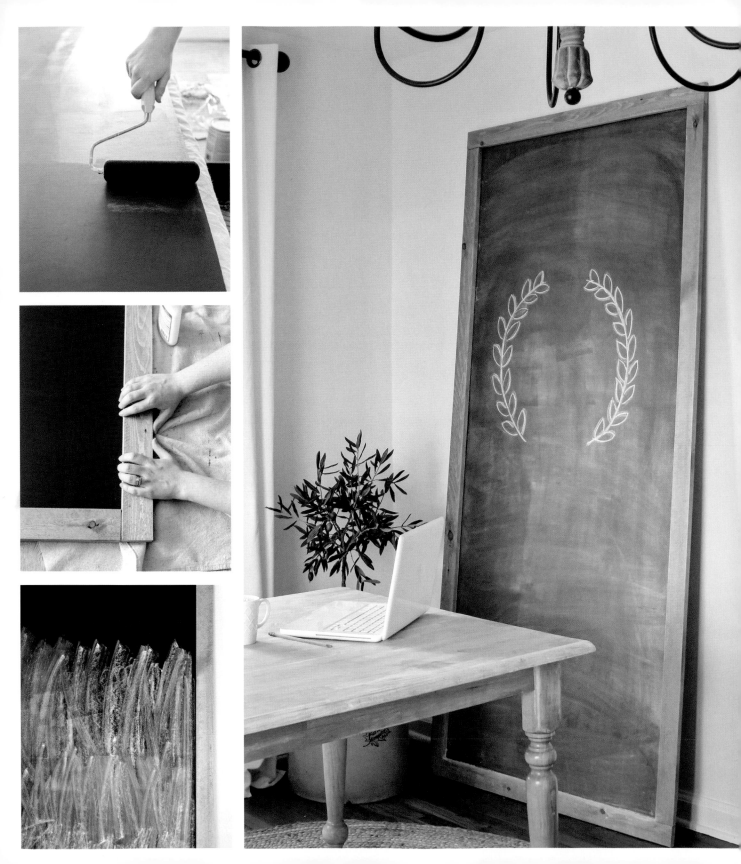

WOOD-FRAMED CHALKBOARD

Chalkboards are fun to decorate with because you can easily change your artwork as often as you like. This super-sized framed chalkboard will make a big impact in a room and can be simply leaned against an open wall. You can adjust these measurements to make a framed chalkboard of any size and add hangers on the back if you would like to hang it on the wall.

Level of Difficulty: Advanced

SUPPLIES

- ¼-inch (6-mm) MDF, 8 feet x 4 feet
- Circular saw
- Tape measure
- Chalkboard paint
- Paint roller
- 3 (1 x 3) boards, 8 feet (244 cm) long
- Wood stain
- Paintbrush
- Clean rags
- Wood glue
- Brad nail gun
- ¾-inch (2-cm) brad nails
- Chalk

DIRECTIONS

Cut the MDF to 80 inches (203 cm) by 36 inches (91.5 cm) using a circular saw. Paint one side of the MDF with 2–3 coats of chalkboard paint, and allow the paint to dry completely between each coat. Follow the instructions on your paint can for specific application details.

Measure and cut two pieces of 1 x 3 to 37 ¼ inches (94.5 cm) long and two pieces of 1 x 3 to 79 inches (200.5 cm) long. Apply stain to the boards using a paintbrush. Allow the stain to penetrate for 5–15 minutes until the desired color is achieved. Wipe the boards with a clean rag to remove any remaining stain, and allow them to dry completely, about 8 hours.

Place the 1 x 3s around the edges of the chalkboard, creating a frame. Attach them using wood glue and ¾-inch (2-cm) brad nails. The ends of the short pieces should butt up to the sides of the long pieces.

To prepare the chalkboard for use, condition the surface by rubbing the side of a piece of chalk over the entire chalkboard. When the surface is thoroughly covered in chalk, erase the board with a dry cloth.

TIP | *MDF, or medium density fiberboard, can be purchased in large sheets at your hardware or home improvement store and is usually found in the same aisle as plywood.*

PLANKED BOOKCASE

Give your bookcase a facelift by adding horizontal planks to the inside. This simple detail will instantly add character and provide a great backdrop to display your favorite reads and accessories. Paint the planks the same color as your bookcase for a classic farmhouse feel or try a different shade for a bolder look.

Level of Difficulty: Intermediate

SUPPLIES

- *Tape measure*
- *¼-inch (6-mm) plywood*
- *Circular saw*
- *Bookcase*
- *Brad nail gun*
- *1-inch (2.5-cm) brad nails*
- *Caulk*
- *Paint*
- *Paintbrush*

ALTERNATIVE | *You can also use beadboard paneling in place of the plywood to get the same planked look.*

DIRECTIONS

Measure and cut the plywood into 4-inch (10-cm) wide planks using a circular saw. Trim the planks to fit inside the bookcase.

Arrange the planks on the bookcase and secure with a nail gun.

Caulk all seams where the plank edges meet the bookcase, and allow the caulk to dry completely, about 30 minutes. Paint the planks and allow the paint to dry completely, about 4 hours.

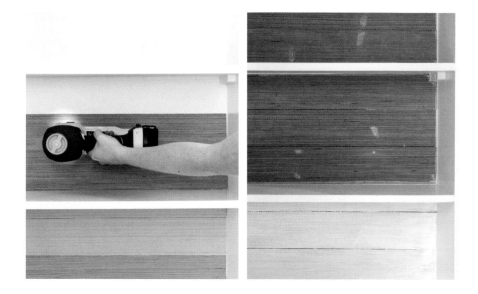

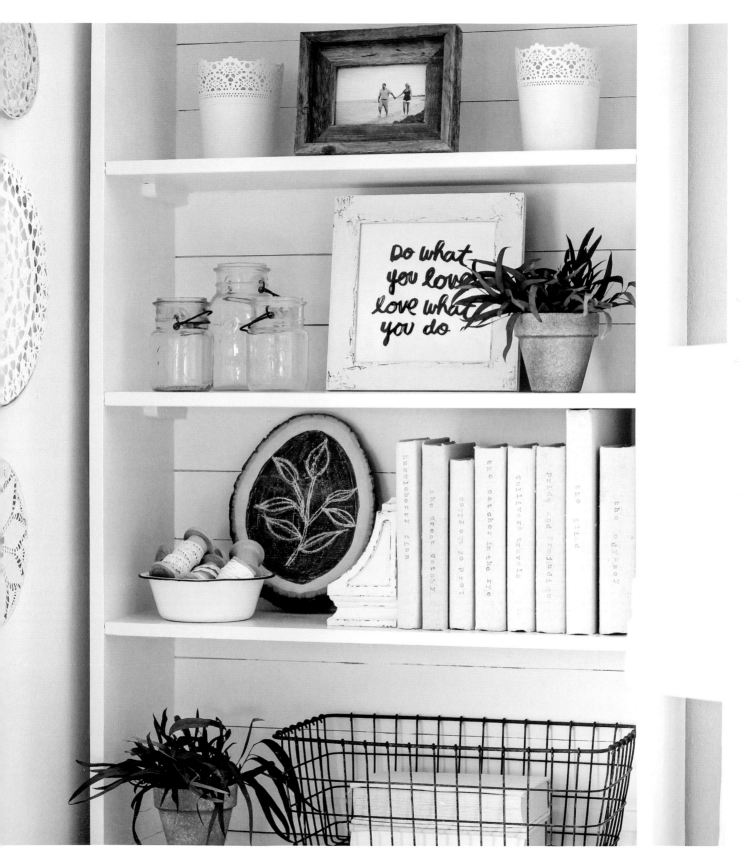

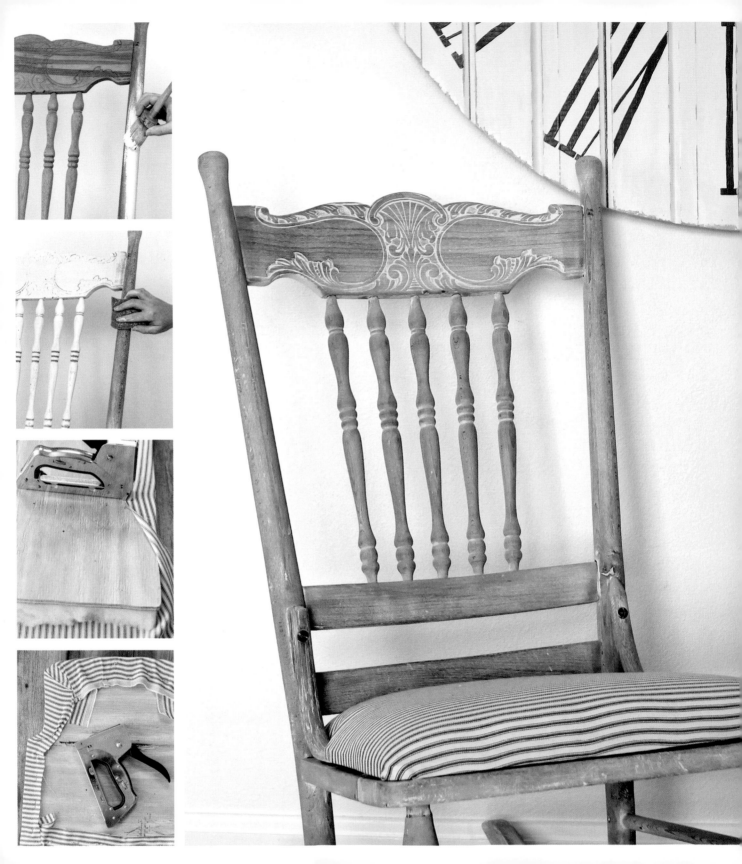

LIME-WASHED CHAIR WITH UPHOLSTERED SEAT

Lime washing was a technique often used by farmers to protect their wood barns from the elements and insects, and it gave the wood a faded, whitewashed look that has become very popular in today's décor. You can easily re-create that look by applying a thin layer of white paint over your wood furniture, then wiping the paint away, leaving a beautiful whitewashed appearance. Wood with an open grain, such as oak, works best for this lime-wash technique, and the more details your piece has, the more cracks and crevices there are for the paint to settle into. Try this technique on tables, dressers, chairs and more.

Level of Difficulty: Beginner

SUPPLIES

- *Wood chair with upholstered seat*
- *Clean rags*
- *White flat-sheen paint*
- *Paintbrush*
- *Sponge*
- *Bucket of water*
- *Pliers*
- *Tape measure*
- *Fabric*
- *Scissors*
- *Staple gun and staples*

DIRECTIONS

Remove the upholstered seat and wipe the entire chair with a damp rag to remove dust. Working in small sections, apply a thin coat of paint to the chair, pushing the paint into the grain of the wood with the paintbrush.

Allow the paint to dry for just a few minutes, then wipe the paint off with a clean rag. You want the paint to remain in the pores of the wood, but not on the main surface. You should be able to see the wood grain again after wiping off the paint. If the paint dries too much and does not wipe off easily, use a damp sponge and a bucket of water to wet the paint. When you finish painting the entire chair, allow it to dry completely, about 4 hours.

To reupholster the seat, remove the old fabric, padding and any staples using pliers. Measure the seat and add about 3 inches (7.5 cm) to each side. Cut a piece of fabric to that measurement and lay it right-side down. Place the chair padding centered on top of the fabric and the seat on top of the padding. Stretch the fabric over the padding and seat and secure with a staple in the center of each side. Continue working your way around the seat, pulling the fabric taut and stapling in place. When finished, reattach the seat to the chair.

TIP | *If the padding in your chair has seen better days, replace it with a new foam pad found at most craft stores.*

TIP | *If your piece of furniture has a lot of small details, try using an old toothbrush to wipe the paint out of tight spaces. Rinse it off in the bucket of water as you go.*

LAYERED PAINT CORBEL BOOKEND

Add interest to your bookshelves with this corbel turned into a unique bookend. If you're lucky, you might be able to find a really old corbel at an antique store, but if you have to purchase one new from the hardware or home improvement store, use this layered paint technique to add some age to it. By layering different paint colors and chipping some of the finish away, you'll end up with a corbel that looks like it's been on an old building for decades. Try this paint technique on furniture, signs or other décor items.

Level of Difficulty: Beginner

SUPPLIES

- *Corbel*
- *Paint in at least three colors*
- *Paintbrush*
- *Sanding block*

DIRECTIONS

Apply the first paint color to the corbel in a thick layer using a paintbrush and allow it to dry completely, about 4 hours. Repeat with the second and third paint colors.

When the corbel is completely dry, use a sanding block to sand the top layer of paint off the corners and edges of the corbel, exposing the colors underneath. Set the corbel on a shelf or table next to a stack of books.

TIP | *You can purchase unfinished wood corbels at hardware and home improvement stores, and the more layers of paint you add to it, the better it will look! Try to find a corbel with lots of details and interesting edges to make the layered paint really stand out.*

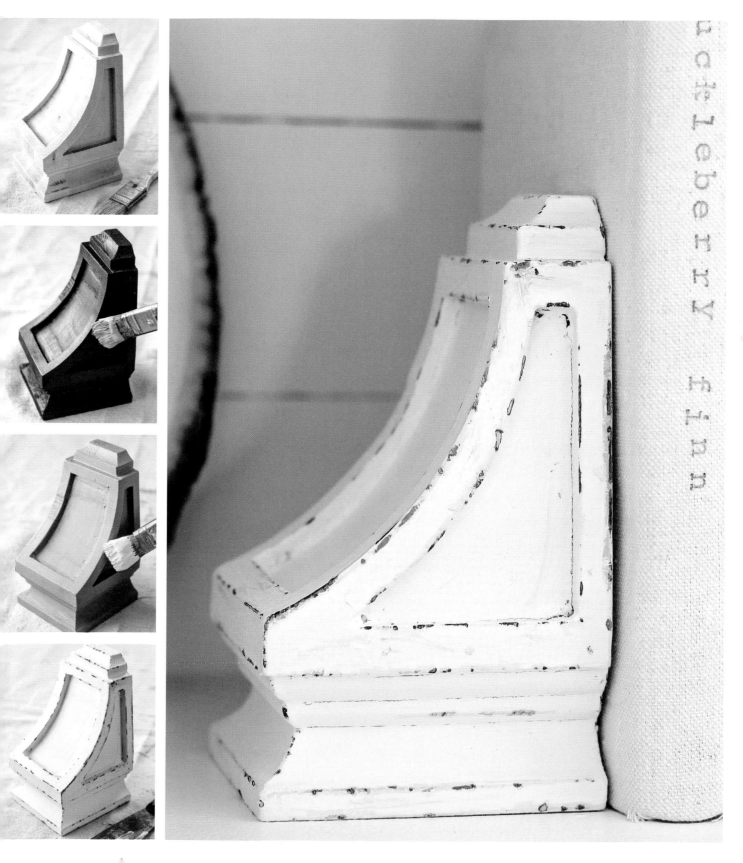

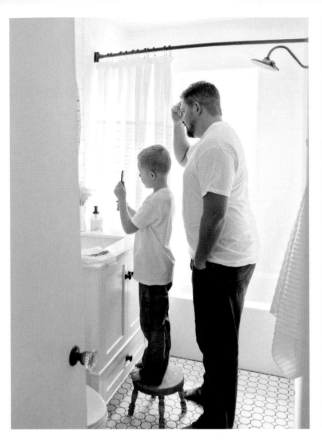
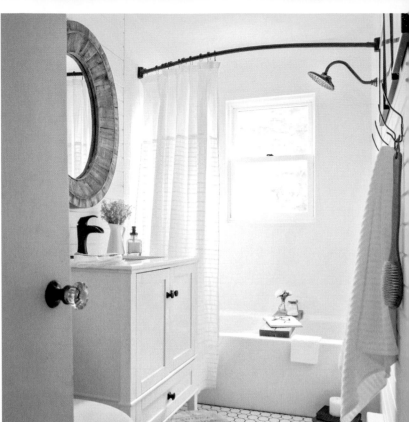
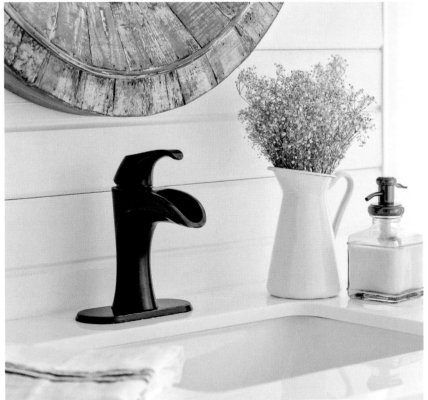
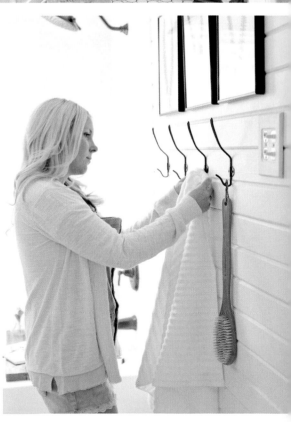

BATHROOM

The bathroom might not be the most exciting place to decorate, but it's a room that you and your family use often and your guests will see as well, so don't forget to add a touch of farmhouse here, too. Bathrooms are generally small spaces, so make the most of every square inch you have. From brushing your teeth in the morning to bathing your kids at night, you probably spend more time in the bathroom than you realize. Give yourself a relaxing retreat that feels clean, bright and cheerful.

We have one bathroom and four people in our little farmhouse, so it was important for me to make this room as open and functional as possible. We replaced the tub and shower and switched out the old vanity for one with more storage. The laminate floor was ripped up and a white mosaic tile was laid using dark gray grout to accentuate the pattern. On the walls we added tongue-and-groove boards and painted them white, which added lots of character and made the room feel cozy and welcoming. A focal point was created with a distressed oval wood mirror hung over the vanity, and large hooks were added to the opposite wall for towels.

In this chapter, I'll show you how to add storage to your bathroom with hanging crates (page 122) and a wood plank tub shelf (page 121) and how to decorate with pressed fern art (page 118) and grain-sack towels (page 126) that you can make yourself! You'll also learn my technique for transferring designs from your computer onto your projects, which you can use on the wood stool (page 125) in this chapter and many other projects throughout the book.

PRESSED FERN FRAMED ART

Inspired by vintage botanical prints, this easy project is a great way to bring a touch of nature into your home and fill up a blank wall. No need to buy expensive artwork, just press clippings from your garden and add them to a picture frame. For a bigger impact, hang a collection of these framed ferns together on the wall.

Level of Difficulty: Beginner

SUPPLIES

- *Fern clippings*
- *Wax paper*
- *Spray adhesive*
- *Thick paper or cardstock*
- *Picture frame*

DIRECTIONS

Place the freshly clipped ferns flat on a piece of wax paper. Place another piece of wax paper on top. Set a heavy object, such as a stack of books, on top of the ferns, and allow 2–3 days for them to dry and be pressed.

Lightly spray the back of each fern with adhesive and arrange them on a thick piece of paper. Gently press the leaves down to make sure they adhere well. Add the paper to a picture frame and hang your work of art.

TIP | Look for fresh, bright-green ferns without any missing leaves or curled, dry edges. Using a variety of shapes and sizes will also make your artwork more interesting! If you cannot find ferns, try pressing flowers such as pansies, peonies or cosmos. Flowers with thin petals work best for pressing!

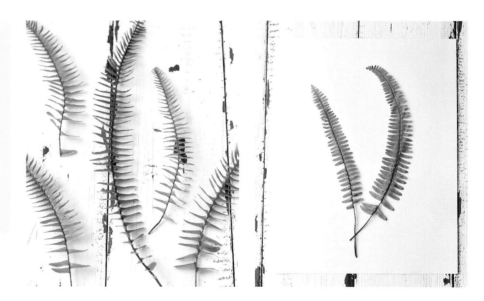

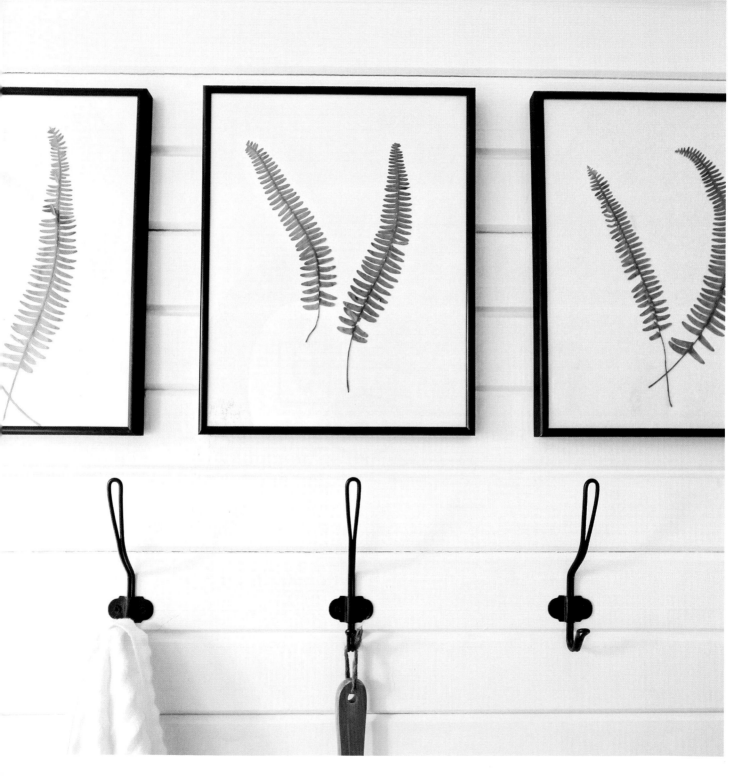

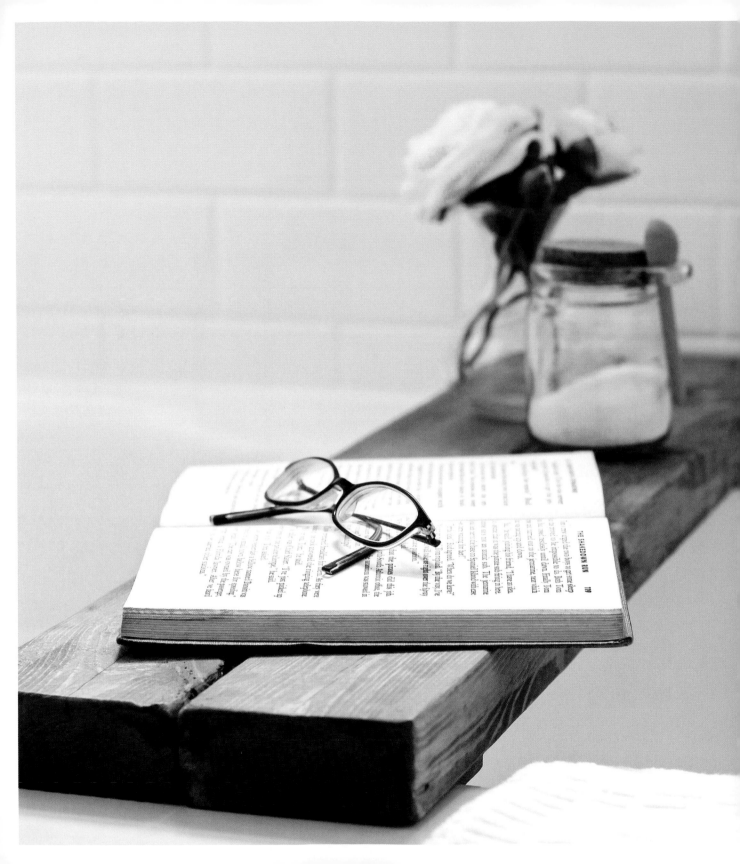

WOODEN PLANK TUB SHELF

When you're taking a relaxing bubble bath at the end of a long day, wouldn't it be great to have a place where you could set a candle, a good book and maybe even a glass of wine? This project creates just that. A few pieces of wood can quickly be transformed into a gorgeous, rustic shelf that fits right over the top of your tub and is easily removed when not in use.

Level of Difficulty: Intermediate

SUPPLIES

- Tape measure
- 2 x 4 board
- Miter or circular saw
- 1 x 2 board
- Wood glue
- Pencil
- Drill
- 1 ½-inch (3.8-cm) screws
- Sanding block
- Clean rags
- Wood stain
- Paintbrush
- Paste wax

DIRECTIONS

Measure the outer width of your bathtub and cut two pieces of 2 x 4 to that length using a saw. Cut two 6-inch (15-cm) pieces from the 1 x 2. Lay the 2 x 4 pieces next to each other, using wood glue in between to hold them together.

Place the shelf on your tub and mark with a pencil where the inside edge of the tub meets the bottom of the shelf on both sides. Place one of the 1 x 2 pieces on each end just inside of your pencil mark. Use wood glue and screws to secure the 1 x 2s to the shelf. The 1 x 2s help hold the 2 x 4s together and also act as a brace so the shelf can't slide off the sides of the tub.

Sand the entire shelf, focusing on the corners and edges to round them slightly. Wipe off dust with a clean rag and apply stain to the wood using a paintbrush. Allow the stain to penetrate for 5–15 minutes until the desired color is achieved. Wipe the wood with a clean rag to remove any remaining stain, and allow it to dry completely, about 8 hours. To seal the wood, apply a layer of paste wax with a paintbrush and buff with a clean rag.

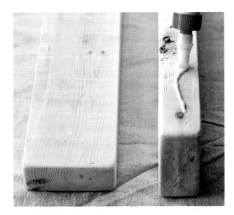
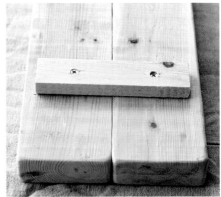

HANGING CRATE STORAGE

Bathrooms often run short on storage space, but these hanging crates make great use of an empty wall, adding storage and plenty of farmhouse charm. You can use them to hold extra towels or toiletries, and these crates would look great in a kids' bedroom or playroom, too!

Level of Difficulty: Intermediate

SUPPLIES

- *D-ring hangers with screws*
- *Wood crate*
- *Screwdriver*
- *Tape measure*
- *Pencil*
- *Level*
- *Drill and drill bit*
- *Wall anchors and screws*
- *Hammer*

DIRECTIONS

Attach two D-ring hangers on the bottom of the crate near the corners using a screwdriver. Measure the distance between your hangers, and mark on the wall with a pencil where you want your crate to hang. Use a level to make sure your crate will hang straight.

Drill two holes in the wall using a drill bit just big enough to fit your wall anchor. Add an anchor to each hole, using a hammer to gently tap them in. Insert a screw into each wall anchor using a screwdriver. Leave the screw sticking out just enough to slide the D-rings onto. Hang the crate on the wall, making sure the D-rings are seated securely on the screws before adding any weight. Repeat the same steps to hang as many crates as you need.

TIPS | *Vintage wood crates are generally easy to find at antique stores, or you can purchase new, unfinished crates from craft stores.*

Use one crate to add storage to a small space, or stack several together to create a large display.

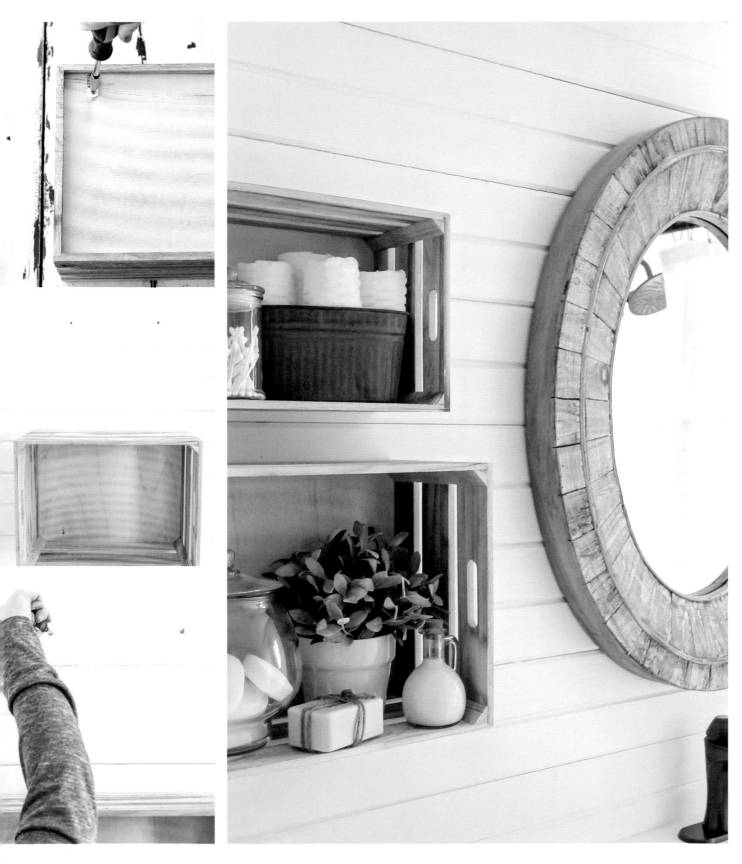

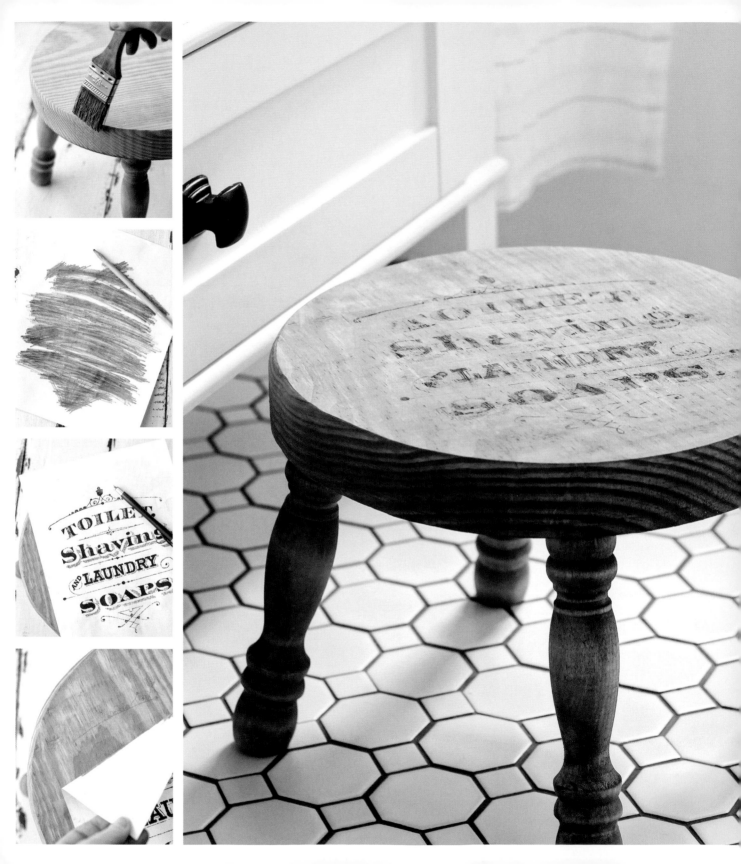

VINTAGE LABEL WOODEN STOOL

This little stool was cute already, but the addition of a vintage soap label on top makes it positively darling. In this tutorial, you'll learn how to easily transfer an image from the computer onto your project without the use of any fancy tools or equipment. See the Family Name Sign, Herb Planter Box, Large Roman-Numeral Clock and Alphabet Chart Art projects on pages 23, 56, 105 and 163 for more ways to use this technique.

Level of Difficulty: Beginner

SUPPLIES

- *Wood stain*
- *Wooden stool*
- *Paintbrush*
- *Clean rags*
- *Computer and printer*
- *White printer paper*
- *Pencil*
- *Tape*
- *Ballpoint pen*
- *Black paint pen or permanent marker*
- *Sandpaper*
- *Paste wax*

DIRECTIONS

Apply stain to the entire stool using a paintbrush. Allow the stain to penetrate for 5–15 minutes until the desired color is achieved. Wipe the wood with a clean rag to remove any remaining stain, and allow it to dry completely, about 8 hours.

Print a vintage label image from the computer onto white printer paper. Flip the paper to the backside and use a pencil to heavily shade over the design. You can hold the paper up to a window to make the image easier to see while you shade.

Center the label image on top of the stool with the shaded side down. Tape the sides of the paper to hold it in place. Carefully trace over the entire label design with a ballpoint pen, then remove the paper. The design should be transferred to the stool in pencil. Use a black paint pen or permanent marker to trace over the pencil marks.

Lightly sand over the design to give it an aged appearance. Seal the wood by applying a layer of paste wax with a paintbrush and buffing with a clean rag.

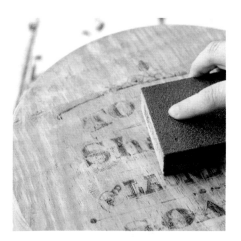

TIPS | *You can often find unfinished wood stools at craft stores or search for a vintage one at an antique store.*

There are some fantastic sources for vintage graphics online, but the one I use most often is TheGraphicFairy.com. Just search for the type of design you're looking for (in this case, a vintage soap label), and print right from the website.

GRAIN-SACK STRIPE TOWEL

*Grain-sack stripes instantly evoke the farmhouse feeling, and this simple tutorial will show you how to easily
add them to a pretty towel for the bathroom. Try this technique on pillow covers, upholstered chair seats
and even furniture.*

Level of Difficulty: Beginner

SUPPLIES

- Iron and ironing board
- Flour-sack towel
- Drop cloth or newspaper
- Painter's tape
- Small bowl
- Acrylic craft paint
- Fabric-paint medium
- Paintbrush

DIRECTIONS

Wash, dry and iron your flour-sack towel to remove any wrinkles, and set it
on newspaper or a drop cloth to protect your work surface. Use thin strips of
painter's tape to create a striped design on the ends of your towel. Press the
edges down firmly to make sure the tape adheres to the towel.

In a small bowl, mix the craft paint and fabric-paint medium in a 2:1 ratio. Check
the instructions on your paint medium to confirm the correct ratio before using.
Carefully apply paint inside the taped stripes with a paintbrush, being careful
not to push paint underneath the tape. After all the stripes are painted, remove
the tape, and allow the paint to dry for 24–48 hours before using.

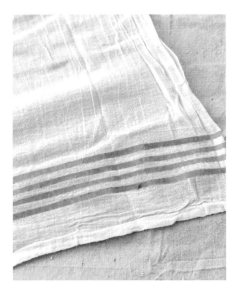
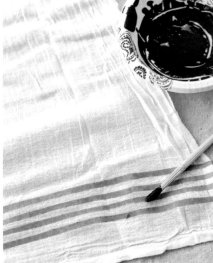

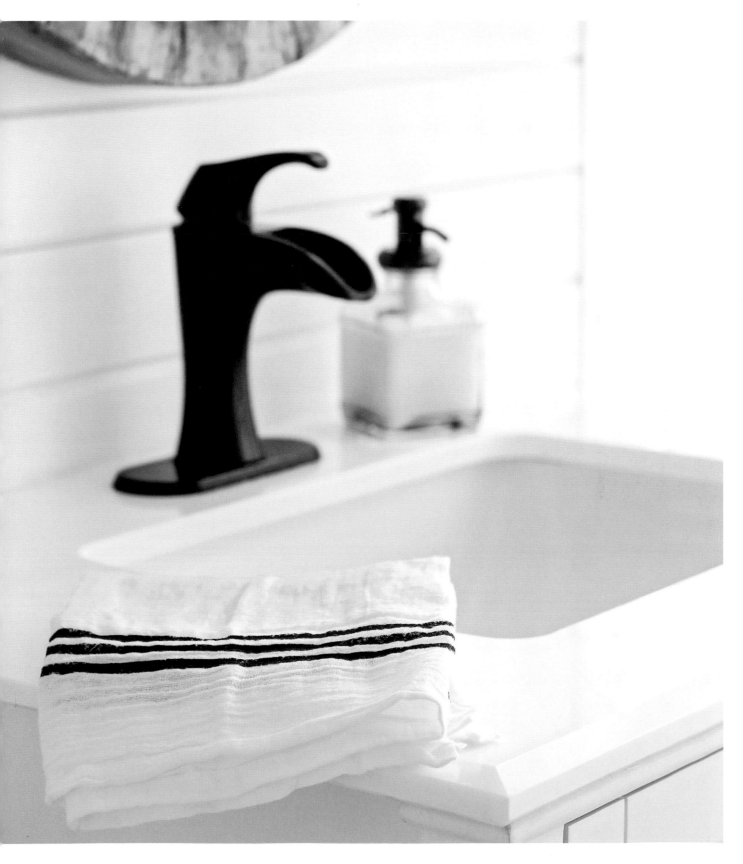

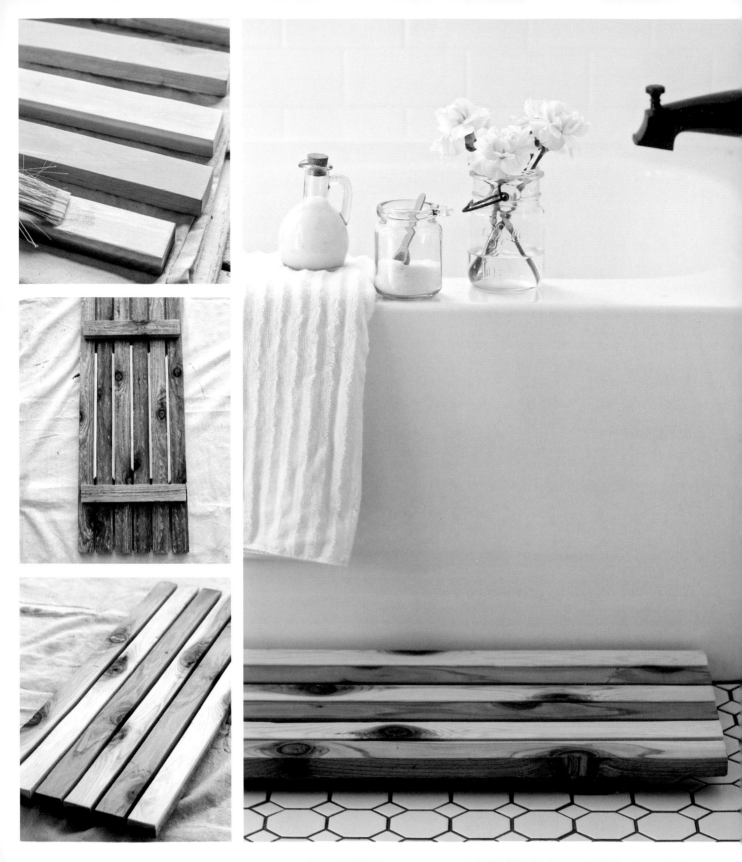

WOODEN BATH MAT

Make your bathroom feel like a luxurious spa retreat with this gorgeous wooden bath mat. Built with cedar boards and sealed with teak oil, this wooden mat holds up well to moisture and adds a great rustic appeal to your space. This tutorial shows you how to create a mat that is 26 x 10 ½ inches (66 x 26.5 cm), but you can easily customize the dimensions to fit your needs.

Level of Difficulty: Intermediate

SUPPLIES

- *Tape measure*
- *2 (1 x 2) cedar boards, 8 feet (244 cm) long*
- *Miter or circular saw*
- *Fine-grit sandpaper*
- *Clean rags*
- *Teak oil*
- *Paintbrush*
- *Wood glue*
- *Brad nail gun*
- *1-inch (2.5-cm) brad nails*

DIRECTIONS

Measure and cut six pieces of the cedar boards to 26 inches (66 cm) long and two pieces to 9 ½ inches (24 cm) long using a saw. Sand each board with fine-grit sandpaper until all the rough spots are gone and the boards are completely smooth. One side of the wood will be rougher than the other, but you will use the rougher side as the bottom of the mat. Wipe the boards with a clean rag to remove dust.

Apply teak oil with a paintbrush in a heavy layer on every side of the boards, using the instructions on the container as a guide. When the teak oil has set, about 30 minutes, place the six long boards next to each other with the smooth side facing down and spaced about ¼ inch (6 mm) apart. Place the two short boards across the long boards about 6 inches (15 cm) in from each end. Apply a small amount of wood glue to the short boards and attach them to the long boards using a brad nail gun and 1-inch (2.5-cm) brad nails.

Flip the bath mat over and place it on the floor in front of your tub or shower.

TIP | *I used two wooden paint-mixing sticks as spacers in between each long board, but you could also use a couple of quarters as spacers.*

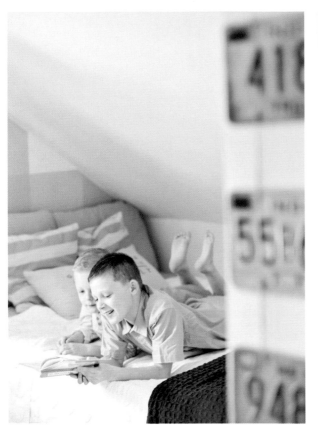
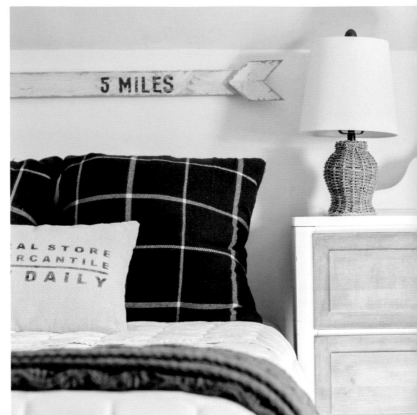
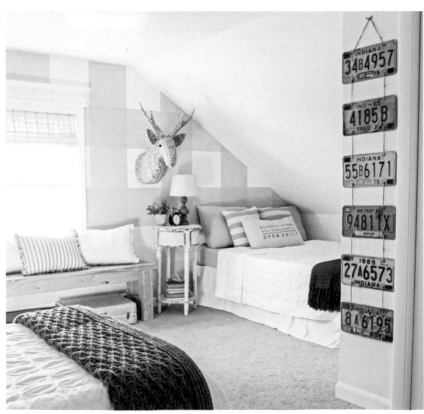
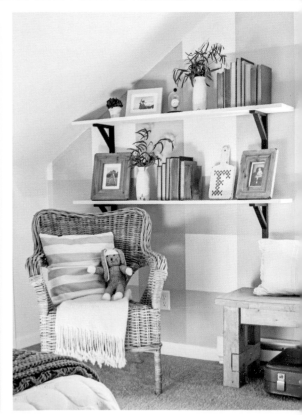

KIDS' BEDROOM

A kids' room is a fun space to decorate because it's where they use their imagination and lay their little heads to sleep at night. You can be more playful with the design and try new things that you might not necessarily want in the main living areas of your home. It's important for the kids to love their room as much as you do, so include them in the design plan, and let them help paint walls and create the artwork. I find that kids take better care of their room and furniture when they know the hard work and time that went into them.

Our boys' bedroom is one of the few rooms in the house that includes color because I know that they don't love neutrals quite as much as their momma does. I painted most of the walls white and added a fun accent wall in a large-scale gingham pattern to give the room some personality and warmth. The boys' bedding is mostly white with accents of color in the pillows and blankets, and I added open shelving along one wall to give them a place for their favorite bedtime stories and trinkets. Baskets and bins hold their stuffed animals and sports equipment, and a wicker deer head adds a touch of rustic whimsy.

In this chapter, I'll show you how to create stenciled pillow covers (page 139), a license plate gallery wall (page 132) and a wooden arrow sign (page 147) to decorate with, along with aged galvanized bins (page 140) and repurposed dresser drawers for storage (page 144). You'll also find out how to whitewash a dresser (page 135) and create an accent wall inspired by a classic farmhouse fabric (page 136).

HANGING LICENSE PLATE GALLERY WALL

Instead of a traditional art display, try a unique gallery of old license plates! By hanging the plates on twine, you save a lot of holes in your wall while adding a ton of rustic charm to your space. For a fun twist, look for license plates from your own home state!

Level of Difficulty: Beginner

SUPPLIES

- *Collection of old license plates*
- *Twine*
- *Scissors*
- *Hammer and nails*

DIRECTIONS

Starting from the bottom of the license plate, thread a piece of twine through the holes on one side of the plate. Tie a knot at the bottom of the license plate to hold it in place. Tie another knot about 3 inches (7.5 cm) up from the top of the license plate and add another plate to the twine. Continue adding license plates and leave about 6 inches (15 cm) of twine at the top of the last license plate.

Use another piece of twine to thread through the holes on the other side of the license plates. Try to keep the plates evenly spaced as you go and leave about 6 inches (15 cm) of twine at the top on this side as well. When you have all the plates threaded with twine on both sides, tie the ends of both twine pieces together in a tight double knot. Add a nail to the wall using a hammer and hang the knotted twine on the nail.

TIP | *You can find old license plates at many antique stores, and I think that the older they are, the better!*

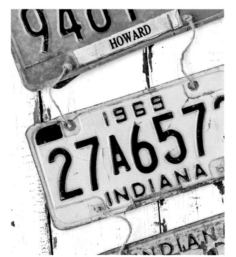
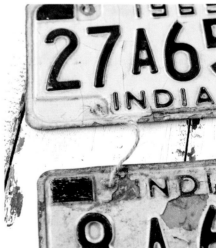

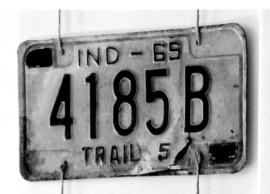

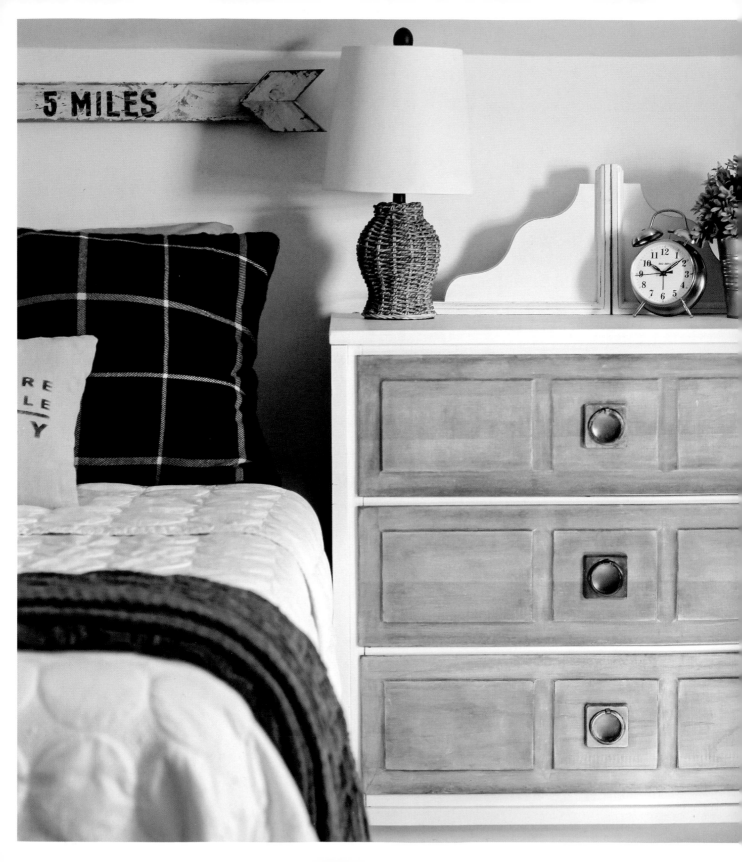

WHITE AND WOOD DRESSER MAKEOVER

Refinishing your existing furniture saves money and allows you to keep family heirlooms that might not match your style. There are endless ways to refinish old furniture, but this technique will show you how to lighten up a dark wood dresser by painting the outside a light, creamy white and whitewashing the wood drawer fronts. By applying a coat of white wax over the drawers, you are able to tone down the dark wood, while keeping the beautiful wood grain underneath.

Level of Difficulty: Beginner

SUPPLIES

- *Dresser*
- *Sanding block*
- *Clean rags*
- *White chalk paint*
- *Paintbrushes*
- *Clear paste wax*
- *Small bowl*

DIRECTIONS

Remove the drawers from the dresser and take any hardware or knobs off the drawers. Lightly sand every surface to prepare it for paint. Wipe the dresser and drawers with a damp clean rag to remove dust.

Paint 2–3 coats of white paint on the dresser, allowing about 2 hours of drying time between each coat. When the dresser is dry, apply clear paste wax with a paintbrush and buff with a clean rag.

For the drawers, scoop a small amount of clear paste wax into a bowl and mix in drops of white paint until the wax turns white. Apply an even layer of the white wax to the drawer fronts with a paintbrush and buff with a clean rag. Reinstall any hardware you took off and place the drawers back inside the dresser.

TIPS | *Chalk paint is a special type of paint that eliminates the need to sand or prime before painting. You can also use regular latex paint, but make sure to apply primer before painting.*

To give the drawer hardware an aged look, apply the same white wax used on the drawer fronts.

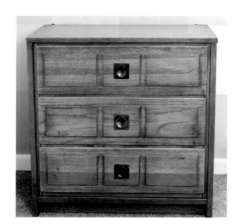
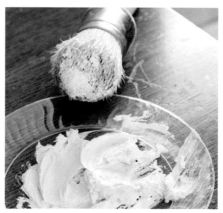

GINGHAM PAINTED ACCENT WALL

Use the pattern of classic farmhouse fabrics on a bigger scale to create a stunning accent wall. This tutorial will show you how to mimic the look of gingham with painted stripes, which creates a super cozy atmosphere for a bedroom or living room. This project takes a few days to complete due to the drying time required, but it is actually a really simple process that will make a big impact in your room.

Level of Difficulty: Intermediate

SUPPLIES

- *Two paint colors (base color and accent color)*
- *Sheet of paper*
- *Tape measure*
- *Painter's tape*
- *Level*
- *Mixing glaze*
- *Paint roller*

DIRECTIONS

Paint the entire wall with your base color choice, and allow it to dry at least 12 hours. Meanwhile, measure the height of your wall and determine how wide you want your stripes to be. Ideally, the stripe width should divide evenly into the height of the wall. (Our wall height was 78 inches [198 cm], so we went with six 13-inch [33-cm] stripes for this room.) Draw a diagram on a sheet of paper to help decide where each stripe should go.

Measure and tape off your horizontal stripes for the accent paint color with painter's tape, making sure to keep the lines level, and press the tape firmly to the wall. Paint inside the tape lines with the base color, and allow the paint to dry, about 4 hours. This will seal the stripe edges and prevent the accent color from bleeding underneath.

Mix two parts mixing glaze with one part accent color paint, and paint the mixture on the horizontal stripes using a paint roller. Peel the tape off as soon as you finish painting, and allow the paint to dry at least 12 hours.

Repeat the same process for your vertical stripes. Measure and tape off stripes in the same width and paint them with the same 2:1 paint mixture used on the horizontal stripes. Peel the tape off as soon as you finish painting, and allow the paint to dry completely.

TIP | *Because the accent color is slightly translucent from the mixing glaze, try to paint as evenly as possible to avoid a splotchy finish.*

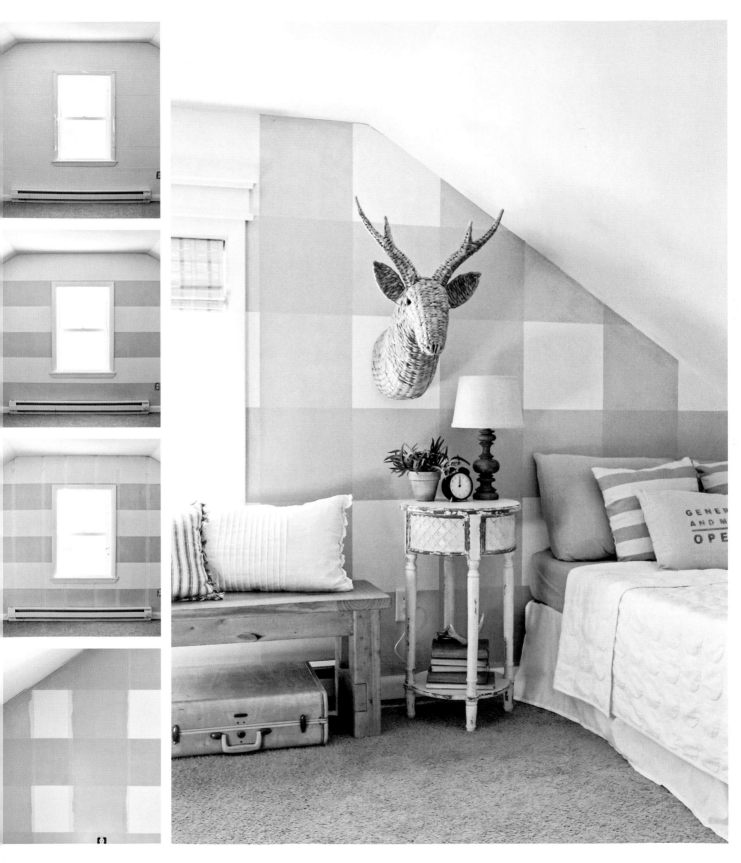

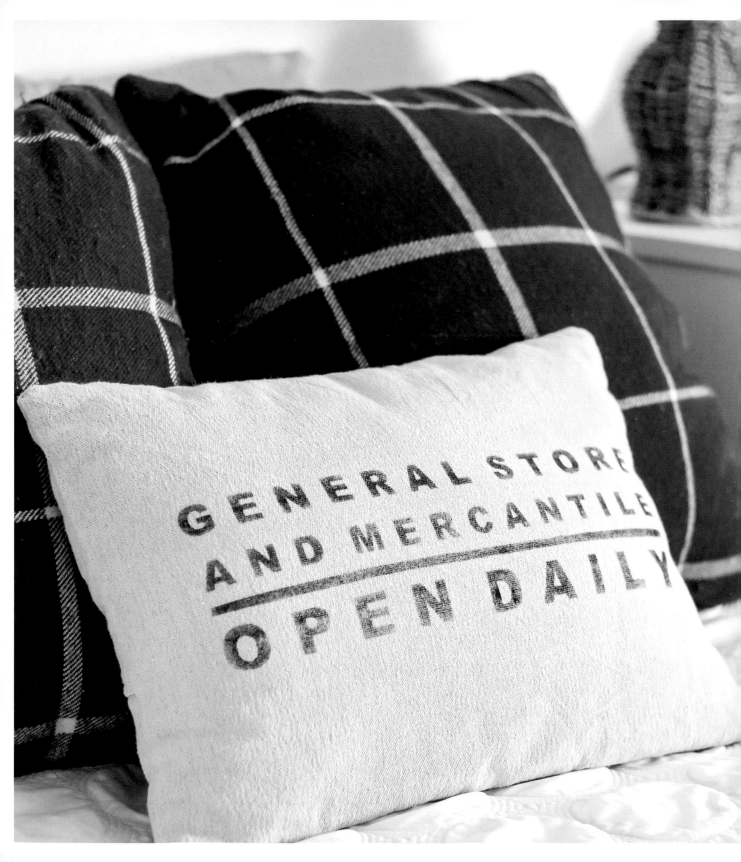

STENCILED LINEN PILLOW COVER

Pillows are an easy way to accessorize your living room or bedroom, and this stenciled linen pillow cover is a quick project that will make your space extra cozy. The neutral linen fabric makes a lovely background for the stenciled letters that look beautifully faded over time. Buy a pillow cover from the store, or make your own from a drop cloth for an inexpensive alternative.

Level of Difficulty: Beginner

SUPPLIES

- *Electronic cutting machine with adhesive vinyl, or alphabet stencils*
- *Linen pillow cover*
- *Small bowl*
- *Acrylic craft paint*
- *Fabric-paint medium*
- *Paintbrush*
- *Paper plate*
- *Pillow form*

DIRECTIONS

Create your own stencil using a cutting machine or use store-bought alphabet stencils. Lay the pillow cover on a flat surface and center your vinyl stencil on the front of the cover.

In a small bowl, mix the craft paint and fabric-paint medium in a 2:1 ratio. Check the instructions on your paint medium to confirm the correct ratio before using. To give the pillow a timeworn look, dip your brush in the paint mixture, and wipe most of the paint off on a paper plate. Dab the paintbrush over your stencil, adding a small amount of paint at a time. Keep adding paint until you can read the lettering, but the fabric is not overly saturated with paint. Remove the stencil, and allow the paint to dry for 24–48 hours before using. When dry, insert a pillow form.

TIPS | *If you do a lot of projects or crafting, investing in a cutting machine will allow you to easily create custom stencils and much more. If purchasing a cutting machine isn't an option, craft stores have a variety of letter and number stencils to choose from! Just trace the outline of the stencils on the pillow cover using a pencil, and fill in the pencil marks with paint.*

If you need to wash the pillow cover, turn it inside out and use the gentle wash setting.

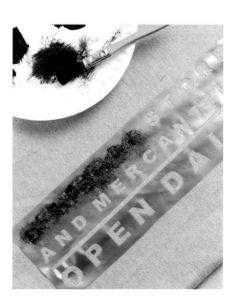

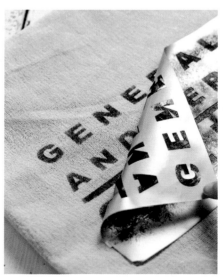

AGED GALVANIZED METAL BIN

Galvanized metal is often used in farmhouse décor, and this easy tutorial will give your shiny, brand-new metal a beautifully aged, rustic patina. Each piece of galvanized metal is different and will have its own unique look, so try this technique on buckets, bins, vases, planters, trays and more!

Level of Difficulty: Beginner

SUPPLIES

- *Galvanized metal bucket or garbage can*
- *Garbage bag*
- *Rubber gloves*
- *Acidic toilet bowl cleaner*
- *Paintbrush*
- *Garden hose*

DIRECTIONS

Take the galvanized metal outside and set it on a large garbage bag to protect the surface underneath. Wearing gloves to protect your hands, squirt the toilet bowl cleaner all over the metal and use a paintbrush to spread the cleaner over the entire piece. The cleaner will slowly corrode the finish on the metal, removing the shininess and giving it a beautiful aged look. Depending on the metal you're using, it may take anywhere from 2–8 hours to age the piece. Reapply the cleaner as needed to achieve the desired look.

When you are happy with the finish, carefully wash the cleaner off the metal with a garden hose. Allow the metal to air dry completely before bringing it inside.

TIPS | *I used Zep Acidic Toilet Bowl Cleaner for this project, but any strong toilet bowl cleaner should work. I would avoid using any natural or chemical-free cleaners, as they may not work as well.*

Try this technique on the Galvanized Metal Flower Bucket (page 51)!

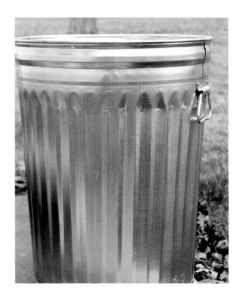
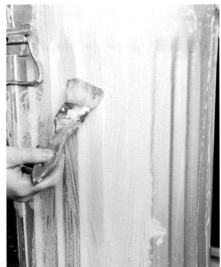

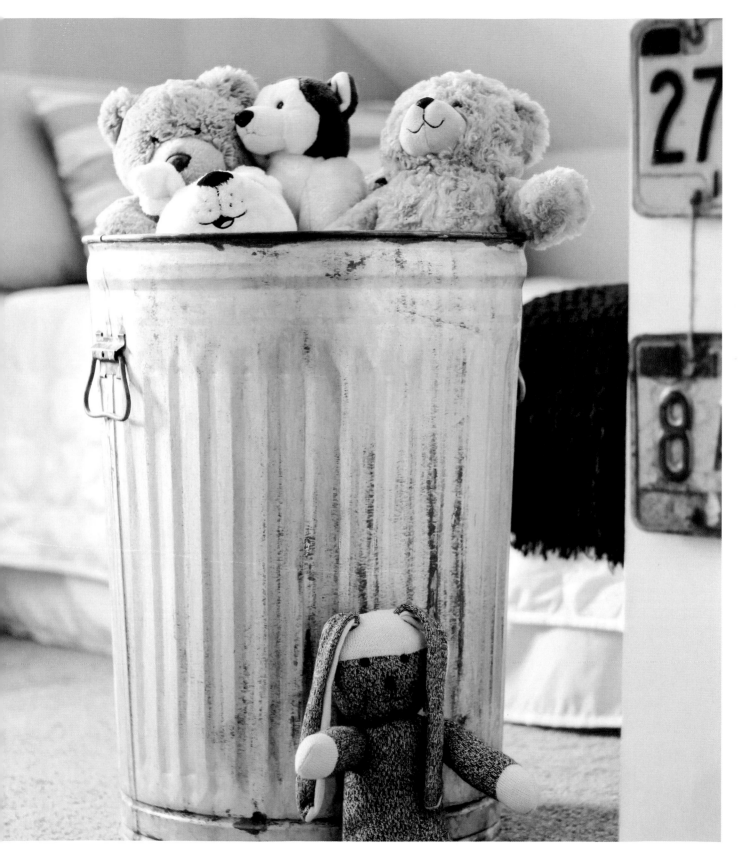

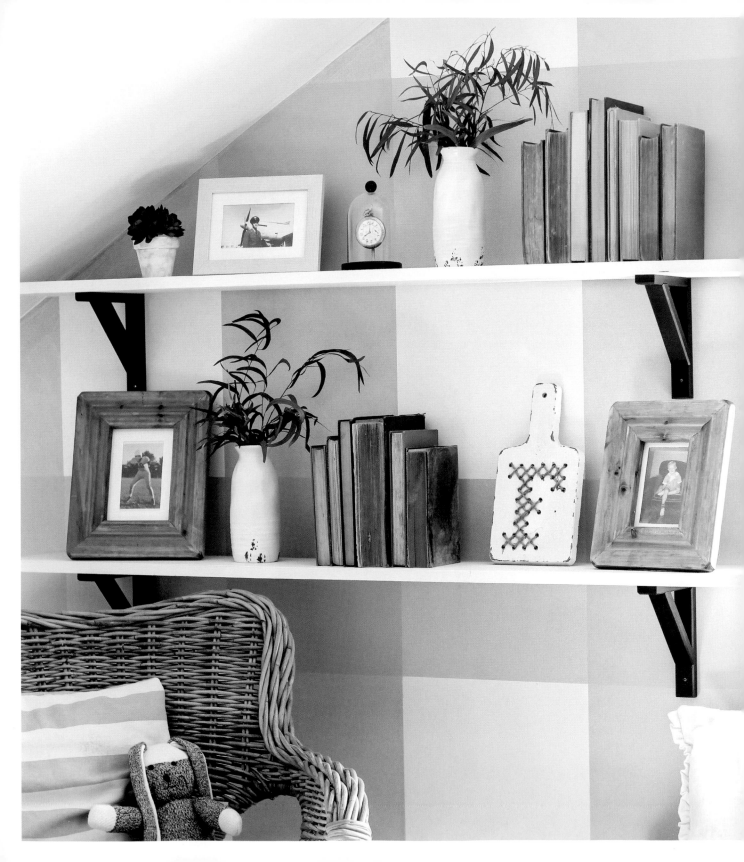

EASY OPEN SHELVING

Open shelving is perfect to store and display items when you want to keep the room airy, yet organized, and it's as easy as buying shelf brackets from the store and adding a wood shelf. Get creative by using barn wood for the shelf or metal brackets for a more industrial look. You can also use these shelves in a kitchen for plates and mugs, in an office for books or in a bathroom for towels.

Level of Difficulty: Intermediate

SUPPLIES

- *Tape measure*
- *1 x 8 board*
- *Miter or circular saw*
- *Paint*
- *Paintbrush*
- *2 shelf brackets*
- *Wall anchors with screws*
- *Drill and drill bit*
- *Hammer*
- *¾-inch (2-cm) screws*

DIRECTIONS

Measure the wall for your open shelving and determine how long your shelves will be. Cut a 1 x 8 board to that length using a saw. Paint all sides of the shelf, and allow it to dry completely, about 4 hours.

Attach your shelf brackets to the wall using wall anchors and screws. Measure so that your brackets will sit about 6 inches (15 cm) in from the shelf ends. Drill a hole in the wall using a drill bit just big enough to fit your anchor. Use a hammer to gently tap the anchor into the hole. Insert a screw through the pre-drilled holes in the bracket and screw it into the anchor using a drill.

When the shelf is dry, place it centered on the brackets. Secure the shelf on the brackets by adding a ¾-inch (2-cm) screw through the pre-drilled hole on the bottom of the bracket underneath the shelf. Add as many shelves as you need to store or display items.

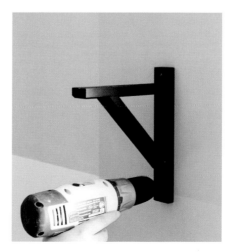
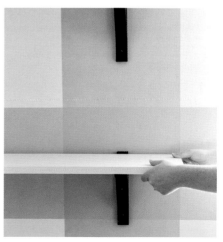

DRESSER DRAWER STORAGE BOX

If you have an old dresser that has seen better days, make sure to save the drawers for this easy storage solution!
Add a few caster wheels to the bottom of the drawers and slide them under a bed for hidden but easily accessible
extra storage.

Level of Difficulty: Intermediate

SUPPLIES

- *Old dresser drawer*
- *Sanding block*
- *Clean rags*
- *Paint*
- *Paintbrush*
- *Paste wax*
- *4 small caster wheels*
- *½-inch (13-mm) screws*
- *Screwdriver*

DIRECTIONS

Remove any knobs or hardware on the drawer, and sand the entire piece with a sanding block to remove the old finish and prepare the drawer for paint. Wipe off dust with a clean rag, and paint both the inside and outside of the drawer. Allow the paint to dry completely, about 4 hours, then seal the wood by applying a layer of paste wax with a paintbrush and buff with a clean rag.

When the drawer is dry, screw a caster into each corner on the bottom of the drawer using ½-inch (13-mm) screws and a screwdriver. Reinstall the knobs, and slide the drawer underneath a bed for easily accessible storage.

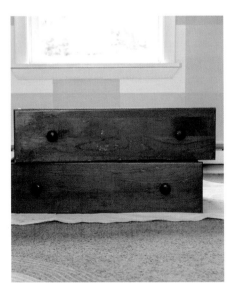 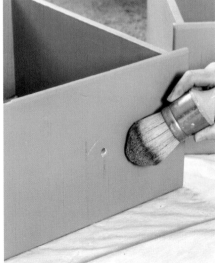

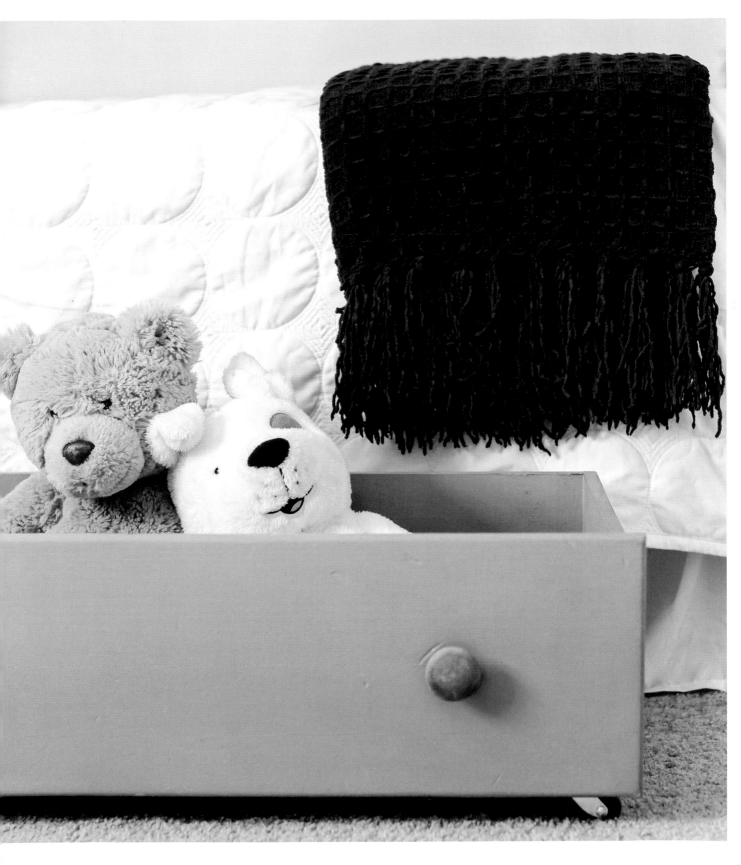

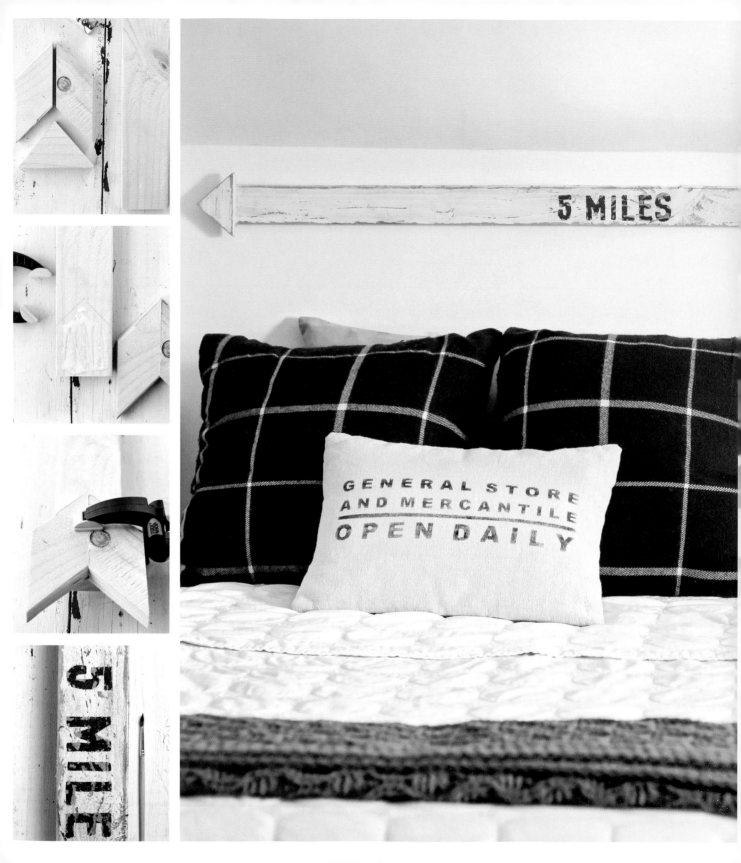

WOODEN ARROW SIGN

Which way to the next town? This wooden arrow sign is the perfect rustic piece to add a touch of whimsy to your walls. You can use it alone or as part of a gallery wall, and the entire thing is made from one small piece of lumber. The narrow design makes this a great piece to add to small spaces above doorways and windows!

Level of Difficulty: Advanced

SUPPLIES

- *Tape measure*
- *1 (1 x 3) board, 6 feet (183 cm) long*
- *Miter saw*
- *Wood glue*
- *Hammer and nails*
- *Clamps*
- *Sanding block*
- *Clean rags*
- *Paint*
- *Paintbrush*

DIRECTIONS

Measure and cut a piece of 1 x 3 to 4 inches (10 cm) long using a miter saw. Cut the ends at an opposite 40° angle, creating a point in the center. This piece will be the tip of your arrow.

Cut another piece of 1 x 3 to 2 ¾ inches (7 cm) long using 45° angles in the same direction. Repeat this step to cut a second piece 2 ¾ inches (7 cm) long. Together, these will become the back of the arrow.

Cut a piece of 1 x 3 to 36 inches (91.5 cm) long using a straight cut. Add wood glue to the tip and back pieces, and attach them to the 36-inch (91.5-cm) 1 x 3 with a hammer and nails. Use clamps to hold the pieces together while nailing everything in place.

Sand all the wood and wipe off dust with a clean rag. Paint the arrow with a paintbrush and allow it to dry completely, about 4 hours. If desired, distress the arrow by sanding areas of paint off the wood.

CROSS-STITCH MONOGRAM

This isn't your grandmother's cross-stitch! This fun piece of art features traditional cross-stitch on a large scale, and you can personalize it whatever way your heart desires. Just drill holes through a piece of wood and thread twine through the holes to create a one-of-a-kind monogram for your space.

Level of Difficulty: Intermediate

SUPPLIES

- *Piece of scrap wood or an old cutting board*
- *Paint*
- *Paintbrush*
- *Scissors*
- *Grid paper*
- *Pencil*
- *Tape*
- *Drill and drill bit*
- *Twine*
- *Large sewing needle*

DIRECTIONS

Paint a small cutting board or piece of scrap wood, and allow the paint to dry completely, about 4 hours. Cut a piece of grid paper the same size as your board. Use the grid lines to draw a pattern for your monogram, using an X where each cross-stitch should go.

Tape the grid paper on top of the board, and use a sharp object (such as a screw or pen tip) to make an indent in the wood at the four points of each X. Remove the paper and drill a hole in each indent using a drill bit just big enough to slide your twine through.

Cut a long piece of twine and tie a knot in one end. Thread your needle on the other end and cross-stitch your pattern starting from the back of the board. When finished, tie a knot to secure the twine on the back of the board, and trim any excess twine with scissors.

> TIP | *Get creative with your choice of wood. I had an old cutting board I wasn't using, but a piece of barn wood or beadboard would be great, too!*

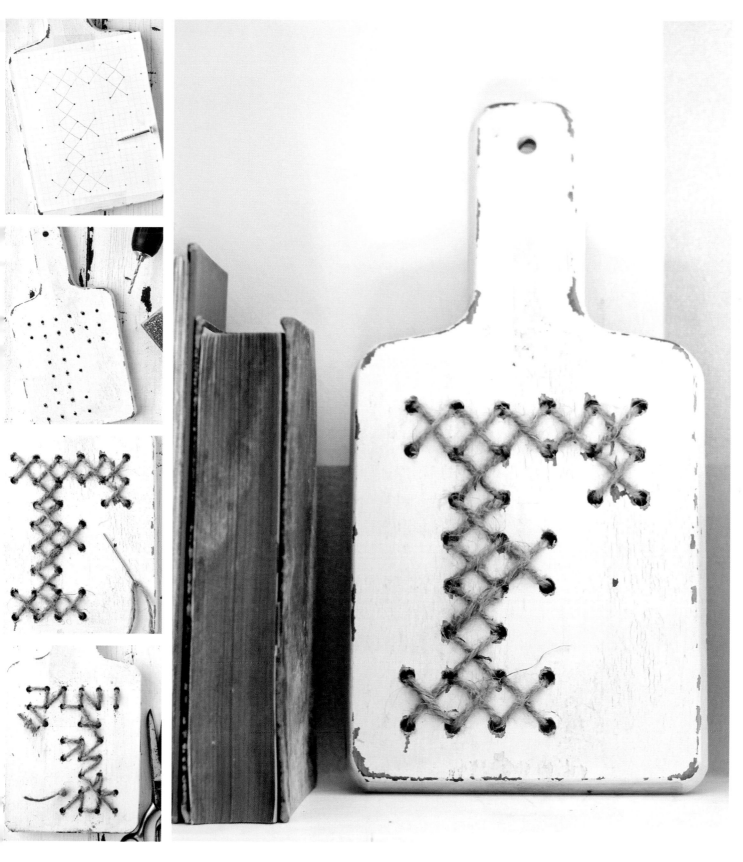

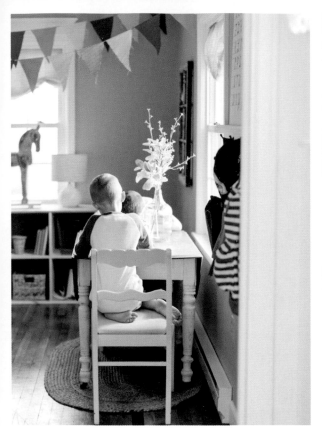

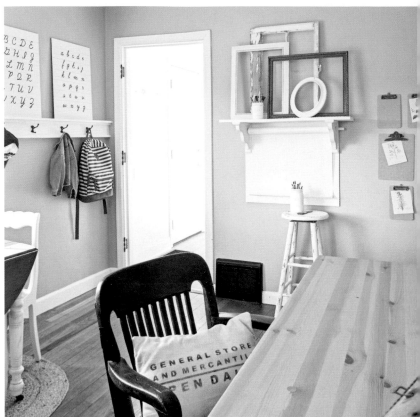

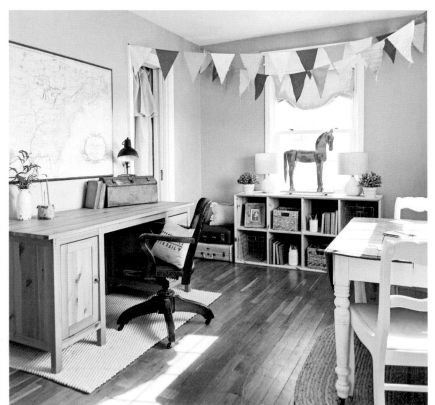

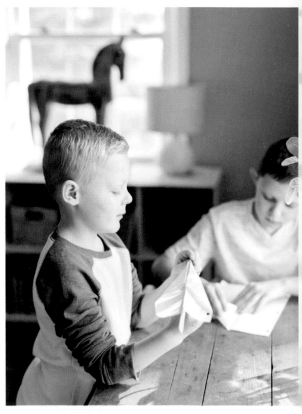

PLAYROOM

Having a separate playroom is a beautiful thing when you have young kids, and it allows you to contain all of their toys in one place. Storage is key in a room like this, but your kids will appreciate plenty of personality added in here, too. Some people would scoff at the idea of putting antiques in a kids' space, but I personally like using antique furniture that is durable and has stood the test of time. If it already has a distressed paint finish, any scratches your kids may add will just increase its character.

In the playroom, we created different zones similar to what we did in my office. There is a desk for homework time, a table by the window for puzzles and games, an art station where they can draw and a bookshelf where they can pick a book to read. This was originally a bedroom, so it has a closet, and we added shelves to it for their toys. Most of their toys fit nicely inside the closet, which leaves the rest of the room as a play space.

I carried the color scheme of blues and greens from their bedroom into their playroom and used vintage pieces like old toolboxes and suitcases to add storage. I also built a custom coat rack on one wall to give them a place for their backpacks and sports bags and hung a colorful pennant banner across the room for a playful touch.

In this chapter, I'll share storage and organizing ideas for your playroom, such as a log pencil holder (page 167) and a custom backpack rack (page 152). I also include a few fun ideas for decorating a kids' space with vintage map art (page 159), alphabet charts (page 163), a window-frame picture display (page 155) and an easy-to-make pennant banner (page 156).

COAT AND BACKPACK STORAGE RACK

Adding hooks on the wall can provide easy storage for towels in a bathroom, coats in an entryway, aprons in the kitchen or clothes in a bedroom. This tutorial shows you how to create a custom wood rack for your hooks that mimics the trim shown in the Farmhouse Window Trim project (page 40). Look for large, unique hooks that have a vintage feel.

Level of Difficulty: Advanced

SUPPLIES

- *Tape measure*
- *1 x 4 board*
- *1 x 3 board*
- *2 (1 x 2) boards*
- *Miter or circular saw*
- *Wall anchors with screws*
- *Drill and drill bit*
- *Hammer*
- *Level*
- *Pencil*
- *Wood glue*
- *Brad nail gun*
- *1 ¼-inch (3-cm) brad nails*
- *Caulk*
- *Paint*
- *Paintbrush*
- *Coat hooks with screws*
- *Screwdriver*

DIRECTIONS

Measure the wall for your coat rack and determine how long you want it to be. Cut one 1 x 4, one 1 x 3, and two 1 x 2s to that length using a saw.

To support the weight of backpacks and coats, you'll need to add several anchors in the wall. First, drill holes using a drill bit just big enough to fit your wall anchor. Add an anchor to each hole, using a hammer to gently tap it in. Hold the 1 x 4 on the wall over the anchors, making sure it is level, and mark on the board with a pencil where each screw will go. Attach the 1 x 4 to the wall by drilling a screw through each mark on the board into a wall anchor.

Attach a 1 x 2 on the top and bottom of the 1 x 4 using wood glue and brad nails. Then attach the 1 x 3 above the top 1 x 2 in the same manner. Caulk the seams between each piece and along ends of the boards. Paint the boards and allow them to dry completely, about 4 hours.

Add coat hooks along the rack using screws and a screwdriver.

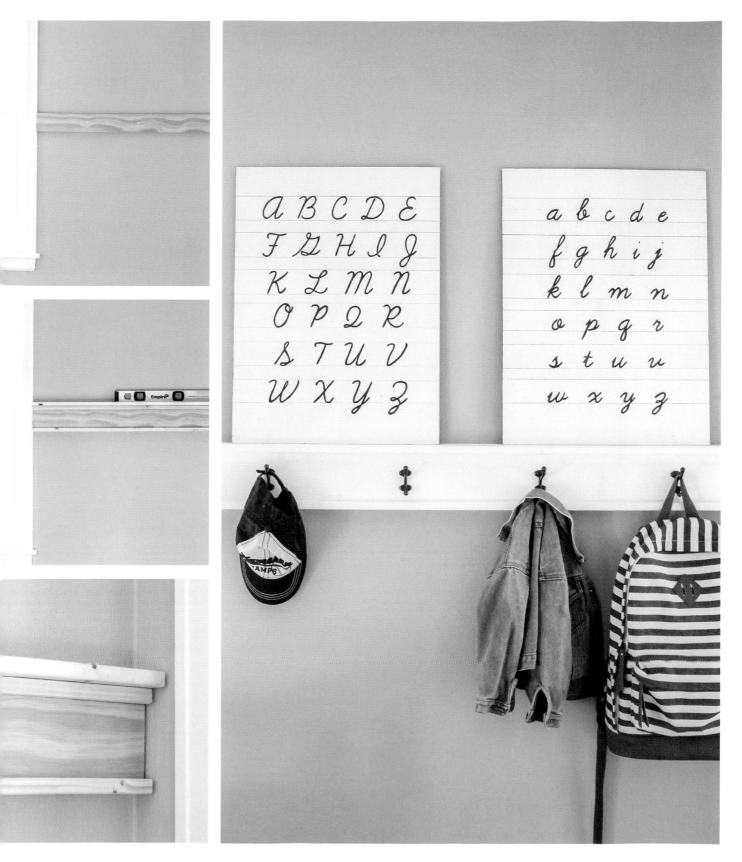

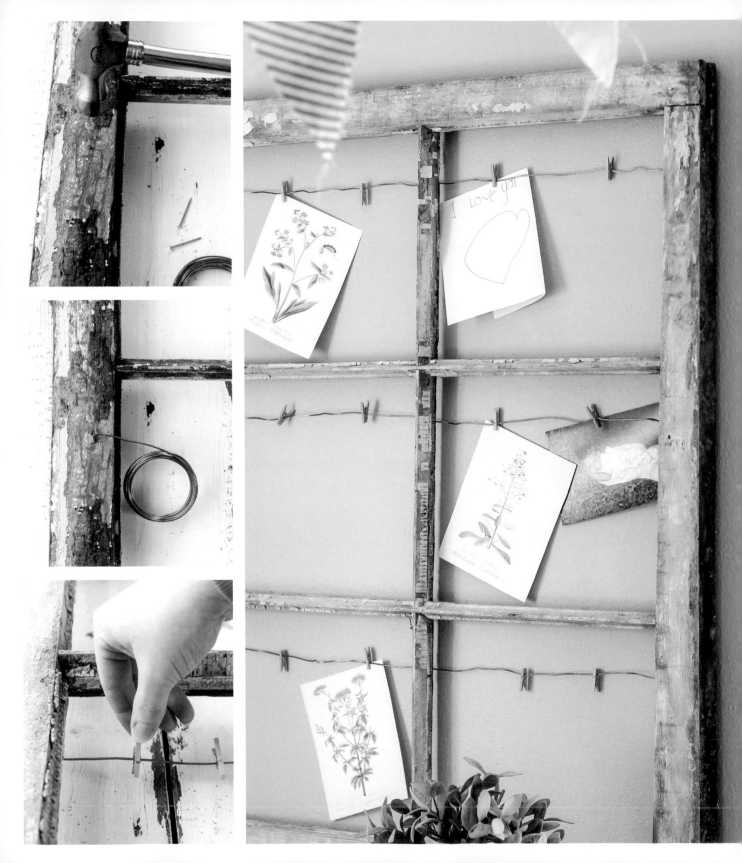

WINDOW-FRAME PICTURE DISPLAY

Ditch traditional frames for your favorite pictures, and use an old window frame to display them! Just wrap some wire around nails on the back of your window and use little clothespins to hang pictures, messages or artwork. Try giving your window frame the finish shown in the Layered Paint Corbel Bookend (page 114) to add some age to it!

Level of Difficulty: Beginner

SUPPLIES

- *Short nails*
- *Old wooden window frame (without glass)*
- *Hammer*
- *Thick jewelry wire*
- *Small clothespins*
- *Sawtooth picture hanger with nails*

DIRECTIONS

Add a nail to the back of the window frame using a hammer. Wrap a piece of wire several times around the nail, and stretch the wire across the window frame to the other side. Add another nail to the frame and wrap the wire several times around that nail to secure the wire in place.

Continue adding nails and wires to the window frame and when finished, clip small clothespins on the wire to hold pictures.

Use a hammer to attach the sawtooth hanger to the back of the frame with nails. Add another nail in the wall, and hang the window frame on the nail.

TIP | *You can find old wooden window frames at antique stores or architectural salvage stores. Typically, window frames with broken or missing glass are less expensive, so keep an eye out for those!*

SHABBY PENNANT BANNER

Pennant banners are really simple to make from scrap pieces of fabric and some twine, and you can use them anywhere to add a touch of playfulness and whimsy. Gather fabrics to match your décor, and try mixing solids with stripes and patterns for interest. Just cut out the pennants from your fabric, glue them to the twine and hang your banner on the walls in a playroom, across the mantel in a living room or along a headboard in a bedroom. To give the pennants a shabby-chic farmhouse feel, fray the fabric edges for a relaxed, casual look.

Level of Difficulty: Beginner

SUPPLIES

- *Cardstock paper*
- *Scissors*
- *Fabric*
- *Pencil*
- *Twine*
- *Hot-glue gun and hot glue*

TIP | *Cut out large pennants to hang around a room or smaller ones to hang along the edge of a mantel or bookshelf.*

DIRECTIONS

Make a template for the pennants by cutting a large triangle out of thick cardstock paper. Lay the triangle on your fabric and trace around the edges with a pencil. Flip the triangle the opposite way to trace another triangle with the short edges butting up to each other. Cut the two triangles out, leaving the line in the center intact.

Continue cutting out pennants until you have enough to make a banner. Lay a pennant open, and place a piece of twine in the center. Apply hot glue along the center and edges of the pennant, then fold the pennant in half, pressing firmly until the glue sets, about 1 minute.

Leave 2 inches (5 cm) of space between each pennant and continue adding pennants along the twine until your banner is finished. Fray the fabric on each pennant by gently pulling loose threads until the edges are as ragged as you would like them to be.

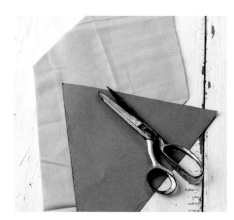
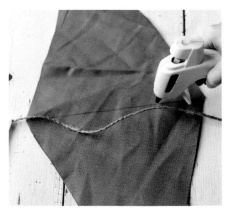

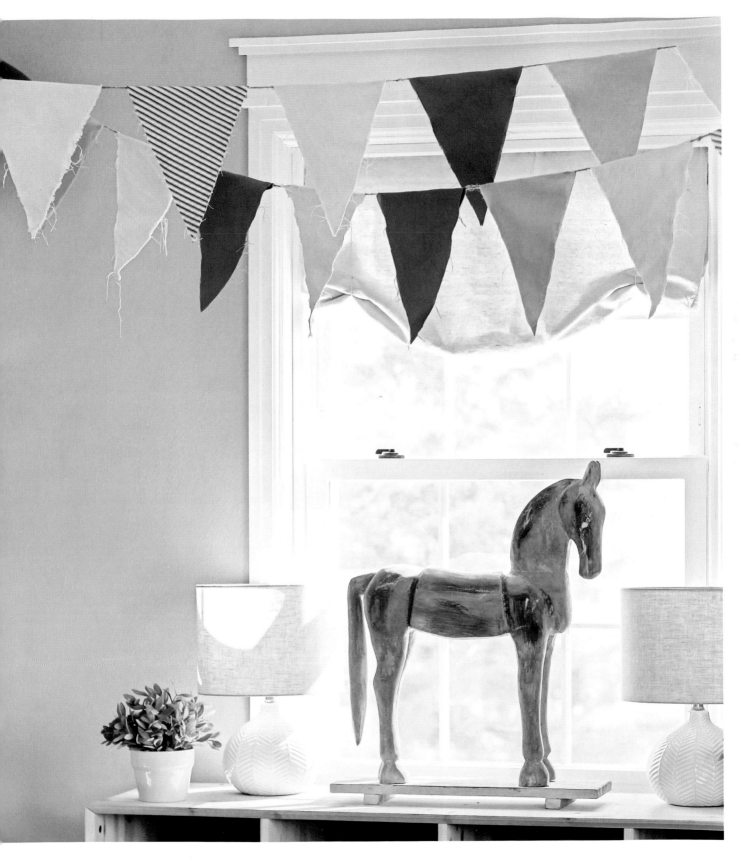

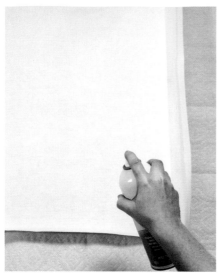

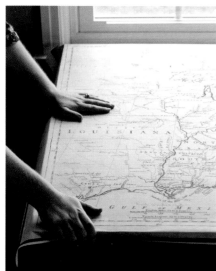

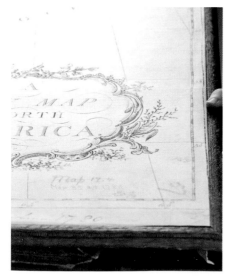

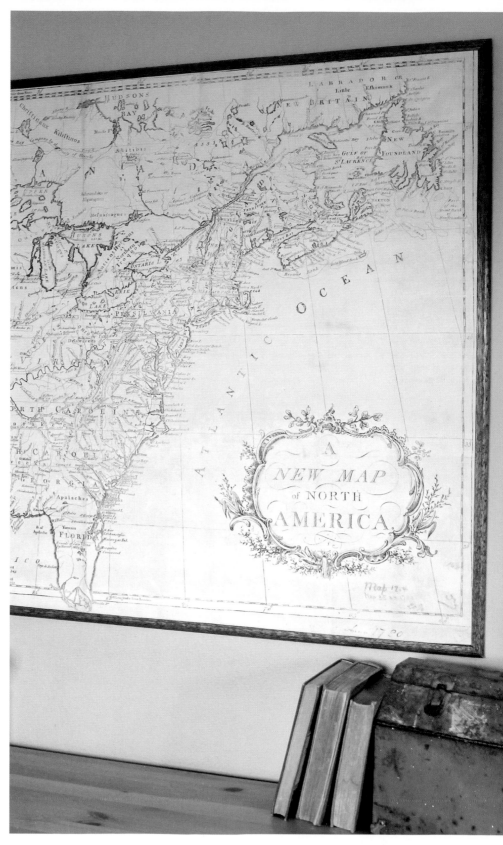

VINTAGE MAP ART

Vintage maps add a great sense of history to a space, but finding a large one can be quite difficult and expensive. This tutorial will show you how to print your own large-scale map and create a custom piece of art that will definitely make a statement on an empty wall.

Level of Difficulty: Advanced

SUPPLIES

- *Tape measure*
- *½-inch (13-mm) MDF*
- *Circular saw*
- *Spray adhesive*
- *High-resolution vintage map, printed to desired size (mine is 36 x 48 inches [91.5 x 122 cm])*
- *½-inch (13-mm) quarter round*
- *Miter saw*
- *Brad nail gun*
- *1 ½-inch (3.8-cm) brad nails*
- *2 D-ring hangers with screws*
- *Screwdriver*

DIRECTIONS

Measure and cut the MDF to 34 inches (86.5 cm) by 43 inches (109 cm) (or your preferred size) using a circular saw. Apply an even layer of spray adhesive on the back of the map print, and place it adhesive-side down and centered on the MDF. Fold the map overhang down along the sides of the MDF.

Cut four pieces of quarter round on a 45° angle using a miter saw long enough to fit around the edges of the MDF, creating a frame. Secure the quarter round to the MDF with brad nails. To hang the map on the wall, screw two D-ring hangers on the back of the map using a screwdriver.

TIP | You can find high-resolution vintage maps online that are free to use. When you find one you like, download it to your computer, enlarge the size and print it at a local printing shop.

KIDS' DRAWING STATION

This DIY drawing station gives your kids a space where they can be creative, and it keeps their beautiful artwork from ending up on furniture and walls. It's made to fit a roll of drawing paper that you can easily replace when it is empty. This drawing station also adds shelf space where you can display their artwork or store art supplies. Hang the drawing station on their bedroom or playroom wall, and watch their creativity come to life!

Level of Difficulty: Advanced

SUPPLIES

- *Tape measure*
- *¼-inch (6-mm) MDF, 4 x 2 feet (122 x 61 cm)*
- *Circular saw*
- *1-inch (2.5-cm) paddle bit*
- *Drill and drill bit*
- *2 (9 x 11-inch [23 x 28-cm]) corbel shelf brackets*
- *Pencil*
- *Jigsaw*
- *¾-inch (2-cm) dowel rod*
- *Paint*
- *Paintbrush*
- *Wood glue*
- *Brad nail gun*
- *1 ½-inch (3.8-cm) brad nails*
- *1 (1 x 12) board, 6 feet (183 cm) long*
- *Wall anchors and screws*
- *Hammer*
- *24-inch (61-cm) roll of drawing paper*

DIRECTIONS

Measure and cut the MDF to 28 inches (71 cm) wide by 24 inches (61 cm) tall using a circular saw. Use a 1-inch (2.5-cm) paddle bit to drill a hole in both shelf brackets near the corner.

Set the shelf brackets on the MDF flush with the top corners. Mark with a pencil on the MDF where the hanging hardware on the brackets sits, then cut out that section of the MDF using a jigsaw. You should now be able to access the hanging hardware on the brackets through the MDF.

Cut a dowel rod to 31 inches (78.5 cm) long using a circular saw. Paint the dowel rod and MDF, and allow them to dry completely, about 4 hours.

Attach the brackets to the MDF using wood glue and 1 ½-inch (3.8-cm) brad nails. Again, the brackets should be flush with the top corners of the MDF, and you should be able to see the hanging hardware from the back.

Cut the 1 x 12 to 35 inches (89 cm) long using a circular saw. Paint the entire board, and allow it to dry completely, about 4 hours. Place the 1 x 12 centered on top of the brackets, and attach them using wood glue and brad nails.

Hang the drawing station on the wall using wall anchors and screws. Drill holes in the wall using a drill bit just big enough to fit your anchors. Use a hammer to gently tap the anchors into each hole. Insert a screw into each wall anchor and leave the screw sticking out just enough to hang the brackets on. Slide the dowel rod through the paper roll, then slide one end of the dowel into each hole in the brackets.

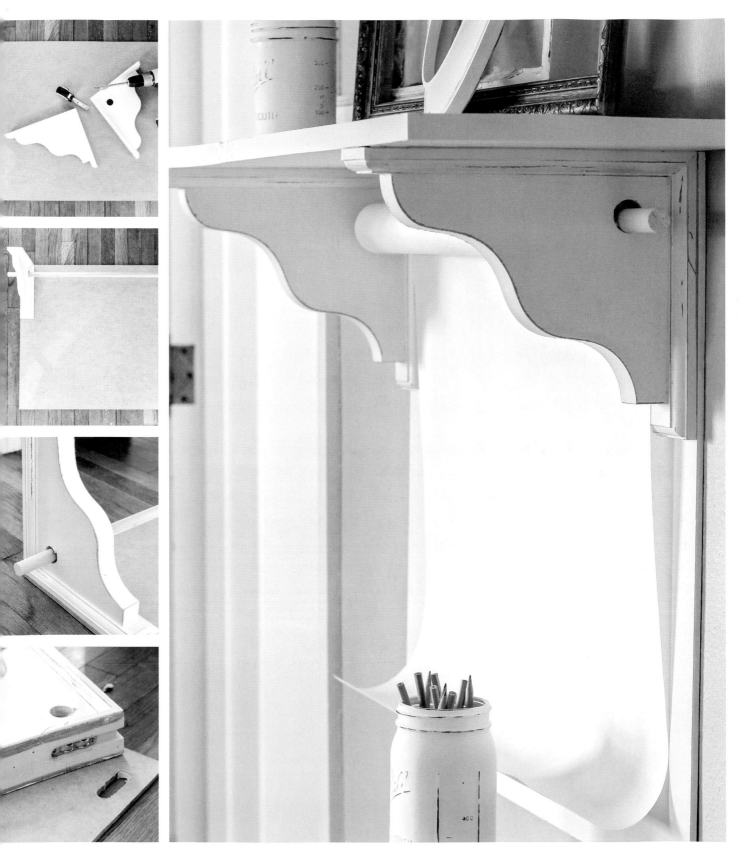

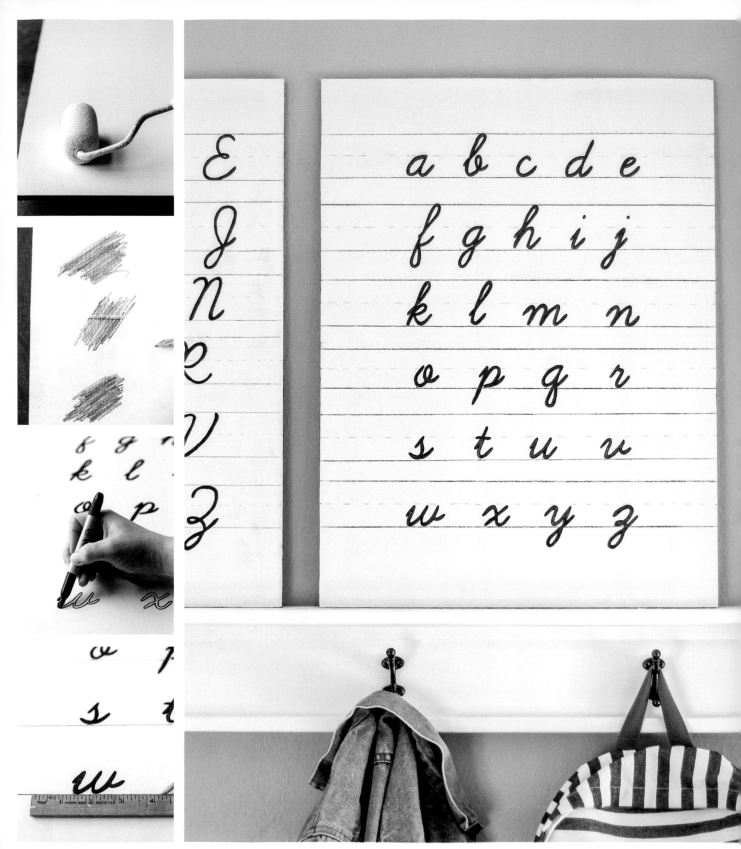

ALPHABET CHART ART

Vintage letter charts are great for decorating kids' spaces, and this handmade version can be done from start to finish in just a few hours. You can customize the chart however you like—with uppercase letters, lowercase letters, cursive, print or even numbers. Try hanging a collection of them together for a fun focal wall!

Level of Difficulty: Intermediate

SUPPLIES

- *Tape measure*
- *¼-inch (6-mm) MDF, 2 x 2 feet (61 x 61 cm)*
- *Circular saw*
- *Black paint*
- *Paintbrush or roller*
- *White paint*
- *Computer and printer*
- *Printer paper*
- *Pencil*
- *Ballpoint pen*
- *Black permanent marker*
- *Ruler*

DIRECTIONS

Measure and cut the ¼-inch (6-mm) MDF to 18 inches (45.5 cm) by 24 inches (61 cm) using a circular saw. Paint the edges of the MDF black to give it the appearance of a frame, and allow the paint to dry completely, about 4 hours. When dry, paint the front of the MDF white using a paint roller, and allow the paint to dry completely, about 4 hours.

Type the alphabet on a computer and print the letters on printer paper. Use the technique described in the Vintage Label Wooden Stool project (page 125) to transfer the printed design onto the MDF. Fill in the letter outlines using a permanent marker. Use a ruler to draw lines above and below the letters with a pencil or marker.

TIP | *Using a permanent marker to fill in the letters is fast and simple, but you could also use black paint, if desired.*

WIRE CLOCHE

Glass cloches are beautiful to decorate with, but this version made out of wire is far less fussy and much less expensive, which makes it perfect for decorating a kids' space. It has a great industrial look that fits in perfectly with farmhouse décor, and you can fill the cloche with a potted plant, some feathers, rolled up book pages or anything else you can imagine. Try setting your cloche on a coffee table or mantel, or you can even group a collection of cloches together as a stunning centerpiece on your dining room table. In a kids' room, these cloches can display sports trophies or their favorite dolls or action figures.

Level of Difficulty: Beginner

SUPPLIES

- *2 x 4-inch (5 x 10-cm) 14-gauge galvanized welded wire*
- *Metal snips*
- *8-inch (20.5-cm) terra cotta pot saucer*
- *Pliers*
- *Thick jewelry wire*
- *Black spray paint (optional)*

DIRECTIONS

Cut a piece of welded wire eleven sections wide (about 22 inches [56 cm]) and five sections tall (about 20 inches [51 cm]) using metal snips. Wrap the wire to form a cylinder, and place it on the terra cotta saucer to make sure it fits inside. Wrap the loose wire ends on one side around the opposite side using pliers to secure the cylinder in place.

Cut the horizontal wires on the top two sections, leaving three full sections on the bottom rows. Bend the top vertical wires toward the center of the cylinder, and wrap the jewelry wire tightly around the bundle of vertical wires to secure them together.

If desired, paint the wire cloche with black spray paint, and allow the paint to dry completely. Set the cloche on the terra cotta saucer.

TIP | *You can use welded wire left over from the Wire Laundry Hamper (page 94) to make this cloche!*

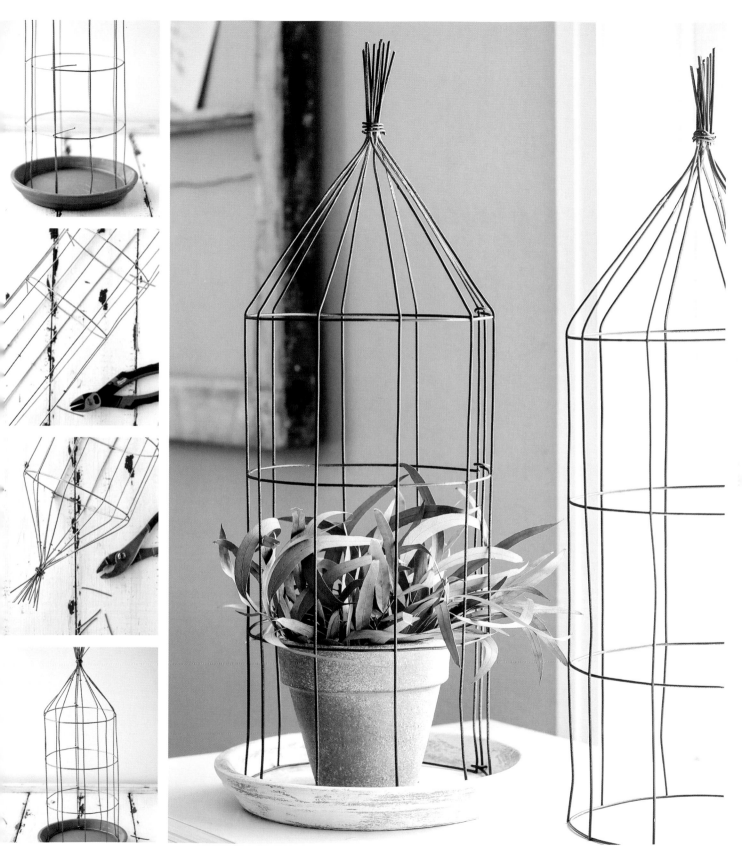

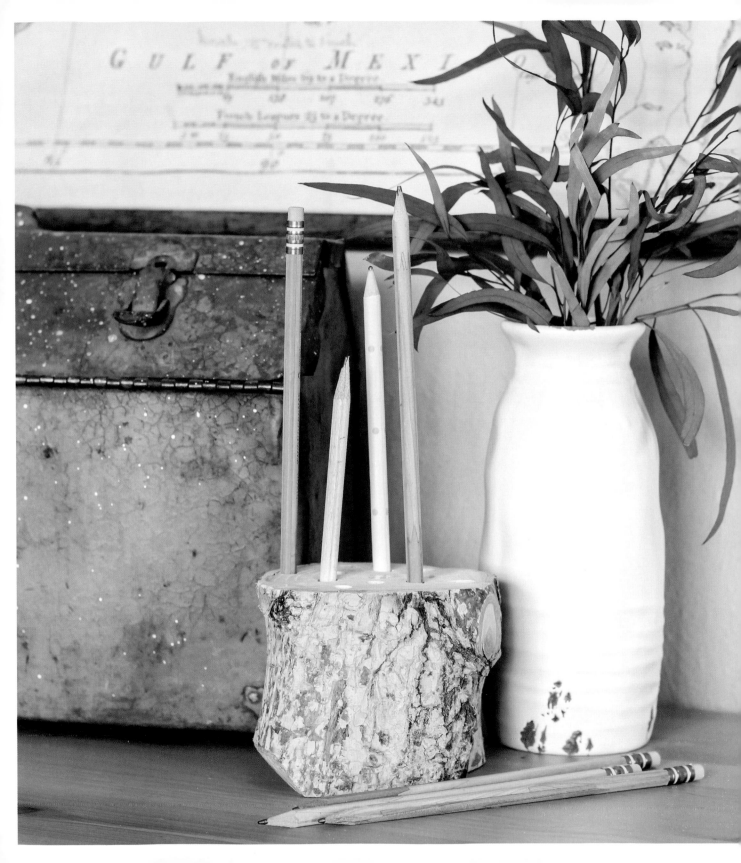

LOG PENCIL HOLDER

This rustic desk accessory takes just a few minutes to make and will help keep your workspace more organized. You might even be able to find the wood in your own backyard!

Level of Difficulty: Intermediate

SUPPLIES

- *Log*
- *Miter or circular saw*
- *Drill*
- *⁵⁄₁₆-inch (8-mm) drill bit*
- *Pencils*

DIRECTIONS

Cut a log about 4 inches (10 cm) long using a saw. Make sure that both ends of the log are flat. Drill holes on one cut side of the log using a ⁵⁄₁₆-inch (8-mm) drill bit. Turn the log upside down to clean any shavings out of the holes, and fill the holder with pencils.

TIP | *You can purchase small logs at craft stores, but this is most likely something you can find in your own yard. Any type of wood will work for this project, just be sure to look for a dry, solid log without any rot. Leave bark on the outside of the log for a more rustic look, or chip some of the bark off for a cleaner look.*

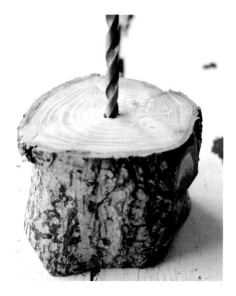
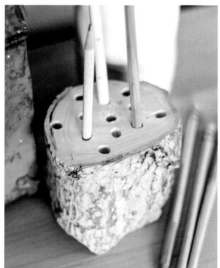

LAYERED FRAME DISPLAY

Sometimes the best way to decorate is also the simplest. To create this layered frame display, pull together a collection of old picture frames of different shapes, sizes and finishes. If you already have a stash of frames you aren't using, this vignette won't cost you a penny, and bonus—you'll make use of all those random frames you've been hoarding.

Level of Difficulty: Beginner

SUPPLIES

- *Photo frames in a variety of shapes and sizes*
- *Paint*
- *Paintbrush*
- *Sanding block*

DIRECTIONS

Gather a variety of photo frames in different shapes and sizes. Dig through closets to find old, unused frames or shop thrift stores and garage sales to find frames for a fraction of the price.

The frames can all be the same color or a mix of colors, wood and metal. If any of the frames have a finish that doesn't match your décor, simply paint them in any color you like. Try using a sanding block to distress corners and details on the frames for a vintage look.

To display the frames, set them together on a table or shelf with larger frames in the back and smaller frames layered in the front. Add interest by hanging a wreath inside one of the large frames or placing a framed mirror among the photo frames. If you are short on table space, try hanging the frames as a gallery wall instead.

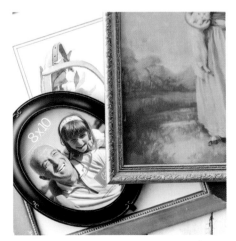 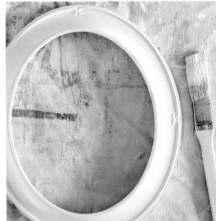

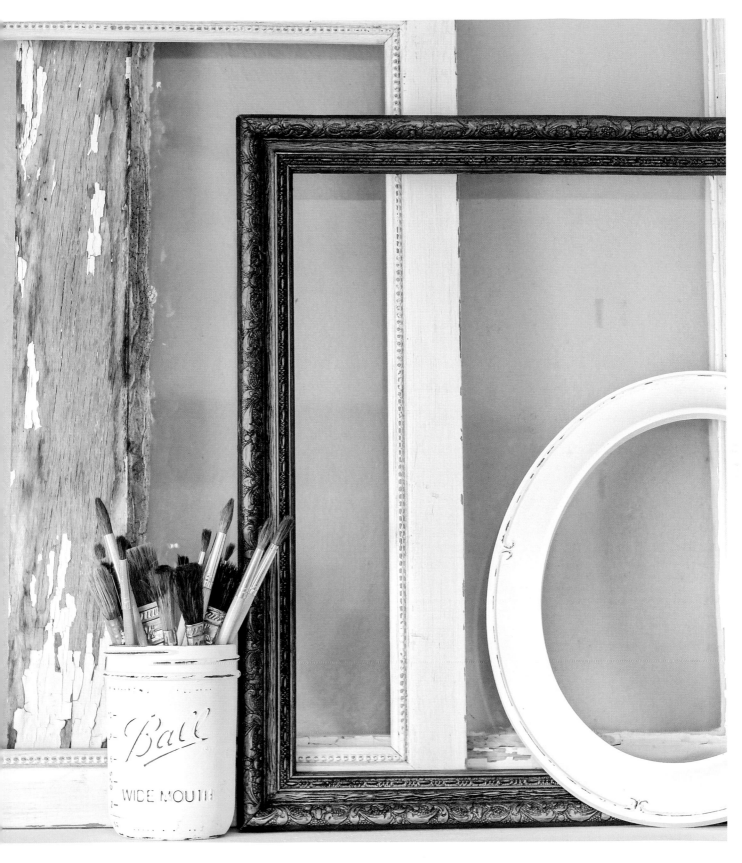

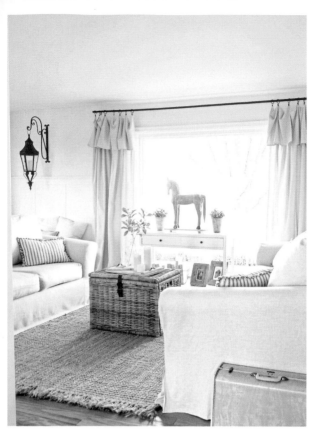

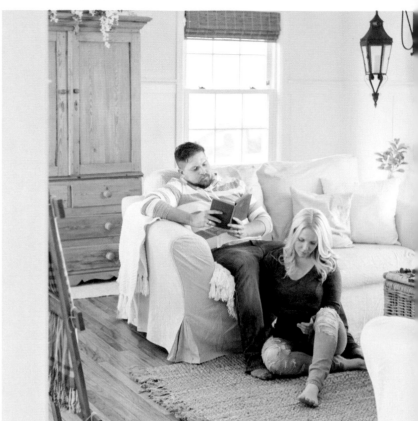

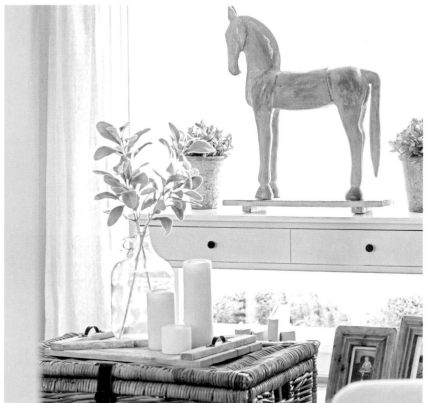

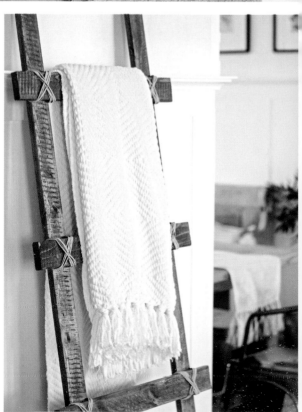

RESOURCES

Get all the details of our farmhouse in one place! Use this resource guide to learn where I found the furniture and accessories for our home, which items are handmade and the paint colors we used.

Living Room

FURNITURE & ACCESSORIES

Sofa slipcovers—Comfort Works

Natural jute rug—Rugs USA *(similar styles at Home Decorators Collection, Ballard Designs and Overstock)*

Wicker trunk—IKEA *(similar styles at Wayfair and Target)*

Striped throw pillows—World Market

Hanging lanterns—Hobby Lobby

Bamboo Roman shades—Home Depot *(similar styles at JCPenny and Overstock)*

White console table by window—Target *(similar styles at Hayneedle and Joss & Main)*

White blanket on ladder—T.J. Maxx *(similar styles at Target)*

Wood picture frames—T.J. Maxx *(similar styles at World Market)*

Glass lamps—Target *(similar styles at Pottery Barn)*

Tray—Rustic Decorative Tray tutorial (page 31)

Cow pillow—Stitched Cow Pillow tutorial (page 28)

Curtains—Easy Drop Cloth Curtains tutorial (page 19)

Ladder—Simple Rustic Ladder tutorial (page 16)

Family name sign—Family Name Sign tutorial (page 23)

Chicken-wire candleholder—Chicken-Wire Candleholder tutorial (page 20)

Framed grain sack—Framed Grain Sack tutorial (page 24)

Greenery wreath—Simple Greenery Wreath tutorial (page 27)

Windowpane mirror—Windowpane Mirror tutorial (page 32)

Farmhouse window trim—Farmhouse Window Trim tutorial (page 40)

ANTIQUES & SECONDHAND FINDS

Large armoire

Vintage suitcases

Glass jug

Horse statue

Wire basket

WALL PAINT COLOR

Du Jour by Valspar

Dining Room & Entryway

FURNITURE & ACCESSORIES

Tufted slipper chairs—Target (*similar styles at Pottery Barn and All Modern*)

Metal tub chairs—Target (*similar styles at World Market*)

Natural jute rug—World Market (*similar styles at Rugs USA and Home Decorators Collection*)

White vases—Hobby Lobby

Iron chandelier—Del Mar Fans & Lighting (*similar styles at Lowe's Home Improvement and Home Depot*)

Bamboo Roman shade—Home Depot (*similar styles at JCPenny and Overstock*)

Faux olive tree—Overstock (*similar styles at Wayfair and Birch Lane*)

Metal olive bucket—Target (*similar styles at Pottery Barn and Magnolia Market*)

Black coat hooks—Menards (*similar styles at Home Depot and Lowe's Home Improvement*)

Woven trunk—T.J. Maxx (*similar styles at Pier 1 Imports*)

Farmhouse dining table—Tutorial on lovegrowswild.com

Dining table bench—Tutorial on lovegrowswild.com

Entryway bench—Tutorial on lovegrowswild.com

Table runner—Fringed Burlap Table Runner tutorial (page 43)

Hanging vases—Rustic Hanging Vase tutorial (page 39)

Window trim—Farmhouse Window Trim tutorial (page 40)

Book-page art—Printed Book-Page Art tutorial (page 36)

Boot tray—Wooden Boot Tray on Casters tutorial (page 48)

Plate rack—Plate Rack tutorial (page 44)

Cutting boards—Vintage Cutting Board tutorial (page 47)

Doormat—Monogrammed Doormat tutorial (page 52)

Flower bucket—Galvanized Metal Flower Bucket tutorial (page 51)

Tied pillow cover—Tied Pillow Cover tutorial (page 81)

ANTIQUES & SECONDHAND FINDS

Wood candlesticks

Market bag

Mounted antlers

White plates

WALL PAINT COLOR

Du Jour by Valspar

FRONT DOOR PAINT COLOR

Rustic Pewter by Rust-Oleum

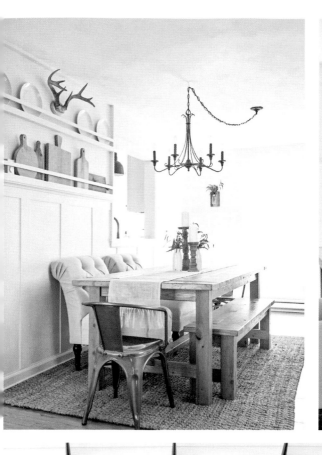
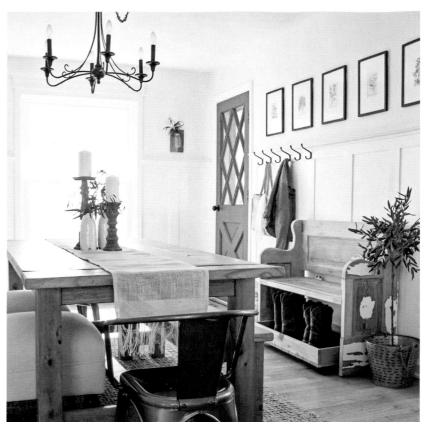
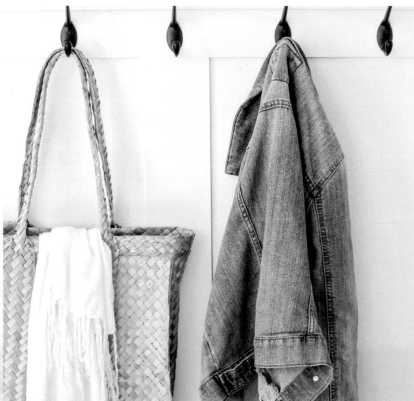
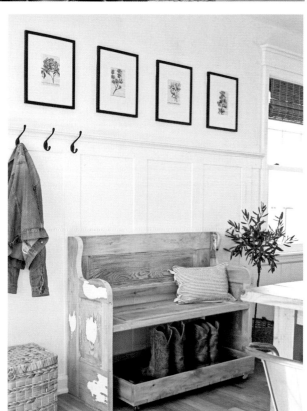

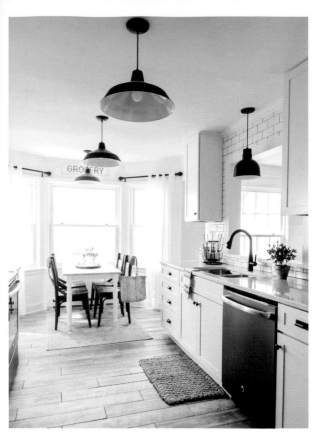

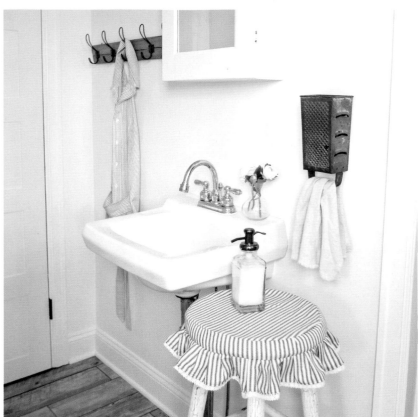

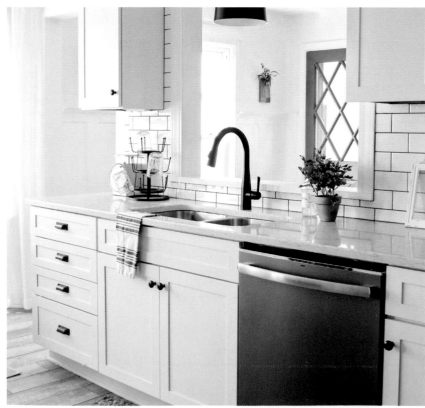

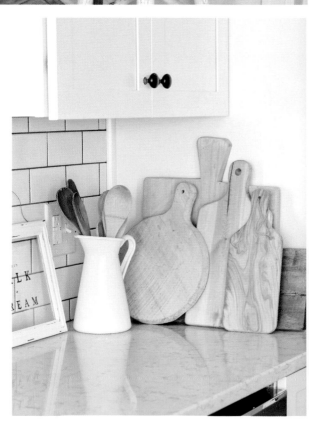

Kitchen

FURNITURE & ACCESSORIES

White cabinets—KraftMaid

Cabinet hardware—Hickory Hardware

Tile floor and backsplash—Lowe's Home Improvement (*similar styles at Home Depot*)

Appliances—GE Appliances

Black pendant lights—Amazon (*similar styles at Wayfair and Barn Light Electric*)

Pendant light over sink—Wayfair (*similar styles at Barn Light Electric*)

Sink faucet—Delta

Dining chairs—World Market (*similar styles at Target and Wayfair*)

Vintage rug—Rugs USA (*similar styles at Overstock*)

Natural jute rug—HomeGoods (*similar styles at Rugs USA and World Market*)

Sheer curtains—Walmart (*similar styles at Target*)

Curtain rods—Walmart (*similar styles at Target*)

Wire drying rack—World Market

White pitcher—IKEA (*similar styles at Pottery Barn and Anthropologie*)

Glass canisters—Target (*similar styles at Bed Bath & Beyond*)

Planter box—Herb Planter Box tutorial (page 56)

Canister label—Chalkboard Canister Label tutorial (page 59)

Terra cotta pot—Aged Terra Cotta Pot tutorial (page 63)

Stool slipcover—Ruffled Stool Slipcover tutorial (page 60)

Cake stand—Wooden Cake Stand tutorial (page 64)

Centerpiece—Simple, Natural Centerpiece tutorial (page 67)

Glass sign—Framed Glass Sign tutorial (page 68)

Stool—Cracked Paint Finish tutorial (page 71)

Paneled door—Paneled Door tutorial (page 72)

Grater towel holder—Antique Grater Towel Holder tutorial (page 75)

Cutting boards—Vintage Cutting Board tutorial (page 47)

ANTIQUES & SECONDHAND FINDS

Dining table

Antique scale

Grocery sign

WALL PAINT COLOR

Du Jour by Valspar

Master Bedroom

FURNITURE & ACCESSORIES

Iron bed frame—Overstock (*similar styles at Target*)

Cream rug—Hayneedle (*similar styles at Rugs Direct and Wayfair*)

Lace curtains—IKEA (*similar styles at JCPenny and Overstock*)

Crystal light fixture—Home Depot

Tufted chair—Target (*similar styles at Pottery Barn and Overstock*)

Swing arm lamps—Lowe's Home Improvement (*similar styles at World Market*)

Nightstands—Sauder

White quilt—Target (*similar styles at Bed Bath & Beyond*)

Cream fringe blanket—Hayneedle

White ruffle throw pillows—IKEA

Woven basket—T.J. Maxx (*similar styles at World Market and Michael's*)

Wicker chair—IKEA (*similar styles at Joss & Main*)

Fabric Roman shade—Home Depot (*similar styles at JCPenny*)

Wooden lamp—Target (*similar styles at Lamps Plus*)

Faux wooden beam—Tutorial on lovegrowswild.com

White planked walls—Tutorial on lovegrowswild.com

Wooden bench—Simple Wooden Bench tutorial (page 82)

Silhouette—Framed Silhouette tutorial (page 86)

Pillow covers—Tied Pillow Cover tutorial (page 81)

Greenery wreath—Simple Greenery Wreath tutorial (page 27)

Serving tray—Round Wooden Serving Tray tutorial (page 89)

Wooden frames—Rustic Wooden Frame tutorial (page 85)

Candleholder—Table Leg Candleholder tutorial (page 78)

Jewelry display—Chicken-Wire Jewelry Display tutorial (page 93)

Step stool—Painted Step Stool with Easy Distressing tutorial (page 90)

Laundry hamper—Wire Laundry Hamper tutorial (page 94)

Window trim—Farmhouse Window Trim tutorial (page 40)

ANTIQUES & SECONDHAND FINDS

White side table

WALL PAINT COLOR

Dove White by Valspar

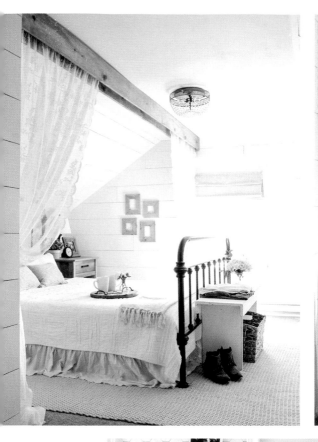
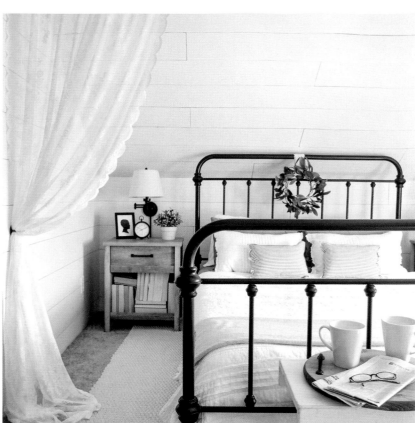
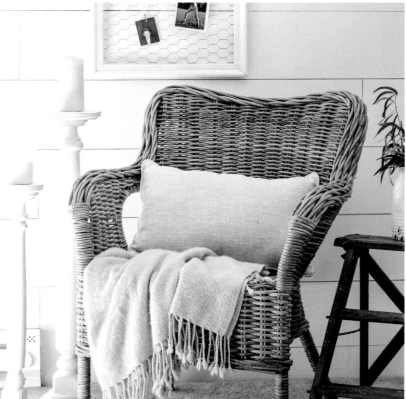
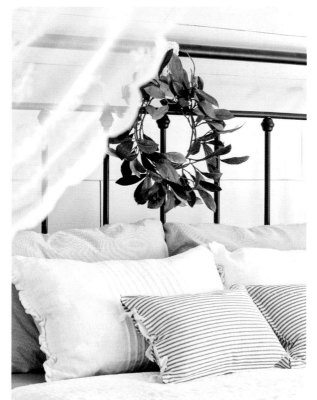

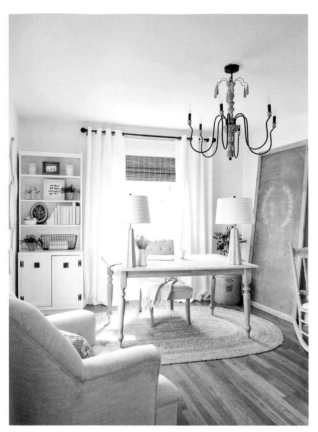
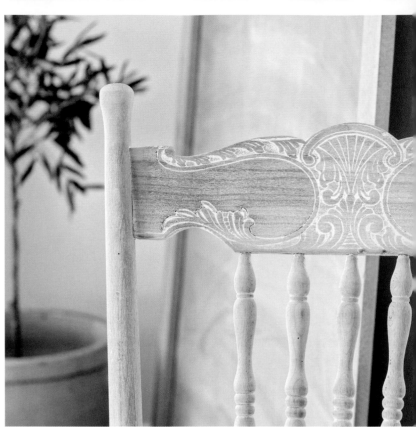
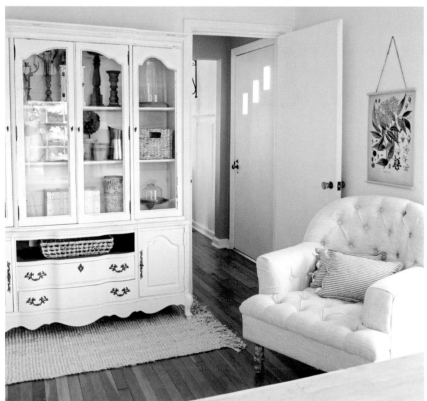
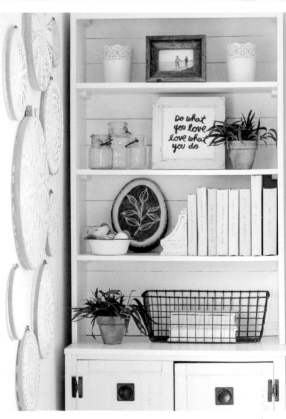

Office

FURNITURE & ACCESSORIES

Oval natural jute rug—Rugs USA (similar styles at Overstock and Hayneedle)

White velvet curtains—Target (similar styles at Pottery Barn and Overstock)

Bamboo Roman shades—Home Depot (similar styles at JCPenny and Overstock)

Concrete lamps—World Market (similar styles at Hayneedle and Lamps Plus)

Wood and iron chandelier—World Market (similar styles at Pottery Barn)

Tufted desk chair—Kirkland's (similar styles at Target and Pottery Barn)

Olive tree—Overstock (similar styles at Wayfair and Joss & Main)

Cream fringe rug—Rugs USA (similar styles at Hayneedle and Rugs Direct)

Clock—Large Roman-Numeral Clock tutorial (page 105)

Chalkboard—Wood-Framed Chalkboard tutorial (page 109)

Bookcase—Planked Bookcase tutorial (page 110)

Corbel bookend—Layered Paint Corbel Bookend tutorial (page 114)

Linen-covered books—Linen-Covered Book tutorial (page 106)

Wood spools—Vintage Wooden Spool tutorial (page 102)

Doily gallery wall—Doily Gallery Wall tutorial (page 98)

Chair with upholstered seat—Lime-Washed Chair with Upholstered Seat tutorial (page 113)

Botanical wall hanging—Botanical Wall Hanging tutorial (page 101)

Window trim—Farmhouse Window Trim tutorial (page 40)

Terra cotta pot—Aged Terra Cotta Pot tutorial (page 63)

Pillows—Tied Pillow Cover tutorial (page 81)

ANTIQUES & SECONDHAND FINDS

Farmhouse table/desk

White cabinet

White hutch with glass doors

Large crock

WALL PAINT COLOR

Du Jour by Valspar

Bathroom

FURNITURE & ACCESSORIES

Sink vanity—Lowe's Home Improvement *(similar styles at Home Depot and Wayfair)*

Sink faucet—Home Depot

White floor tile—Lowe's Home Improvement *(similar styles at Home Depot)*

Oval mirror—Target *(similar styles at Pottery Barn)*

White shower curtain—Target *(similar styles at Kohl's and Wayfair)*

Bathtub and shower—Bath Fitter

Shower head and faucet—Moen

White pitcher—IKEA *(similar styles at Pottery Barn and Anthropologie)*

Glass soap dispenser—Target *(similar styles at Walmart and Wayfair)*

Black towel hooks—IKEA

White bath towel—Target

Grain-sack stripe towel—Grain-Sack Stripe Towel tutorial (page 126)

Wooden stool—Vintage Label Wooden Stool tutorial (page 125)

Tub shelf—Wooden Plank Tub Shelf tutorial (page 121)

Crate storage—Hanging Crate Storage tutorial (page 122)

Fern art—Pressed Fern Framed Art tutorial (page 118)

Bath mat—Wooden Bath Mat tutorial (page 129)

WALL PAINT COLOR

Bright White by Dutch Boy

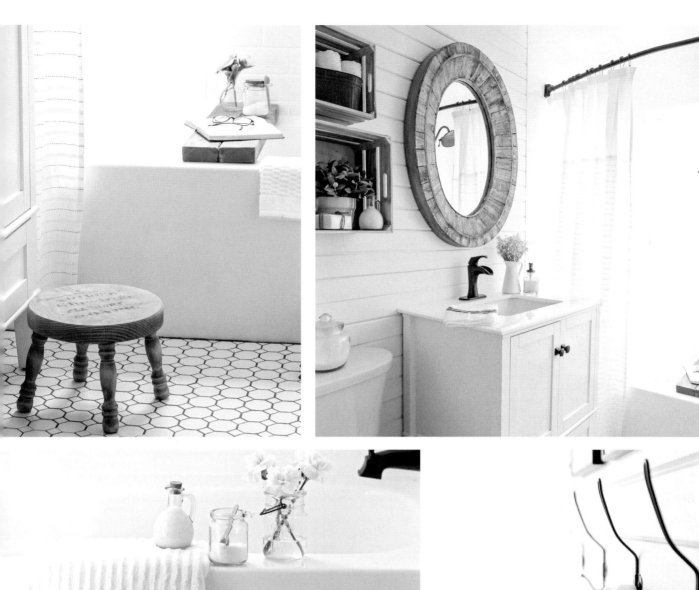

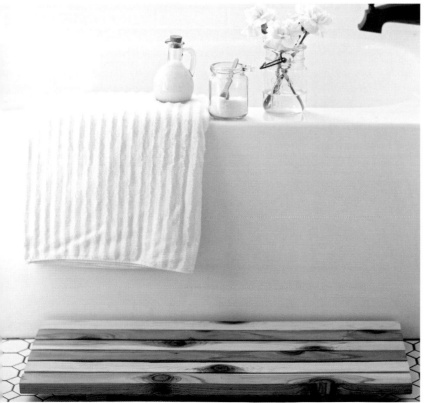

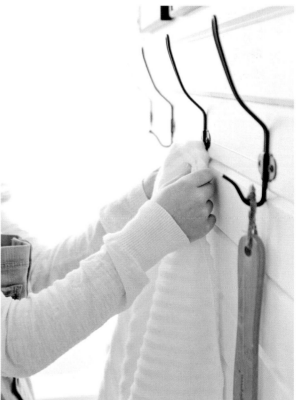

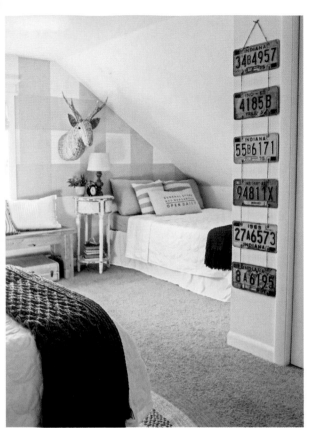
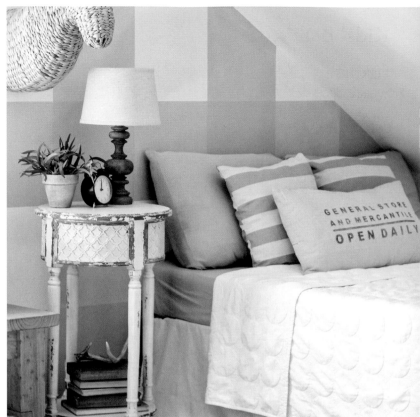
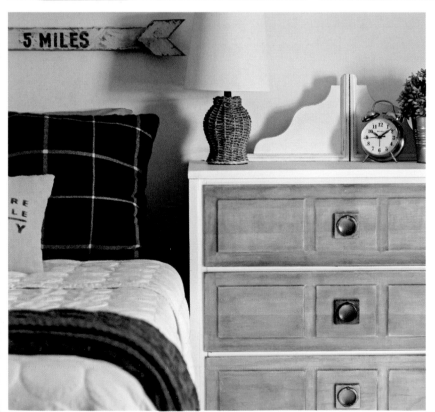
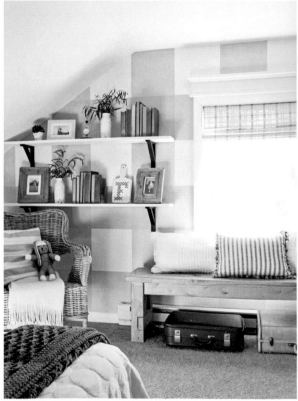

Kids' Bedroom

FURNITURE & ACCESSORIES

White comforter—Target (*similar styles at Bed Bath & Beyond*)

Olive-green throw blanket—Target (*similar styles at Macy's and Hayneedle*)

Navy-blue throw blanket—Target (*similar styles at Overstock and All Modern*)

Blue plaid throw pillows—Target

Natural woven lamps—Kirkland's (*similar styles at Lamps Plus and Wayfair*)

Wicker chair—IKEA (*similar styles at Joss & Main*)

Cream fringe throw on chair—Hayneedle

Wooden picture frames—T.J. Maxx (*similar styles at World Market*)

White ruffle throw pillow—IKEA

Striped throw pillow—World Market

Deer head—Target

Wooden lamp—Target (*similar styles at Lamps Plus*)

White side table—Hobby Lobby

Metal clock—Target (*similar styles at Wayfair and Hayneedle*)

Wooden bench—Tutorial on lovegrowswild.com

Stenciled pillow—Stenciled Linen Pillow Cover tutorial (page 139)

Dressers—White and Wood Dresser Makeover tutorial (page 135)

Wooden arrow—Wooden Arrow Sign tutorial (page 147)

Open shelving—Easy Open Shelving tutorial (page 143)

Cross-stitch monogram—Cross-Stitch Monogram tutorial (page 148)

Accent wall—Gingham Painted Accent Wall tutorial (page 136)

License plate gallery wall—Hanging License Plate Gallery Wall tutorial (page 132)

Metal bin—Aged Galvanized Metal Bin tutorial (page 140)

Dresser drawer storage box—Dresser Drawer Storage Box tutorial (page 144)

Window trim—Farmhouse Window Trim tutorial (page 40)

ANTIQUES & SECONDHAND FINDS

Gray stripe pillows

Vintage suitcases

WALL PAINT COLOR

Du Jour by Valspar + Woodsmoke Gray by Sherwin-Williams

Playroom

FURNITURE & ACCESSORIES

Desk—IKEA *(similar styles at Sauder)*

Cream rug—Hayneedle *(similar styles at Rugs Direct and Wayfair)*

Desk lamp—Target *(similar styles at Walmart and Wayfair)*

Bookshelf—IKEA

White lamps—Target *(similar styles at Lamps USA and Hayneedle)*

Oval jute rug—Rugs USA *(similar styles at Overstock and Hayneedle)*

Map—Vintage Map Art tutorial (page 159)

Log pencil holder—Log Pencil Holder tutorial (page 167)

Pennant banner—Shabby Pennant Banner tutorial (page 156)

Window-frame display—Window-Frame Picture Display tutorial (page 155)

Storage rack—Coat and Backpack Storage Rack tutorial (page 152)

Alphabet chart art—Alphabet Chart Art tutorial (page 163)

Drawing station—Kids' Drawing Station tutorial (page 160)

Layered frames—Layered Frame Display tutorial (page 168)

Wire cloche—Wire Cloche tutorial (page 164)

Stenciled pillow—Stenciled Linen Pillow Cover tutorial (page 139)

Tied pillow covers—Tied Pillow Cover tutorial (page 81)

White stool—Cracked Paint Finish tutorial (page 71)

ANTIQUES & SECONDHAND FINDS

Desk chair

Green toolbox

Vintage suitcases

Horse statue

Drop-cloth shades

Antique drop-leaf table

Dining chairs

Clipboards

WALL PAINT COLOR

Woodlawn Colonial Gray by Valspar

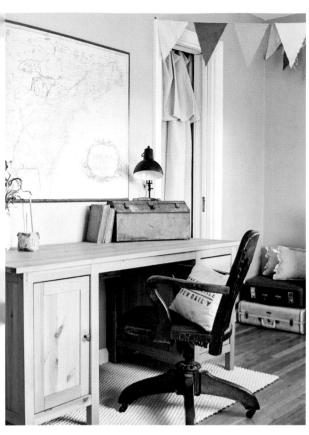
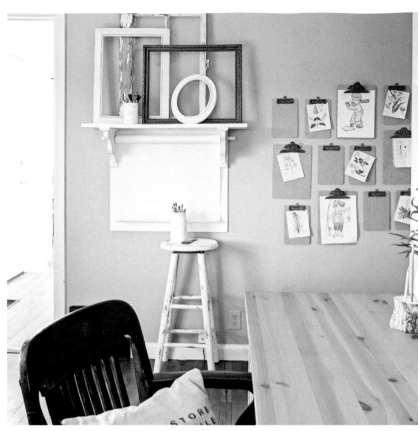
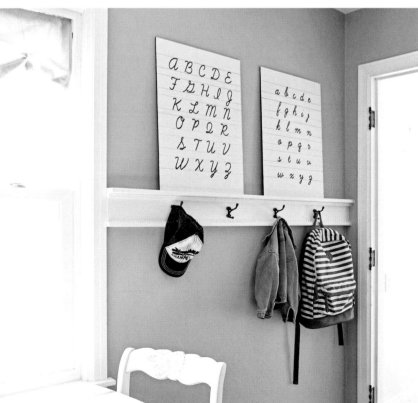
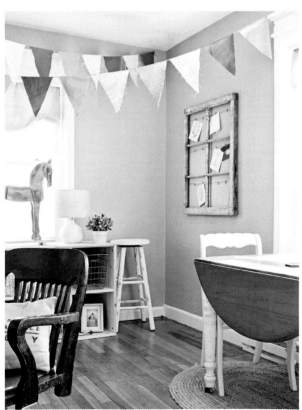

THANK YOU

To Jeremy—You most likely deserve an award or something for being married to me. When we first met, I think you probably assumed you had found the perfect farm wife. I would spend the rest of our days together raising babies, bringing meals out to the tractor, keeping track of the farm bookwork and running to the store for parts if the combine broke down mid-harvest.

But then I went and started a blog that turned from just a dream in my head to a fun, part-time hobby to a full-time job to an up-and-coming career that is growing even faster than I can keep up with at times. All of these things happened because of what you have taught me in the last eight years we've been together: Work hard. Don't give up. Go against the grain and make your own path if the one laid out for you isn't good enough. Don't settle for anything less than you're worth, and don't be afraid to try something new . . . even if it terrifies you.

I might be the name and face in front of Love Grows Wild, but I couldn't do any of it (well, most of it) without you. You taught me how to use a drill when you got tired of me asking for things to be hung on the wall. Then you taught me to be really awesome at covering holes in the wall when I decided to move everything the very next week. You have moved more pieces of furniture, picked up more pizzas for dinner and installed more light fixtures in the last six months of me writing this book than you probably have in your entire lifetime. Thank you for letting our home be my blank canvas and for supporting me every step of the way. I love the home, family and beautiful life we are building together. And just for the record, I'll try my hardest to still be the farm wife you've always imagined I would be. I think I owe it to ya.

To my boys—Mommy loves you to the moon and back. Thank you for always knowing how to bring a smile to my face and for watching my favorite design shows with me. When you walk in the house after school and get just as excited as I am about a piece of vintage furniture I brought home from the antique store or a new furniture arrangement in the living room, it makes my heart so happy. Even if you couldn't really care less about all this home decorating stuff, you care about how much I love it, and for that I love you more than you'll ever know. I hope one day you get just as excited to build a house for your own family. P.S. Did you have fun busting through that wall in the kitchen?

To my Mom—Where do I start? Thank you for being my dish fairy when I work too much, my child-wrangler when I need a few hours of peace and quiet and my never-ending pillar of love and support. You taught me how to work hard and that men shouldn't be the only ones with a fully stocked toolbox. I still use that pink tool set you bought me when I first moved out on my own. Most of all, thank you for all the laughter you bring into my life. I love you.

To my Dad—Thank you for always supporting me no matter how crazy my ideas were . . . even when I chose blogging as a career over the cosmetology schooling you paid for. You let me make my own decisions, make my own mistakes and learn how to clean up my own messes when things went bad. Without those experiences, I wouldn't be the tough cookie I am today.

To my sister—We grew up together and survived to tell the tale. You are my best friend . . . my "person," as Meredith Grey would say. Thank you for showing me what quiet strength looks like. I'm still working on the quiet part.

To my in-laws—Thank you for giving me free reign in your farmhouse. This book wouldn't have been possible without you!

To the numerous family members and friends throughout the years—Thank you for your endless support! Who knew this small-town girl from Coal City would become a published author?

To my amazing Love Grows Wild readers . . . you are the whole reason this book happened. Every blog post you read, comment you leave and email you write encourages me to keep doing what I love to do. I've made lasting friendships with readers on the other side of the globe and even right in my own backyard here in Indiana. Thank you for following me on this crazy journey.

To my amazingly talented fellow bloggers who are also on this journey with me . . . thank you for your wonderful advice and for understanding things no one else in the world does. I feel so lucky to be in a community as supportive and awe-inspiring as this one.

To the many people who helped make this book possible, my thanks goes to:

Emily Layne, for capturing the beauty of our farmhouse and the people who live inside.

Lindsay Hipp and Lowe's of Kokomo, Indiana, for helping us design the perfect farmhouse kitchen.

Heath Keeling and the crew from RHK Contracting, for building us our dream farmhouse kitchen.

Will and Sarah from Page Street Publishing, for allowing me to share our little farmhouse with the world.

ABOUT THE AUTHOR

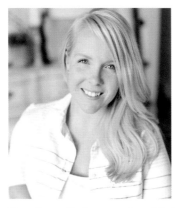

Liz Fourez lives with her husband and two boys in Indiana on a fourth-generation family farm. She created the popular home and lifestyle blog Love Grows Wild in 2012 and has been sharing her passion for homemaking ever since. Liz gives her followers a front-row seat as she renovates and decorates her 1940s farmhouse by sharing project tutorials, room makeovers and design ideas, all with her signature farmhouse style.

Liz's keen eye for photography and intuitive decorating style have earned her features on *The Today Show*, *Redbook*, *Country Living*, and Huffington Post websites, as well as a spread in *American Farmhouse Style* magazine. Liz has shared hundreds of decorating tutorials on her blog and has gained a loyal following of fellow homemakers who are inspired by the creative yet attainable beauty Liz demonstrates in her home.

Follow her journey at: http://lovegrowswild.com
Instagram: http://www.instagram.com/lizlovegrowswild
Facebook: http://www.facebook.com/LoveGrowsWild
Pinterest: http://www.pinterest.com/lovegrowswildlf
Twitter: http://twitter.com/LoveGrowsWild

INDEX